Menopause Matters

Menopause Matters

Your Guide to a Long and Healthy Life

JULIA SCHLAM EDELMAN, M.D., F.A.C.O.G.

THE JOHNS HOPKINS UNIVERSITY PRESS
Baltimore

Notes to the reader: This book is not meant to substitute for medical care and advice, and decisions about medical treatment and other matters should not be based solely on its contents. Instead, decisions must be developed in a dialogue between the individual and her physician. This book has been written to help with that dialogue.

Drug dosage: The author and publisher have made reasonable efforts to determine that the selection and dosage of drugs discussed in this text conform to the practices of the general medical community. The medications described do not necessarily have specific approval by the U.S. Food and Drug Administration for use in the diseases and dosages for which they are recommended. In view of ongoing research, changes in governmental regulations, and the constant flow of information relating to drug therapy and drug reactions, the reader is urged to check the package insert of each drug for any change in indications and dosage and for warnings and precautions. This is particularly important when the recommended agent is a new and/or infrequently used drug.

© 2010 Julia Schlam Edelman
All rights reserved. Published 2010
Printed in the United States of America on acid-free paper
9 8 7 6 5 4 3 2 1

The Johns Hopkins University Press
2715 North Charles Street
Baltimore, Maryland 21218-4363
www.press.jhu.edu

Library of Congress Cataloging-in-Publication Data
Edelman, Julia Schlam, 1954–
   Menopause matters : your guide to a long and healthy life / Julia Schlam Edelman.
   p. cm. — (The Johns Hopkins Press health book)
   Includes bibliographical references and index.
   ISBN-13: 978-0-8018-9382-7 (hardcover : alk. paper)
   ISBN-10: 0-8018-9382-8 (hardcover : alk. paper)
   ISBN-13: 978-0-8018-9383-4 (pbk. : alk. paper)
   ISBN-10: 0-8018-9383-6 (pbk. : alk. paper)
   1. Menopause—Popular works. I. Title.
   RG186.E29 2009
   618.1'75—dc22   2009007045

A catalog record for this book is available from the British Library.

Special discounts are available for bulk purchases of this book. For more information, please contact Special Sales at 410-516-6936 or specialsales@press.jhu.edu.

The Johns Hopkins University Press uses environmentally friendly book materials, including recycled text paper that is composed of at least 30 percent post-consumer waste, whenever possible. All of our book papers are acid-free, and our jackets and covers are printed on paper with recycled content.

Contents

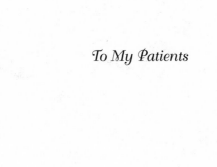

To My Patients

Acknowledgments

First I would like to thank my patients. It is a privilege to participate in your care. You kept asking me why you hadn't heard this information before and wondering where you could read more.

Literary agent John Riina championed this project from the time the initial ideas for the book were generated and contributed wisdom gained through decades of publishing experience. Jacqueline Wehmueller, executive editor at the Johns Hopkins University Press, believed this book would make a difference in women's health and navigated it through the entire publishing process from the manuscript's acceptance to its final publication. Martha Murphy was a pleasure to work with and made a major contribution to the editorial development of the book. The entire team at the Johns Hopkins University Press, including Juliana McCarthy, managing editor, Maria denBoer, copy editor, and Mary Lou Kenney, production editor, contributed valuable expertise to this book.

Additional support came from many quarters, including family, friends, and staff, ranging from playing the role of sounding board to providing technical assistance. Particular thanks to long-term office staff members: Anne-Marie Dexter, for her ongoing dedication to patient care, and Michelle Leonard, for her technical support.

My parents, Martin and Florence Schlam, a dynamic duo, set an example of dedication to their respective professions, engineering and medicine, and they continue to model a lifelong enthusiasm for learning. Younger brothers, Randy Schlam and Everett Schlam, are always fun to speak with as friends as well as colleagues who provide high-quality "curbside consults" in their respective specialties, radiology and family medicine. Sons Abe and Eric Edelman, both good writers, provided honest feedback on select passages when requested and shook their heads at early drafts, inspiring me to do better. My husband, Paul, offered insight, encouragement, and support in too many ways to enumerate here.

Introduction

You probably picked up this book because you are in some stage of menopause, and you are looking for current, reliable information to help you optimize your health during or after "the change." Maybe your symptoms have begun interfering with your normal life, or maybe you are not experiencing any discomfort at all but are concerned about your long-term health. Whether or not your body reminds you of the fact on a daily basis, it is going through a major transition, and you are entering a new phase of your life that brings with it new health concerns and responsibilities.

It's true that menopause is natural, and it's also true that our grandmothers handled it without a lot of medical tests and medications. On the other hand, our grandmothers led lives very different from our own, and their life expectancy was shorter. The women of our generation will be spending more than one-third of their lives in postmenopause. We owe it to ourselves to find out what the implications are.

For you to be as healthy, energetic, and productive as you can be, for as long as possible, form an alliance with a doctor who is well informed about women's health. Being fully in control of your own health does not mean avoiding the doctor's office. Nor does it mean that you must become your own doctor. It means taking an active role in protecting your well-being. The best place to start is by reading this book, then scheduling an appointment with your doctor.

This book is unique. While my credentials and experience as a board-certified gynecologist, certified menopause clinician, and member of the North American Menopause Society allow me to address your concerns, one of my strongest qualifications is what I have learned from my patients. Over the past 25 years, they have brought me their insights, concerns, and questions. As I have been researching the answers to their questions, I have been focusing my medical practice on gynecology and menopausal women. As a gynecologist, mother, wife, and postmenopausal woman myself, I have read countless medical studies to gather the most up-to-date, useful, and scientifically sound information about the most effective tests, procedures, medications, and lifestyle choices for women like us.

When is it a good idea to take hormones? What are the long-term consequences? Are nonprescription alternatives as effective? How does perimenopause affect memory? What is the best possible approach to osteoporosis? To heart disease? To sex? What are the best screening and diagnostic tests for women over age 40? What diseases can mimic the symptoms of perimenopause?

I am excited to share my knowledge and perspective with you. In this book you will find chapters devoted to the specific health issues associated with menopause, including hot flashes, bleeding, bone strength, weight management, sex after 40, cancer prevention, and more. Although you may want to jump to a particular chapter right now if you have a specific concern, I encourage you eventually to read the book from beginning to end. In every chapter, you'll find practical tips for monitoring and maintaining your health, and case histories about women like you. These cases are composites: each is a blend of hundreds of women with similar symptoms. Chapters also contain a list of resources providing additional information about each topic.

One of my most important messages is this: even if you look and feel good, you will benefit from preventive care, especially if you are over the age of 40. Many of the medical problems we associate with aging are, in fact, a result of unhealthy lifestyle choices. It is never too late to modify your lifestyle to enhance your health. Further, changes in our physical health that take place after age 40 are not always obvious. In our twenties, it was safer to assume that if we felt healthy we *were* healthy, but the same does not hold true beyond age 40. For us, choosing to "do nothing" sets in motion serious health consequences that rise dramatically after age 50 and with the onset of postmenopause.

For example, as your bones thin, there is no telltale pain to alert you. While broken bones are painful, bone thinning is a silent process that is all too common. Subtle changes in your metabolism may signal diabetes or another metabolic problem predisposing you to obesity. Your cholesterol may be high, due to lifestyle or heredity or both. If you have high cholesterol, you are at greater risk for heart disease. If you are *aware* of this, you can take steps to lower your high cholesterol with lifestyle changes or medication or both, allowing you to avoid heart disease. But unless you have a cholesterol blood test, you may never know you have a problem until you have a heart attack.

Age-related illnesses not only affect your later decades but also have an impact on your life in your forties or fifties. Whether you are 35 or 75, it is not too early (or too late) to learn what preventive measures are available for you. After you read this book and have learned more about the changes that are happening in your body, schedule an appointment with your health care provider. The last chapter of this book will help you get the most out of your doctor visits. Actually, this information will help you and your family members get the best medical care for *any* health condition. With his or her help, you and your doctor will be able to determine the current state of your health, address any apparent or hidden issues, and take precautions to safeguard your well-being into your eighties and beyond. We have the gift of many more years than our grandmothers had, so let's use it wisely and enjoy those years to the fullest as we stay mentally sharp, physically active, and well.

Julia Schlam Edelman, M.D., F.A.C.O.G.

Menopause Matters

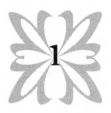

1

You and Your Doctor: The Health Alliance

I t's a tough time to be menopausal. Information about scientific advances in women's health care is more accessible than ever before—through television, the Internet, newspapers, and magazines. But despite this abundance of information, women have less peace of mind. New concerns about menopause arise daily as women are bombarded with "facts." Some are not accurate and others are presented out of context, troubling women with what appears to be flip-flopping medical advice. For example, my patients, my colleagues in gynecology, and I are still coping with the misconceptions caused by the results initially published by the Women's Health Initiative, released in July 2002. Some of my patients became so alarmed by what they read and heard in the news about hormone therapy that they immediately stopped taking their medications—even though the study showed that in some circumstances this was not necessary or even advisable.

Research into menopause has blossomed in the past two decades. Fifty years ago, the medical community had little to offer women at this time in their lives. Now there are many options—but it is difficult to sort out which ones benefit which women. A principal goal of this book is to clarify which medical options may be safest and most advisable for you, depending upon the phase of menopause you are in.

"My Grandmother Never Went to the Doctor. Why Should I?"

The average age for achieving postmenopause in North America today is 51 years. This age has remained constant since the Roman Empire. Postmenopause is more significant now, however, than even just 100 years ago, because of the dramatic increase in longevity. An American woman in 2009 has an average life expectancy of 84 years. For many women, this means 30 years or more spent in postmenopause.

We are much less active than our mothers and grandmothers were. We travel more, but walk less. Cars, planes, buses, and trains move while we sit still for hours. We have time-saving devices that spare us from the backbreaking labor of the past. These conveniences also "save" us from moving or using our muscles. Laundry is no longer scrubbed vigorously, then wrung out and hung to dry. Few of us plant, grow, or harvest what we cook for dinner—if we cook at all. Even watching television is a more passive pursuit than it was 20 years ago; with the advent of remote control, it is no longer necessary to get up to change the channel!

Our modern lifestyle, while more comfortable, puts us at a greater risk of osteoporosis, obesity, diabetes, and heart disease as well as breast, ovarian, and uterine cancer. Today, many women live into their eighties and beyond, but this increase in life expectancy does not come with a warranty that ensures good quality of life. The choices you make now set the stage for your health and well-being during the last third of your adult life. You have options to consider in the areas of nutrition, dietary supplements, exercise, stress management, and screening for hidden medical problems. Even if you are over 65, you can still benefit from making better-informed choices.

Visiting your doctor and taking preventive measures will save you time, expense, and hassle. In the long run, you will make fewer trips to the doctor, and spend less time waiting in reception areas for visits to treat high blood pressure, diabetes, osteoporosis, and advanced cancer. Embracing preventive care will lighten your financial burden as well: you will avoid paying for expensive medications and making more frequent visits to your doctor to monitor your more fragile state of health.

Women who reject preventive care strategies miss opportunities to be proactive about their health. They can expect to have more numerous and more severe health problems. The most devastating consequence of this adverse medical status can be the loss of independence.

"But I Feel Fine!"

Many "apparently" healthy women have told me: "I feel well, so I must be healthy. I don't want to have expensive tests when I feel fine!" Some of these women dislike the time, expense, and experience of the tests themselves, and some of them dislike the notion of taking medications and are concerned about side effects. The hazards of taking hormones and the perils of other prescription medications have been overemphasized in the media. Many women have simply concluded it is safest to tough out the perimenopause transition without a doctor's input and to "let nature take its course" during postmenopause. If they feel fine, why should they have tests done?

All of our lives, most of us have relied on doctors to treat acute problems, like a broken leg. I find that people are very accepting of "fix-it" medicine. If they develop a urinary tract infection, they will take antibiotics. If they break a hip, they will have surgery to repair or replace it. You may have the mindset, "I won't fix it if it isn't broken." Good medical care today, however, *must* include good preventive care.

Neglecting your health is never a good idea, but as you get older the consequences can become grave. It can be difficult for a woman to care for herself during perimenopause and beyond because she is often juggling the demands of elderly parents as well as her own partner, children, and grandchildren. I know what it is like to be a member of the "sandwich generation." Even if you have a very busy life (and even if you feel fine), please take time to meet with your doctor and have a checkup. You may have invisible health problems that should be addressed, and the sooner you identify and deal with them, the better. On the other hand, if you get a clean bill of health, you can take comfort knowing you are on the right track. Find the time now to see your doctor and consider your medical options based on your age and menopause status. The old adage is still true: "An ounce of prevention is worth a pound of cure!"

⚔ LENORE'S STORY ⚔

"I'm Through with Menopause!"

At age 60, Lenore thought she was through with menopause. "I felt fine and had no bleeding or hot flashes, so I decided I no longer needed to keep going to the doctor on a regular basis.

"One day, while I was gardening, I was bitten by a tick. Then several days later, I developed a fever and muscle aches. When I went to my family doctor, he ordered a blood test to check for evidence of Lyme disease. Since I was overdue for a complete physical examination, he ordered additional blood work as well.

"When the lab results came back, it was clear I had not only Lyme disease, but also very high cholesterol, which, he explained, dramatically increased my risk of heart attack and stroke. My doctor prescribed antibiotics for the Lyme disease and talked to me about exercising and modifying my diet. He told me that if these lifestyle changes did not have a great enough effect, he would recommend a type of medication called a statin to further lower my cholesterol and reduce my risk of heart attack and stroke."

Lenore had weathered the storms of perimenopause but she had not continued to take care of her health. Her Lyme disease turned out to be a blessing in disguise, as it ultimately led her to take control of her cholesterol.

Hidden Threats Your Doctor Can Evaluate

Women who have hot flashes, urinary problems, vaginal dryness, or other concerns are more likely to find their way to a doctor's office because they are looking for relief. But even women with none of these physical discomforts still need special care. The body's hidden needs do not correlate with hot flashes, night sweats, or menstrual irregularities. Relying on these symptoms to gauge whether or not you need care can be misleading. One goal of this book is to familiarize you with the hidden threats to your health that you may not be monitoring. They include:

- *Cardiovascular disease,* including heart attack and stroke. Your risk of heart disease rises after you enter postmenopause, especially after age 50. Cardiovascular disease is women's largest silent killer. In the United States, one out of every two women over age 50 will die of heart disease! This exceeds the combined death rate of women from all types of cancer.
- *Weight gain.* As you age, your metabolism slows, making weight gain an issue, even as early as age 35 or 40. Excess weight strains your heart, increases your risk of cancer, stresses your joints, and puts you at risk of developing diabetes.
- *Diabetes.* Obesity and diabetes are rapidly growing concerns; more than 60 percent of the U.S. population is now overweight, and the incidence of diabetes has reached epidemic proportions. The onset of Type 2 diabetes is linked to obesity and is a huge factor in heart disease and heart attack, among other serious conditions.
- *Osteoporosis.* Rapid bone thinning occurs early in postmenopause when estrogen levels plummet. Thin bones put you at risk for fracture, and serious fracture, such as of the hip, can put you at risk for pneumonia and other complications of being bed-bound.
- *Cancer.* It looms large in nearly every woman's mind. Your risk of breast cancer continues to increase every year of your life until you reach roughly 80 years old. For men and women, the incidence of colon cancer (easily avoided by following preventative measures) increases at age 50 and beyond.

These hidden threats are more common and more threatening to your well-being at this stage of your life than they were when you were younger. The good news is that treatments are available that may preserve your lifestyle and independence, and even save your life. Working with a doctor to prevent problems and catch disease early means you will enjoy better health than if you wait until a hidden problem, normally amenable to medical treatment, becomes obvious but difficult to treat.

At this stage, your gynecologist can play a key role in helping you maintain or achieve all-around good health, since so many aspects of your health are linked to your hormone levels. If you are experiencing the hot flashes, night sweats, and irregular periods that can go along with perimenopause, you may take them all in stride, assuming they are all part of "getting old." I encourage you to avoid the temptation of identifying perimenopause on your own rather than seeing a doctor to diagnose your symptoms. Self-diagnosis may result in overlooking problems that need to be addressed. You may miss the opportunity to discover a disorder that can be treated—and that may or may not be related to menopause. Different symptoms that resemble the problems of menopause can actually be caused by other health disorders. For example, many of the symptoms associated with perimenopause and postmenopause can be caused by a thyroid abnormality. In those instances, appropriate diagnosis and treatment of the underlying thyroid imbalance can put an end to the symptoms.

Similarly, it is not safe to assume that if you are a postmenopausal woman who is not having sex, you do not need gynecologic exams. Whether or not you are currently sexually active, it is still important to have regular gynecologic exams to stay healthy.

⚘ ALICIA'S STORY ⚘

A Sluggish Thyroid

Alicia is 46 years old. "I was distressed by a recent 15-pound weight gain and hot flashes. My nails had stopped growing, and my hair was falling out in clumps when I shampooed. I missed six menstrual cycles in seven months, but based on the experience of my friends with similar issues, I thought it was just part of perimenopause. When I discussed my symptoms with my doctor, he wanted to see whether my thyroid gland was functioning normally.

"A blood test revealed that my thyroid was underactive. My doctor said its function was sluggish, so my metabolism 'went into slow motion.' He prescribed a thyroid medication, to be taken orally once a day. Eight weeks after I started taking it, my hot flashes were gone. And after six months, my hair had stopped falling out and my nails began to grow back. My menstrual cycles became more predictable, and I was finally able to shed the excess weight I had gained."

What Stage of Menopause Are You In—and Why Does It Matter?

It's important not to assume you are postmenopausal when you are still in perimenopause. Postmenopause is a permanent phase that follows perimenopause. Postmenopause marks the end of your fertile years. Once you enter the postmenopause phase, you remain in it for the rest of your life. These two distinct phases affect your health differently. For example, postmenopausal women cannot conceive; perimenopausal women can and do. The ability to conceive is just one example of the differences between them.

Treatment options differ by phase of menopause. The risks, benefits, and safety profiles of a given hormone, medication, supplement, or surgical procedure may be drastically different for a postmenopausal woman than they are for one who is perimenopausal. Measures that maintain or restore health in one phase can be detrimental in another. For example, a perimenopausal nonsmoker who is experiencing severe hot flashes may benefit from taking a low-dose birth control pill. The hormones in the pill might relieve her symptoms. On the other hand, even a low-dose birth control pill is not suitable for a postmenopausal woman over 50. The hormone levels are too high for her system. Moreover, the pill delivers hormones in a cyclic pattern that does not match a postmenopausal woman's biology. Since she no longer has a menstrual cycle, her hormones stay constant.

Even if your body behaves the same way in postmenopause as it did in perimenopause, there are significant differences to note. For example, if you are perimenopausal, bleeding is expected. If you are postmenopausal, even a small amount of bleeding is a warning sign. It can signal that there is a problem in the uterus. While 9 out of 10 times that problem is not due to cancer, one out of 10 times the postmenopausal bleeding *is* due to cancer. In postmenopause, a single episode of bleeding may be a woman's only warning sign.

The term "menopausal" can be misleading because it means different things to each of us. For example, if a man says, "My wife is menopausal," to me that indicates she no longer has menstrual periods, so she is postmenopausal. However, if the next sentence is, "She is driving me crazy!" he probably means that his wife is experiencing mood swings associated with perimenopause. This language mix-up is problematic. Perimenopause and postmenopause are not the same thing and the terms are not interchangeable. Women can be perimenopausal or postmenopausal, but not "menopausal," and it is important to know which you are. Your doctor will help you find out.

Changing Hormone Levels

The role of the ovaries changes over time, from birth to the postmenopause years. When puberty arrives, the ovaries become the conductor of the childbearing orchestra. They produce key female hormones (estrogen and progesterone) and are responsible for releasing eggs. Throughout life, the ovaries also produce the male hormone testosterone, which contributes to a healthy woman's sex drive. Even in postmenopause the ovaries continue to produce small amounts of testosterone.

The ovaries in a female fetus can contain up to two million follicles, tiny cysts that may develop into eggs. Some follicles dissolve before a baby girl is born, but the majority of follicles remain in her body. At birth, a female infant begins releasing eggs from her ovaries. She cannot conceive, however, until her body goes through puberty and is primed for her first menstrual period—somewhere between ages 9 and 16 years. This marks the beginning of her reproductive years, when her biology is geared to conceiving children. After menstruation is established, follicles can be released as eggs during ovulation. Eggs released during ovulation are available for fertilization by male sperm. Eggs that are not fertilized by sperm dissolve in the pelvis or abdominal cavity.

While the ovaries play an important role in releasing eggs and manufacturing hormones, they do not act alone. Other organs, such as the hypothalamus (in the brain), also influence their performance.

The most regular menstrual cycles occur in a woman's twenties and early thirties, with a recurring pattern each month that includes mid-cycle ovulation when the ovary releases an egg. During each cycle the ovaries make predictable amounts of the female hormones, estrogen and progesterone, in a set sequence. Levels of estrogen and progesterone rise and fall in a natural rhythm that repeats itself about every 28 days, and women know what to expect. Progesterone released after ovulation is responsible for shedding of the uterine lining, usually two weeks later, with the menstrual period.

Hormones in Perimenopause: Unpredictable Fluctuations

Wider fluctuations in estrogen and progesterone levels occur during the menstrual cycles of women in their late thirties, forties, or fifties. By the time a woman is age 40, the ovaries are starting to shrink and have fewer follicles to release. They continue to shrink in size over the next 20 years or so. As the ovaries begin to show signs of age, hormones no longer rise and fall in a smooth, predictable pattern over a four-week cycle. Ovulation still occurs, but it is less frequent and more erratic. During perimenopause, ovary hormones fluctuate wildly and move away from the regular, predictable patterns established in the childbearing years. Irregular menstrual cycles are common, and changes in your body's level of estrogen and progesterone can be difficult to endure.

Estrogen levels are erratic in perimenopause. It is a common misconception that the discomforts of perimenopause are all caused by lack of sufficient amounts of estrogen. In fact, during perimenopause, estrogen levels often are too high. Some of the hallmarks of perimenopause, such as heavy bleeding, are a result of excess estrogen.

Your body makes different types of estrogen. The most potent, estradiol, is made by your ovaries during the reproductive and peri-menopausal years. If your estradiol levels are high, taking extra estrogen during this time may make you feel worse. During the reproductive years, estrogen levels rise and fall smoothly like gentle hills and valleys. During the perimenopausal years, the pattern becomes erratic with sharp spikes. The spikes represent rapid, unexpected shifts from very high to very low estrogen levels. This jagged see-saw pattern creates a rocky perimenopause for many women. After rising too high, estrogen levels can plummet, sinking too low. Periodically, estradiol levels sink so low that they trigger a hot flash or night sweat. Unpredictable and erratic estrogen levels can also wreak havoc in the form of mood changes and abnormal bleeding.

Women usually spend anywhere from 2 to 10 years in perimeno-pause. For some women this is a trying time. The erratic hormone shifts may produce debilitating hot flashes and night sweats, irregular menstrual periods, disturbing mood changes, and poor sleep quality. For other women, these changes are mild and barely noticeable. For a fortunate minority the transition is invisible. Twenty percent of women do not experience any hot flashes or night sweats.

During perimenopause, levels of progesterone, the other female hormone made in the ovaries, are also erratic and often too low. They may be too low to effectively counterbalance the high estrogen levels. Bloating, irritability, and breast tenderness may result. Some women with erratic hormone fluctuations benefit from additional progesterone—not estrogen!—to balance their estrogen peaks (more information on this can be found in Chapter 3). Imbalances of estrogen, progesterone, or both are characteristic of the perimenopausal years. When there is no ovulation for a cycle, little or no progesterone is released and the monthly shedding of the lining does not take place, often resulting in a missed period.

Hormones in Postmenopause: Low and Steady

Steady, low estrogen levels do not appear until postmenopause. Once they are established, they are maintained for the rest of a woman's life. This can be a relief to women who suffered with the erratic peaks and valleys of perimenopause.

Estradiol is no longer the dominant estrogen in your body when you become postmenopausal. There is another type of estrogen that plays an even more important role at this time: estrone, a weaker form of estrogen. Estrone becomes the dominant form of estrogen in your body in postmenopause, and it is not made in your ovaries. Your body's fatty tissues, also called adipose tissue, manufacture estrone. There is a reason for the extra belly fat that none of us can seem to avoid at this age. It is helpful to have a modest amount of extra fat in postmenopause to maintain your supply of estrone, which helps you to maintain your bone strength. As in life, there can be too much of a good thing. Women with a great deal of adipose tissue produce excess amounts of estrone that may cause abnormal bleeding and increase the risk of breast and uterine cancer.

FERTILITY AND PERIMENOPAUSE

Perimenopause represents the transition a woman's body undergoes when it changes from childbearing status to non-childbearing status. Fertility gradually declines for women in their thirties and continues to diminish until their fifties, depending on their personal biological schedule. Many women think that the signs of perimenopause mean that they are no longer fertile. In reality, fertility persists until postmenopause. Women in their forties have unplanned pregnancies at a rate second only to that of teenagers. Postmenopausal women cannot become pregnant. Perimenopausal women can and *do*.

⚡ DORIS'S STORY ⚡

Pregnant at 46

"I began to have hot flashes when I turned 45 and then missed four menstrual periods in a row. I assumed I was in postmenopause and told my husband to cancel his appointment for a vasectomy. We had decided on a vasectomy for him because we had recently sent our youngest child off to college and did not want to risk an unplanned pregnancy.

"I was actually perimenopausal and had missed menstrual periods because I was pregnant. Subsequently, I miscarried. After we weathered

the stress of the unplanned pregnancy and miscarriage, my husband rescheduled his appointment to have a vasectomy. I continued to have irregular menstrual periods. It wasn't until I was 55 that I had gone 12 consecutive months with no bleeding. At that time my doctor confirmed I had entered postmenopause and was no longer fertile."

MENSTRUAL BLEEDING AND PERIMENOPAUSE

Irregular menstrual periods are the most frequent sign of perimenopause. Ninety percent of women experience changes in their menstrual cycle for 4 to 10 years preceding postmenopause. Menstrual cycles in perimenopause often disappear, only to reappear without warning. I have heard horror stories about the sudden, unexpected return of a menstrual period that can involve bleeding through clothes in a public setting. If this happens to you, rest assured: you are not alone!

During perimenopause, your menstrual flow may become lighter or heavier. You may bleed for longer or shorter periods of time. You may miss periods or bleed more often. Even though each woman's experience is unique, there are medical guidelines doctors use to determine if something is not right. The more information you are able to share with your doctor about what your version of "normal" bleeding has been, the easier it will be to recognize anything abnormal. I ask all of my patients to keep a record of their bleeding patterns so I can see at a glance when something changes.

HOW LONG DOES PERIMENOPAUSE LAST?

"When will this end?" is a question I am asked daily. You have a right to know, but neither you nor your doctor has a way to tell until after the fact. The end of perimenopause is still determined by looking back, after the fact, at *12 consecutive months without any menstrual bleeding.*

When my patients pose this question, I can't help thinking how ironic it is that we live in a world that can send an astronaut to the moon but still has not pinpointed when perimenopause begins, how long it will last, and when it will end.

Perimenopause can last as long as 10 years. Unfortunately, there is currently no blood test to confirm that you are definitely in perimenopause, nor is there a test that accurately predicts when your perimenopause will end. New testing is in the works but is not yet available, reliable, or accurate. At this time, perimenopause is usually established by taking a careful medical history.

In my experience, the most frequently requested test for perimenopause is a blood test for follicle-stimulating hormone (FSH). FSH is reputed to tell you whether you are perimenopausal or not, and when you can expect to enter postmenopause. In fact, FSH usually *cannot* give you this information. Here's why.

If you are in perimenopause, your levels of FSH are still fluctuating widely. So a single blood test result showing elevated FSH could represent just one part of a given menstrual cycle. I will tell you what I tell my perimenopausal patients: you can have your blood drawn one day and get an FSH result that looks like a 20-year-old's (a low number), yet on another day that same week you could get a result that looks like a 60-year-old's (a high number). These erratic results may reflect your perimenopausal status, but do not predict whether postmenopause is imminent. In postmenopause, FSH is consistently elevated, but this rise does not begin until one year after your final menstrual period. We need a better test.

Recently it was found that a woman who missed three menstrual periods in a row could expect to enter postmenopause within the next few years. Postmenopause was farther away for women who only skipped one menstrual period at a time or continued to have regular cycles.

In addition to blood tests of certain hormone levels, which you can get through your doctor, mail-order companies offer saliva tests to measure estrogen, progesterone, and testosterone. You can order the kit to do your own saliva testing and then get the results by phone, email, or a mailed report. This may appeal to you for several reasons. You can avoid the unpleasant experience of having your blood drawn; you can do the saliva test yourself in the privacy of your home without a doctor's visit; and you are taking charge of your own care. Unfortunately, the accuracy of these saliva tests is not established. Hormone levels in saliva are not biologically meaningful. It is not possible to test for the concentration of free unbound hormone in the saliva. Further, there is no biological relationship between salivary sex steroid hormone concentration and the amount of free hormone in the blood. There are large differences in salivary hormone concentrations between individual women that are not understood, as well as variability for individual women at different times during their menstrual cycle and during different phases of menopause. Salivary hormone levels will also vary with diet, the time of day of testing, and the specific hormone being tested. In the future, there will, no doubt, be better tests. Testing levels of inhibin, a hormone that plays a role in the timing of postmenopause, shows promise. Levels of inhibin are elevated in postmenopause, but not in perimenopause. The timing and accuracy of this blood test are still being investigated, so it is not yet available for clinical use.

Diagnosing Postmenopause

Postmenopause begins when a woman has had 12 consecutive months with no menstrual bleeding. In postmenopause, menstrual cycles are no longer possible and fertility ends. The ovaries have released their last follicles and there are no eggs remaining. Postmenopause is a permanent state.

Each woman is born with a certain number of eggs and uses them up at her own rate. Women who have had two full-term pregnancies enter postmenopause later than those who do not. During full-term pregnancies, ovulation is suspended, so eggs are not used up as quickly. You also have a break from ovulation during the time you spend nursing your infant.

The average age for postmenopause in North America is 51 years old, although women commonly reach this milestone seven years before or after this age. So, the normal age range for entering postmenopause is 44 to 58 years old.

Usually perimenopause precedes postmenopause. But postmenopause can occur rapidly when the ovaries are surgically removed or are inactivated by infection, radiation, chemotherapy, or, rarely, severe stress.

Although the postmenopausal ovaries have retired from child-bearing, they still have other functions. A common misconception is that the ovaries stop making hormones in postmenopause. In fact, ovaries continue to make testosterone. Postmenopausal ovaries also continue to make estradiol; they just make it in drastically reduced amounts, and it is released slowly and steadily. This is a stabilizing, tranquil time for many women after they have weathered the storms of perimenopause.

Sometimes it can be hard to tell whether you are postmenopausal or just experiencing a longer gap between menstrual cycles in peri-menopause. If you suspect that you are postmenopausal, ask your doctor to confirm it. He or she will perform a physical exam, update your personal medical history, and perhaps order lab work to con-firm that you are truly in postmenopause.

Once you establish steady, low levels of estrogen and progester-one in postmenopause, you will maintain steady, low levels of these hormones for the rest of your life. They will not fluctuate each month. This means that monthly mood changes are a thing of the past. If your moods vary, you and your doctor should look for other causes, such as depression, stress, or anxiety.

Postmenopause may be associated with discomforts such as vagi-nal dryness or pain with sexual intercourse. Another medical issue that can arise is unexpected urine loss. Hot flashes may persist into the postmenopausal years, but they are not likely to begin then.

EARLY POSTMENOPAUSE

While the average woman in North America becomes postmenopausal at age 51, younger women may be postmenopausal for many different reasons. Women who become postmenopausal in their early forties, between ages 40 and 44, are referred to as having early postmenopause.

There are a number of factors that influence the timing of prema-ture menopause and postmenopause:

- *Premature menopause* refers to the cessation of menstrual peri-ods and the end of fertility before the age of 40. This can occur naturally or as a consequence of radiation or chemotherapy. Survivors of childhood cancer are more likely to experience premature menopause.

- *Surgical menopause* occurs when a woman's ovaries are surgically removed before she has made the transition into postmenopause on her own. (If the ovaries are surgically removed after age 55, for example, and a woman is already postmenopausal, she has not experienced a surgical menopause.)
- *Cigarette smoke.* Smoking is toxic to the ovaries and almost doubles the chances of premature menopause. It is also associated with postmenopause arriving up to two years earlier than it would have in the same woman if she did not smoke.
- *Early onset of menstruation.* A woman whose first menstrual period occurs at age 13 or younger is more likely to have premature menopause or early postmenopause.
- *The Pill.* Using oral contraceptives or birth control pills lowers the risk of early menopause. This is probably related to the fact that ovulation is suppressed while a woman is on oral contraceptives. This conserves follicles for later release.
- *Genetic predisposition.* Some women have several family members who enter postmenopause by age 40, suggesting a hereditary pattern. Genetic mutations may explain some of these cases.

Surgical Menopause

Surgical menopause is a cloudy concept because the term "hysterectomy" is loosely used to describe several different operations. In my experience, the most common misconception is that a "total hysterectomy" results in instant menopause. In surgical terms, a total hysterectomy represents the surgical removal of the uterus and the cervix. It does not indicate the status of the ovaries—which is what determines postmenopausal status. The surgical procedure that produces postmenopause is a *bilateral oophorectomy,* or the removal of both ovaries. You could have a "total hysterectomy" at age 42, but if you have healthy ovaries and they are not surgically removed, you will not become postmenopausal at that time. The ovaries will continue to make normal amounts of estrogen and progesterone and to release follicles that are absorbed into the abdominal cavity. As long as you have even one functional ovary remaining, you are still perimenopausal. The remaining ovary will take over and continue to manufacture hormones, including estrogen, progesterone, and testosterone.

In this case you cannot judge your menopausal stage by your menstrual periods, since you will not have any periods after your uterus is surgically removed.

☙ PETRA'S STORY ❧

Total Hysterectomy without Oophorectomy

"I was 43 years old when I found out that I had a large uterine fibroid. The size was comparable to a four-month pregnancy. I had been experiencing pelvic pressure and abdominal bloating. I also had heavy menstrual bleeding and clots and had become anemic. My doctor recommended a hysterectomy and told me he planned to conserve both of my ovaries if they appeared normal at the time of surgery. He said he expected them to continue to function normally, providing me with adequate levels of hormones. If my ovaries were abnormal, he said he would remove them and prescribe estrogen so I wouldn't experience sudden 'surgical menopause.' Fortunately, my ovaries were normal and were left in place. I didn't notice any hormonal shifts or mood changes that were different from what I was experiencing before surgery. My doctor explained that I was perimenopausal at the time of surgery and still am. My ovaries are still functioning. Since the operation, I really have only two significant changes: I can no longer become pregnant, and I no longer have any menstrual bleeding."

How Your Doctor Can Help You

I do not have a crystal ball to see your future, but I am well equipped to identify your risk factors for cardiovascular disease, osteoporosis, and diabetes. Extensive research has shown me what to look for when I analyze your personal medical history and family history. I know what to check during your physical examination, which tests to order, and how to interpret the results. Your own doctor has the same experience and skills.

In order to customize prevention strategies that suit your needs and preferences, your doctor needs your input. An effective prevention strategy meets two criteria: it helps you stay healthy and it consists of recommendations that you are willing to follow.

Many people become motivated to get more exercise, improve their nutrition, or take preventive medication only after their first heart attack or stroke, or after they have been diagnosed with diabetes, or after fracturing their backbone or hip. Others will be proactive and embrace preventive measures before they have a medical crisis.

Even if you feel fine, don't let a hidden problem catch you by surprise. By the time it comes to your attention, it will be much harder to correct. Every year, fine-tune your prevention and treatment regimens with your doctor. He or she can help you decide if your current approach is best or if it is time to incorporate the results of a new medical breakthrough or newly available natural remedy.

Your doctor wants you to be healthy. While some illnesses cannot be prevented, many can. It is sad to see patients whose lives become limited by preventable illnesses. It is heartening to see active, energetic, motivated patients who take control of their health and future.

RESOURCE

The Menopause Guidebook, 6th edition, October 2006. Published by the North American Menopause Society, this 64-page manual is an overview of all aspects of menopause, including perimenopause and early menopause. It can be ordered and viewed online (www.menopause.org/edumaterials/guidebook) or obtained in print.

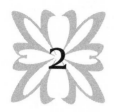

2

Handling Hot Flashes
without Hormones

Hot flashes themselves are harmless, provided they are not disruptive. Often they can be managed without hormones using the approaches discussed in this chapter. Lifestyle changes are simple, effective, and affordable, and have few side effects. Some over-the-counter remedies are worth trying, while others have side effects or are not safe long term. Finally, there are non-hormone prescription medications that were designed for other purposes but are effective in reducing hot flashes.

Hormone solutions for hot flashes are discussed in the next chapter. Healthy perimenopausal women who are nonsmokers also have the option of a low-dose oral contraceptive to control their hot flashes or night sweats (for more information, see Chapter 8).

What Is a Hot Flash?

A hot flash is sudden, temporary warmth, with flushing and perspiring. In other words, you become hot, red-faced, and sweaty! Some women refer to hot flashes as "power surges."

Certain physical changes occur during a hot flash. First, the body's core temperature goes down, producing central cooling. Then heat is lost through the skin. Skin temperature measurements show that the skin gets several degrees warmer as a hot flash takes place.

Perspiring and evaporation cause additional rapid heat loss. A chill may follow the hot flash.

Who Gets Hot Flashes?

One hundred years ago, women spent less time in post-menopause. Their life expectancy was decades shorter, and hot flashes were not a major issue. Today, about 75 percent of women experience hot flashes—and about 25 percent do not.

Hot flashes are the second most common sign of perimenopause, after irregular vaginal bleeding. Even though no one understands exactly what causes hot flashes, there is an increasing awareness of the benefits of lifestyle choices, including the role of diet and exercise, to alleviate them.

Vegetable-based diets are associated with less frequent, milder hot flashes. Vegetarians in the United States, as well as those in other parts of the world, report fewer hot flashes.

Those who exercise regularly, or are physically active, have fewer, less intense hot flashes. Women who walk daily report fewer hot flashes.

In Japan, women eat mostly vegetables, have a more active life-style, and are seldom overweight. Fewer than 25 percent of Japanese women have hot flashes. In fact, the Japanese language does not include a word for hot flashes. Women in certain African tribes also meet these criteria and, similarly, have fewer hot flashes.

Diet and exercise may only partially explain why women in other cultures enjoy a smoother midlife transition, with fewer medical concerns. Middle-aged women in Japan, the Mayan culture, and some Arabic and African nations are more highly regarded during midlife and beyond. Their status in society increases with their seniority. They gain more respect from society and their families as they age. These women welcome the end of childbearing responsibilities. For them, this time of life is associated with attaining the highest status possible, equal even to that of a respected male member of society. I suspect this is a positive incentive to weather the changes of perimenopause and postmenopause, and it may decrease the stress levels of women living in these societies.

Contrast this situation with the messages North American women receive. We live in a youth-centered culture. Many women mourn the end of their childbearing years as well as the loss of their youth. A quick glance at the magazines in any newsstand illustrates the message clearly: look young, banish wrinkles, and attain a thinner, more youthful body, at any cost. Whatever it takes: creams, Botox, liposuction, plastic surgery—or, in Madonna's case, a grueling exercise routine reported to exceed six hours a day. The price is never too high.

The first general menopause book I read was Gail Sheehy's *Silent Passage*, published decades ago. The author laments aging in a youth-centered culture. Despite her insights, our society's view of our adult female citizens has not matured. In a room full of older women, few have gray or white hair, and many perimenopausal and postmenopausal women are still reluctant to reveal their age.

It can help women to see how their roles change in interesting ways as they leave their childbearing years. The "empty nest" involves more than the departure of offspring—it brings a different perspective on life. When it coincides with postmenopause, it is also relief from the relentless biology of reproduction and a quieting of the hormone storms of perimenopause. As our hormones are shifting, our "wiring" also shifts, and we end up with a different emotional perspective on the world when we cross the threshold into postmenopause. How would we feel if we were given increased respect and consideration as we aged? What if we were encouraged to share our life experience rather than our repertoire of techniques to look younger?

Hot Flashes Vary

The intensity and frequency of hot flashes varies dramatically between individual women. Hot flashes also vary over time for each woman as she progresses from perimenopause to postmenopause. For some women, the hot flashes come and go over days, weeks, or months. Some women experience hot flashes for a brief time before the flashes disappear, never to return again. Some women get hot flashes or night sweats while they still have periods; others get them when their periods are infrequent or after they have stopped. And although it is not as common, some women find hot flashes troublesome for decades.

You may be comfortable during the day but awaken every hour or two during the night with night sweats. Night sweats are identical to hot flashes, except for their timing. It is possible to have only daytime hot flashes, only night sweats, or both. It is not clear why hot flashes or night sweats plague some women and not others.

Mild or infrequent hot flashes do not have to be treated at all. Hot flashes are harmless unless they compromise your ability to function in daily life. Frequent or severe night sweats can disrupt sleep, causing sleep deprivation, irritability, and memory loss. They are life threatening if they make you sleepy enough during the day to be at risk of falling asleep at the wheel of your car.

Contrary to popular belief, hot flashes do not predict when perimenopause ends or when postmenopause begins. As stated, hot flashes can come and go, without warning, over a period of days, months, or years. In some women, they resolve spontaneously without any intervention; other women only find relief with treatment. Hot flashes and night sweats may be easily tolerated or debilitating. At one point, your hot flashes may be mild or infrequent, causing little or no disruption in your routine. At another time, you may suffer from intense hot flashes that recur every hour, compromising your ability to function effectively at home or work. If your hot flashes are not incapacitating, it is best not to feel smug too soon. Over time they could become debilitating.

A postmenopausal woman whose hot flashes have completely resolved for more than a year without medication can expect them not to return. If they *do* return, your doctor will want to determine why. Causes for hot flashes that are not related to postmenopause include certain prescription medications, some over-the-counter supplements, as well as common medical conditions, including thyroid disease, high blood pressure, and hepatitis. Niacin, which is given to reduce cholesterol, and Lupron, an injection given to shrink fibroids or control endometriosis, also cause hot flashes. Tamoxifen,

given to reduce the risk of breast cancer (or the risk of recurrent
breast cancer), and Evista, given to build bones, are prescription
medications that can be associated with hot flashes. More unusual
medical conditions that cause hot flashes include tuberculosis and
sarcoid, a lung disease. With a medical history, exam, and lab tests,
your doctor can identify why you are experiencing hot flashes.

Hot Flashes Due to Thyroid Problems

Thyroid disease is the most common cause of hot flashes
other than menopause. Sometimes hot flashes may be caused by a
combination of thyroid disease and perimenopause. An underactive
thyroid may cause hot flashes and night sweats, weight gain, and irregular menstrual periods. When the thyroid condition is treated, all
of these symptoms may vanish. So, it is important to check whether
thyroid disease is present before deciding a woman is experiencing
solely perimenopause.

Blood tests check the thyroid function and reveal if it is sluggish
or overactive. While hot flashes due to perimenopause may be simply watched, thyroid disease must be identified and treated to avoid
serious complications affecting the rest of the body.

The thyroid is a soft, butterfly-shaped gland located in the neck, in front of the trachea (windpipe). The thyroid gland regulates metabolism, telling the body how fast to think and move and process food and waste. Thyroid function affects hair health, including breakage, texture, rate of growth, and rate of loss. It affects nail health and growth. It affects reflexes (which may become too fast or too slow) and the quality of sleep.

Thyroid disease is very common, especially in women. For every man with a thyroid problem, there are 10 women with thyroid disease. Thyroid disease also is more common with increasing age. Although thyroid disease runs in families, it is often identified in those with no family history of the problem.

Thyroid disease shows up in different ways. Hyperthyroidism, or an overactive thyroid, is associated with racing thoughts, unintended weight loss, poor sleep, and a rapid heart rate as well as increased sweating. In contrast, hypothyroidism, or an underactive thyroid, may cause sluggishness of thought and motion, depression, and unplanned weight gain without any changes in eating or exercise. Both types of thyroid disease can cause hot flashes and irregular menstrual periods.

It is possible to have hot flashes that are caused by thyroid disease before, during, or after perimenopause. Thyroid disease can be detected by a careful medical history and then confirmed with a blood test. Sometimes a woman may have troublesome symptoms but her thyroid blood tests are only mildly abnormal. These individuals may have subclinical hypothyroidism. Additional specialized blood tests can show that thyroid gland function has been disturbed. In the past, people with subclinical thyroid problems have not always received medication to treat the imbalance. In England, a group of patients was so upset about not being treated for subclinical hypothyroidism that they formed a patient advocate group that petitioned the medical community to be more aggressive about diagnosing and treating subtle thyroid disorders.

Rarely, thyroid disease can be present with normal laboratory results. This requires specialized blood work or an ultrasound of the thyroid to check for nodules that may disrupt the metabolism.

It is uncommon to develop hot flashes for the first time during postmenopause. If you do, get tested for thyroid disease, another cause of hot flashes.

⚥ BETH'S STORY ⚥

Hot Flashes due to a Thyroid Problem

"Nine years ago, when I was 55, I had a total hysterectomy with the removal of both ovaries. I began using a hormone patch after the surgery and was free of hot flashes. But after the extensive media coverage of the negative effects of hormones in July 2002, I became concerned about the risks of estrogen and stopped using the patch. I felt well for six months, but then the hot flashes—severe and frequent—returned. My doctor suspected a thyroid problem because the hot flashes had already resolved when I was off estrogen. She said that because I was in a stable postmenopausal state, my estrogen levels should not be fluctuating. The thyroid blood test showed that I had become hypothyroid. My sluggish thyroid was causing the hot flashes. My doctor prescribed thyroid medication and, after three months, my hot flashes are now gone."

Handling Hot Flashes with Paced Respiration

Paced respiration is a new behavior modification technique that can decrease the frequency of hot flashes by 80 percent. It is promoted by the North American Menopause Society, as well as by the American College of Obstetricians and Gynecologists. When I tell patients about this technique, I emphasize that it is free and has no side effects. Paced respiration also helps treat high blood pressure naturally, in some cases lowering it into the normal range. Paced respiration involves breathing slowly and deeply. You breathe only 5 to 7 times per minute—much slower than the normal breathing rate, which averages over 12 breaths a minute.

To practice paced respiration, count slowly to yourself, up to four or five, while inhaling slowly. Then exhale slowly while counting to four or five. After inhaling fully and deeply, start to slowly exhale; do not hold your breath in between. It is helpful to silently say "one thousand" in between each count. So the counting process is: "One, one thousand; two, one thousand; three, one thousand; four, one thousand; five, one thousand," while breathing in slowly and deeply. Then start to exhale slowly, counting back down: "Five, one thousand; four, one thousand; three, one thousand; two, one thousand; one, one thousand." Those who find it too difficult to breathe slowly enough to count to five while inhaling may start by counting slowly to three or four at first. Others find it easier to start by exhaling first, then inhaling. Often women remember to breathe deeply but they forget to breathe more slowly than normal. *Don't forget to breathe more slowly.* Breathing deeply and quickly won't work. Quick, deep breaths are not successful in reducing hot flashes or high blood pressure.

To master paced respiration, practice the technique until you can perform it for 10 to 15 minutes, continuously, to get comfortable with it. This trains your body to breathe more slowly than normal on command. After you master the technique, it will not take more than a few minutes for it to be effective. After you are able to sustain the slow, deep breathing for 10 to 15 minutes, I suggest you do paced respiration for 5 minutes each morning before leaving your house, and for 5 minutes each evening before going to bed. Keeping up the technique on a regular basis will keep you in practice. The technique is most effective if used when you get a hot flash or night sweat. Any time a severe hot flash or night sweat arrives, begin doing paced respiration. The hot flash or night sweat should vanish or subside within minutes.

Handling Hot Flashes with Lifestyle Modifications

Hot flashes can arrive hourly, daily, weekly, or monthly. Although hot flashes may occur in a cyclic pattern, they don't always appear on cue.

We don't understand exactly why hot flashes occur, but there are common triggers—behaviors, circumstances, or substances that commonly induce hot flashes. Hot or spicy foods were once thought to induce hot flashes; recent research does not support this idea.

On the other hand, caffeine and alcohol definitely can trigger hot flashes. So can an upcoming period.

Avoiding your triggers reduces the number and severity of hot flashes. At times, avoiding or eliminating triggers erases the need for other lifestyle modifications, natural remedies, or prescription medication.

REDUCE YOUR STRESS

Stress is a trigger for many women, although it is not clear why stress triggers hot flashes. There are a variety of strategies to reduce stress and to help you cope with it.

Decreasing the number of stressful situations you face each day at home and/or work may decrease the number of hot flashes you have. Can you:

- delegate tasks to others?
- reduce your commitments?
- change your priorities?
- shorten your work hours?
- eliminate a long or stressful commute?
- change to a different type of work that is less stressful?

Stress reduction techniques are taught by psychologists, social workers, and other mental health professionals. These may include relaxation tapes, meditation, or other approaches.

AVOID ALCOHOL

Whether it is consumed in the form of beer, wine, hard liquor, or a mixed drink, alcohol is almost certain to bring on hot flashes or night sweats. Alcohol also disturbs the quality of one's sleep. Although it may be easy to fall asleep after having a drink or two, the deepest, most restful part of sleep, called rapid eye movement (REM) sleep, is compromised. Decreasing the amount of alcohol consumed improves the quality of sleep, in addition to reducing the frequency and severity of hot flashes and night sweats.

⚬ HEIDI'S STORY ⚬

Hot Flashes and Red Wine

"I was going through perimenopause smoothly. I had been experiencing hot flashes but they resolved after I cut down my daily coffee from an extra-large (24 ounces) to 8 ounces a day. I also practiced paced respiration faithfully. One February, my hot flashes returned, so I went to see my doctor. As we chatted, I mentioned that my brother was staying with me for a month. He is a wine connoisseur, and his way of repaying my generosity was to bring home different wines for us to have with dinner every night. This was not my usual routine. My doctor thought the wine was causing the hot flashes and suggested that I try eliminating it. As soon as I did, my hot flashes were once again under control."

CUT BACK ON COFFEE

Coffee is an especially common trigger, and it's a beverage that is more popular than ever. The number of specialty coffee shops is multiplying, and the coffee cups are getting larger—an extra-large Dunkin' Donuts cup of hot coffee is 24 ounces; a "Venti" at Starbucks is 20 ounces. The more coffee you drink, the longer it takes to eliminate the caffeine from your body. Half the caffeine in a cup of coffee consumed by a healthy, non-pregnant adult is eliminated in six hours. If you drink a large cup of coffee (which may have 200 milligrams of caffeine) at 4:00 p.m., 100 milligrams of caffeine will be eliminated from your body by 10:00 p.m., leaving another 100 milligrams in your body that evening. This will disrupt your normal sleep pattern and promote night sweats. For some women, the caffeine in chocolate also induces hot flashes.

Most hot flash/night sweat sufferers are relieved to hear that it is not necessary to give up coffee entirely. Even a modest decrease in coffee consumption may banish the hot flashes and night sweats.

Abruptly eliminating coffee from your routine is not advised, as doing so produces severe headaches. To taper off your regular java, decrease the amount by just two ounces the first week. Pour off two ounces every day, before taking your first sip. If you still have severe hot flashes the second week, pour off two more ounces of coffee (now you'll be at four ounces less each day). Continue the process until the hot flashes are bearable or gone. After two or three months with no hot flashes or night sweats, it's often possible to add back some coffee slowly, in small increments, without the hot flashes returning.

Keep Cool

Hot weather triggers hot flashes, as does a warm room. Sometimes even slight increases in your body's core temperature can trigger a hot flash. Here are some suggestions for keeping cool:

- Set the thermostat at a lower temperature.
- Open a window.
- If you're feeling hot, sip a cold drink.
- Wear layers of light clothing. A sleeveless cotton shell under a shirt, sweater, or jacket works well. The outer layer can be peeled off, then replaced if a chill follows.
- Choose loose-fitting cotton clothing, which breathes and is more comfortable.
- Try using a personal fan, whether electric or hand-held.
- Be Kool Strips® are another option. The small strips adhere to the skin and provide local cooling for about eight hours. They may be purchased over the counter at a pharmacy.

Eat More Vegetable-based Meals

Eating more vegetable-based meals helps reduce hot flashes, and it isn't necessary to become a vegetarian to get the benefit. Decreasing the size of each meat portion and serving meat less frequently may lessen hot flashes. Recently, another research study showed that those whose daily intake includes 30 grams of fiber had fewer hot flashes than those who did not. Vegetable-based meals, in addition to consumption of soy foods, may be responsible for the dramatically lower rate of hot flashes in Asian women.

The Potential Role of Soy Foods

Some plants, including soy, contain compounds called phyto-estrogens, which are plant-derived estrogen-like substances. Phy-toestrogens are biologically active compounds that are similar to the estrogens in a woman's body, but not identical. They do not act the same way in the body, and in general they are weaker.

There are different types of phytoestrogens. Isoflavones are the type used most often to relieve menopausal symptoms. The two most prominent isoflavones in soy are genistein and daidzein. Iso-flavones attach to receptors in the human body but do not behave the same way a woman's own estrogen would. Some behave similarly to estrogen but with less effect. Others are anti-estrogens and be-have in a way opposite to estrogen.

No doubt you have read at least one article promoting the role of soy foods and phytoestrogens as a method of handling hot flashes. But to date, there is no definitive data about their effectiveness. Studies about eating soy have produced contradictory findings. Soy foods have been shown to decrease the frequency and severity of hot flashes in some studies, but not others. And there are a few concerns. The safety of soy supplements has not been established. Soy foods are preferable. One concern about soy that has not been resolved is its effect in women who have had breast cancer. At this time, women who have had breast cancer are advised not to take soy supplements. Consuming one or two servings of food that con-tains soy on a regular basis is not thought to be harmful, but more data is needed. Asian women consume more soy foods than North American women and have a lower rate of breast cancer.

The second area of complexity that may contribute to the con-tradictory findings about soy is that phytoestrogens possess both estrogen-like properties and anti-estrogen properties. That is to say, in some ways they may act like estrogen, alleviating hot flashes, and in other ways, they may act as estrogen-antagonists and behave ex-actly opposite to the way estrogen would behave. A caution for all women, regardless of health history: *avoid taking soy supplements.* Although some women prefer the ease of taking a soy supplement as a pill or tablet, it may be detrimental—and there is no evidence that it is beneficial. In addition, the additives used to manufacture the supplements may not be healthy. Further, some supplements may contain too much of a particular type of soy, even more than the body can use or eliminate.

Soy supplements are not well studied or understood, but we do know that to make soy supplements, soy must be extracted and processed, which affects the amount of isoflavone that remains in the product. Sometimes, removing the fat or taste or color of natural soy to turn it into a supplement product removes the beneficial isoflavones. If the beneficial isoflavones are removed, the soy supplement may not provide the benefits found in foods such as tofu, soybeans, soymilk or soy cheese, and other types of beans.

Get Regular Exercise

Regular exercise decreases the frequency and severity of hot flashes. Exercise can "reset" the body's thermostat in addition to reducing stress. It can be as simple as walking or dancing, or it can be an exercise class or a class with a specific relaxation component such as yoga or T'ai Chi (for more information on the role of exercise on your overall health, see Chapter 12).

Handling Hot Flashes with Natural Remedies

For those women who do not get adequate relief from hot flashes with the lifestyle strategies mentioned so far, there are more options to consider. These various remedies merit a discussion with your doctor, as they may have an impact on your health in other ways. There is not sufficient space here to discuss every natural remedy being touted as beneficial for hot flashes or other menopausal symptoms; what follows are the handful that receive the most attention in the media, and therefore attract the most interest from women seeking relief without hormones.

Unlike the measures discussed in the previous section, these remedies may interact with medications or supplements you take. And they may not be advisable if you have certain medical conditions.

I would like to be able to tell you that natural remedies are safer and better for you, but proof is lacking for most of the options currently available. Some remedies, such as flaxseed, look more encouraging than others where studies have not been able to show a benefit.

As a group, these remedies have not been studied rigorously, so they may also have side effects that are not well known or understood. That is why it is important to tell your doctor about *all* the supplements you take, as well as your prescription medications, before you try these remedies.

While prescription medications approved by the U.S. Food and Drug Administration (FDA) go through a rigorous testing and review process, over-the-counter remedies do not. The testing and review process in place for FDA-approved prescription medicines is designed to test for safety and effectiveness and to determine whether the medication will help the person who takes it with the fewest possible side effects. The process checks that manufacturing is reliable and uniform and that pills or capsules are made to a precise standard. Without this type of safety check, a given pill or capsule can have no active ingredient in it at all. Or, there can be too much of an active ingredient, which could cause harmful side effects. The FDA checks that the side effects of a medication are studied and described so that it is not taken with something else that is not compatible, and this information must be included when the product is advertised and sold. Although the FDA process is not foolproof, it is rigorous.

Unfortunately, natural preparations and nutritional supplements in the United States have none of these safety precautions in place. As a result, one can purchase a remedy that contains too much of an ingredient in one dose and too little of an active ingredient in another dose. They also are not required to list side effects or warnings about use or possible interactions with other products or prescriptions. This leads to the false impression that they are safer.

Further, if there is a precaution, such as sun sensitivity, the manufacturer of an over-the-counter remedy is not required to disclose it on the packaging.

Just because a natural remedy does not have any precautions written on the package, it does not mean that there are no safety considerations. For example, St. John's wort is an over-the-counter remedy that relieves mild depression. Studies have shown that it is effective. It can cause abnormal bleeding, however, when taken by those on oral contraceptives (birth control pills). Further, St. John's wort is not safe to take at the same time as a prescription antidepressant medication such as Prozac or Paxil.

Manufacturers of over-the-counter remedies are not required to prove that the remedy produces the desired effect. While a prescription medication must include the percent of individuals that can expect to benefit, the over-the-counter remedy does not have to show any proof that it works, how often it works, or in whom it works best. Nor do manufacturers have to specify who should avoid these remedies. When you read the material included with a natural remedy, you may be reading the equivalent of a television commercial.

In addition, the length of time that it is safe to take natural remedies is not well established with sound research. Aside from issues of safety, there is lack of proof that some of the natural remedies actually work; proof of the remedy's effectiveness is not required to sell it, as long as it is not classified as a drug.

Some natural remedies *are* both safe and effective, such as the B vitamin folate, which lowers the risk of birth defects. Solid research is still needed to learn which natural remedies are best suited to which individuals, in what quantity, and for what duration. As this information becomes available, natural remedies can be used with more confidence, by more individuals, with greater safety.

Wild Yam Cream

Wild yam cream is sold as a natural remedy to help reduce hot flashes. It is thought to work by supplying natural progesterone to the body. Although it is true that progesterone is helpful in reducing hot flashes, yam cream is not effective because humans do not have the enzyme necessary to convert the plant compound it contains into active progesterone in the body. The manufacturer is not required to disclose this information. To date, research data indicates that short-term treatment with topical wild yam cream by women seeking relief from menopausal symptoms did not cause any harmful side effects, but neither did it have any effect on menopausal symptoms, including hot flashes.

BLACK COHOSH

Black cohosh preparations are made from the underground stems of *Cimicifuga racemosa*. The plant is native to North America and was used by Native Americans for hundreds of years. Europeans have been using it for more than 50 years, and in 1989 the German Kommission E, a federal institute, approved the use of black cohosh for menopause-related symptoms.

Studies of black cohosh have only evaluated its short-term use, for six months or less. The mechanism of action is not known. In addition, there are many different preparations of black cohosh available, and they are not interchangeable. One preparation may be less effective than another, and side effects may differ. This can be attributed to the unique processing and dosing of each preparation as well as to the different types of ingredients from the various sources being used for each product. Even Remifemin™, a popular formulation of black cohosh in this country, has a different preparation from 40 years ago, when the initial study of its effectiveness was done. At that time, a study showed the original preparation was effective, but that may not apply to the product in use today, with its different formulation.

Black cohosh should not be taken at the same time as other hormone preparations, such as oral contraceptives or hormone prescriptions. Women with hormone-sensitive conditions should probably avoid black cohosh until its effects on breast tissue are better understood. The safety of its long-term use has not yet been established.

Black cohosh may be harmful to the liver for certain people, and those with liver disease should exercise caution. While millions of people have taken the herb without incident, there is at least one published case of a woman who needed a liver transplant three weeks after starting black cohosh. (There were no other reasons for her liver failure.) Be alert for signs of liver disease and see your doctor if you experience dark urine, nausea, vomiting, unusual tiredness, and/or yellow skin or eyes.

Dong Quai

The root of this plant, which is a member of the celery family, has been used in Eastern medicine for thousands of years. It has not been well studied in the West, but one research study indicated that using dong quai alone did not relieve hot flashes better than a placebo. Practitioners of complementary medicine advise that dong quai be used with other herbs, not alone. These preparations have not been formally studied, so more data is needed. A known side effect of dong quai includes making the user more sensitive to sunlight, so wearing sunglasses and a hat or visor is important. Dong quai can trigger heavy uterine bleeding, so women with fibroids should not try it. In addition, women on blood thinners should also avoid it, as should women with bleeding problems or other blood clotting problems.

Red Clover

Red clover is another source of isoflavones. Six different studies looking at two different preparations of red clover concluded that it did not help to reduce hot flashes. Because there is no evidence that it has a significant effect on hot flashes, and because it contains processed isoflavones that do not have a track record for being safe or effective, I do not recommend red clover.

Flaxseed

A small study by the Mayo Clinic indicates that flaxseed may be effective in treating hot flashes. In the study, women suffering from hot flashes (at least 14 hot flashes a week) who added four tablespoons of crushed flaxseed a day to their diet for six consecutive weeks *halved* their number of daily hot flashes. In addition, the intensity of their hot flashes dropped by 57 percent. The women in the study also reported improved mood. While some consider it premature to strongly recommend flaxseed, this option looks promising and, so far, no adverse effects have been reported. Flaxseed also contains healthy omega-3 fatty acids, giving it heart-health benefits as well. It is easily added to cereal, juice, yogurt, or fruit dishes, so most women do not find it difficult to introduce it into their daily meals.

VITAMIN B$_6$ SUPPLEMENTS

Vitamin B$_6$ may provide some relief from hot flashes in doses of 50 milligrams by mouth, once a day. It is important not to exceed the recommended dosage. Taking more than 100 milligrams of vitamin B$_6$ daily may cause irreversible nerve damage. Be certain to check the label of the multivitamin supplement that you take as well as other vitamins, such as B-complex, which may contain additional vitamin B$_6$, so that you do not exceed the recommended dose in your combined supplements.

VITAMIN E SUPPLEMENTS

While some studies suggest that vitamin E may help relieve hot flashes, others do not. Trying up to 400 international units per day of vitamin E is safe for most. Women on blood thinners such as Coumadin™ or aspirin (including low-dose aspirin), nonsteroidal anti-inflammatory drugs such as Ibuprofen or Naproxen, dong quai, evening of primrose oil, garlic or ginger supplements, or ginkgo biloba should avoid taking extra vitamin E, as it may prolong bleeding. It interferes with platelet function and impairs normal clotting. Women who have active bleeding with ulcers, brain hemorrhage, heavy vaginal or uterine bleeding, rectal bleeding, or a history of a bleeding disorder should also avoid vitamin E.

ACUPUNCTURE

Acupuncture has been shown to reduce the number of hot flashes a woman experiences. Although there are not a large number of studies, it is reasonable to try this technique to relieve hot flashes as long as it is performed by a licensed practitioner and the needles are sterile.

Handling Hot Flashes with Non-hormone Prescription Medications

If you continue to have troublesome hot flashes despite making lifestyle and dietary modifications, you may benefit from a non-hormone-based prescription medication. There are a variety of options that may provide relief. Some medications, commonly prescribed for other medical conditions such as high blood pressure, depression, or nerve pain, have been shown to diminish hot flashes and night sweats.

Not all medications in a given category will help hot flashes. For example, many antidepressants and the majority of medications available to treat high blood pressure do not affect hot flashes.

The advantage of using these types of medications is that they are not hormones, so they do not increase a woman's risk of blood clots, stroke, heart disease, breast cancer, or uterine cancer. Discuss these options with your doctor and consider these medications if:

- You choose not to take hormones but you need relief from hot flashes and have already tried the lifestyle modifications described in this chapter.
- You are a breast cancer survivor or the survivor of a stroke or heart attack.
- You need to stop hormone therapy.
- You have both hot flashes and another medical condition that requires one of these types of medications.
- You are taking a low dose of hormones but you have not obtained complete relief of your hot flashes or night sweats, and you want additional relief without taking a higher dose of hormones.
- You are older than 59 years old, and more than 10 years from your last menstrual period.

ANTIDEPRESSANTS

Low doses of certain antidepressants such as Paxil, Prozac, Effexor, or Lexapro can be used to decrease hot flashes. In some cases, the dose is lower than the dose used to treat depression. Antidepressants are not associated with a risk of breast cancer or uterine cancer.

Antidepressants should not be stopped suddenly. As the hot flashes become more manageable, or subside completely, taper off the medication under your doctor's supervision to avoid unnecessary side effects.

Each antidepressant medication will affect each individual differently. If one antidepressant is associated with unacceptable or unpleasant side effects (for example, weight gain or sexual problems), a sister antidepressant medication may provide relief from hot flashes without the same difficulties. You may end up trying several different medications before you find the one that is best for you.

⚡ Evelyn's Story ⚡

Hot Flashes and Antidepressant Medication

Evelyn, 52, is postmenopausal. "I have been on hormones for a year. That includes two prescription hormones, daily: Prometrium, a plant-based FDA-approved progesterone, and Menest, a plant-based FDA-approved estrogen. My doctor explained that taking estrogen alone, without progesterone, could lead to uterine cancer. Unfortunately, I had a suspicious finding on a routine mammogram, and subsequently, the breast biopsy showed cancer. My doctor did not attribute the breast cancer to hormone use, since I had used them for only one year. But she did tell me to stop taking hormones. After I did, I developed severe night sweats. My gynecologist suggested a low dose of Effexor, an antidepressant that works through the nervous system to reduce hot flashes. She also cautioned me not to take any synthetic soy preparations, such as soy powders, pills, or supplements, as the effect on breast cancer is still unknown. Thankfully, I've gotten dramatic relief on Effexor. And my gynecologist has assured me that I can taper off this medication over time once the hot flashes have subsided."

BLOOD PRESSURE MEDICATION

Clonidine (or Catapress) is a medication that helps to lower high blood pressure by working through the central nervous system. It also helps to decrease hot flashes and night sweats. In some cases, a woman's primary care physician, internist, or family doctor may be able to prescribe Clonidine to control high blood pressure and simultaneously reduce hot flashes.

Some women need more than one type of medicine to control high blood pressure, and Clonidine may be selected as one of the prescriptions. A woman on Clonidine would then benefit from its dual effects in reducing her hot flashes and lowering her blood pressure.

❦ PENNY'S STORY ❦

Hot Flashes and High Blood Pressure

"At age 49, I didn't expect to be diagnosed with high blood pressure. After all, as a school nurse, I know a lot about health. But I had to admit I was overweight, and I know that contributes to hypertension. At the same time, I shared with my doctor that my hot flashes have never subsided. My doctor put me on Clonidine, a blood pressure medication that also helps hot flashes. It really helped. After I was able to start exercising, I also modified the way I ate and lost the extra weight I'd gained over the past few years. When my blood pressure remained at a healthy level, I was able to stop the Clonidine, and my hot flashes did not return."

NERVE ADJUSTMENT MEDICATION

Neurontin (gabapentin) is a medication prescribed to decrease nerve pain. Recent research shows that it also decreases hot flashes. In some cases, even in the absence of nerve pain, neurontin may be a good choice to decrease hot flashes; you'll want to discuss this with your doctor to determine if it might be a good choice for you. It is usually prescribed to be taken at bedtime. At first the doctor may prescribe a lower dose, and then increase it every few weeks until you get relief from your hot flashes. It can also help you sleep better.

⚒ ALICE'S STORY ⚒

Hot Flashes and Neurontin (Gabapentin)

"I'm 68 and have been postmenopausal for 12 years. I stopped taking hormones in August 2002 after the media coverage of the Women's Health Initiative. Now I have hot flashes that are annoying and inconvenient. Night sweats interrupt my sleep, and I feel tired during the day. Neither I nor my gynecologist preferred that I restart hormones. We discussed my options. She recommended that I try Neurontin and also instructed me in paced respiration. The combination of the two reduced the frequency and severity of the hot flashes and night sweats enough to make them tolerable."

If none of the interventions in this chapter works for you and your hot flashes are still debilitating, you may have the option of taking hormones. Those options are discussed in the following chapter. I recommend that you familiarize yourself with them before discussing your choices with your doctor.

RESOURCES

American Academy of Family Physicians (www.familydoctor.org). This professional organization has excellent resources for medical professionals and the public about menopause and more general health topics.

American College of Obstetricians and Gynecologists (www.acog.org). This site has Patient Education Pamphlets for the major topics in women's health and preventive care.

Mayo Clinic (www.mayoclinic.com). This is a world-class medical center with resources for the public on its website. They also publish a newsletter about general health topics of interest to men and women.

Menopause Flashes® E-Newsletter. This is a free monthly email newsletter for consumers containing information about all aspects of menopause and available therapies, both traditional and complementary, to ease symptoms and preserve long-term health. You may preview an issue and subscribe at www.menopause.org/newsletter.aspx.

National Center for Complementary and Alternative Medicine (http:// nccam.nih.gov/). This site has objective reviews of studies showing the benefits and risks of complementary and alternative strategies. It is also helpful to look at what has not been studied completely and what is not known.

North American Menopause Society (www.nams.org). In addition to the newsletter available online, there are print brochures on special aspects of menopause, including early menopause (The Early Menopause Guidebook). They also publish *Pause*, a print journal available quarterly through your gynecologist's office. Book reviews and other resources are also featured.

Taking Hormones
in Menopause

For more than 40 years, middle-aged women were encouraged to take prescription medications containing female hormones to replace the hormones their bodies were no longer making at youthful levels. Hormone therapy (HT) was prescribed to ease the troublesome symptoms of menopause, and it was thought to confer other benefits as well. HT was believed to help preserve memory; maintain young-looking skin; control hot flashes and night sweats; improve sleep and moods; ease vaginal dryness; prevent weak bones, heart disease, and Alzheimer's disease; and lower the risk of colon cancer. Some of these assumptions have turned out to be incorrect, while others are still true for certain groups of women.

Now that additional research has been done, taking hormones has become increasingly controversial. A woman who is thinking about using hormones needs to take into account multiple factors, such as her age, her stage of menopause, whether she has had a hysterectomy, whether she has heart disease, any history of breast cancer, and so on. Each woman is unique, with her own individual profile. The information in this chapter will help you clearly understand the risks and benefits of hormone therapy so that you'll be able to ask your doctor the most appropriate questions and work together to find the best approach for you.

Your preferences, too, are an integral part of the decision process. If you are against certain lifestyle changes or medications, they cannot improve your health. But even if you are certain that you would never take hormones or other prescription medications, stay informed about the risks and benefits. The benefits will increase and the risks will diminish as newer, better medications are developed. Also, with time, your risk for age-related conditions such as osteoporosis, stroke, and heart disease will increase. Review your health with your gynecologist regularly and be on the lookout for new treatments that may become available.

Currently, the pendulum has swung away from hormones. So you may wonder why I am going to discuss them. Here's why: startling headlines, inaccurate and incomplete assessments of research results, and important information reduced to sound-bites have not helped the discussion of what's best for women's health from perimenopause on. My goal is to help you sort through the confusing barrage of information and be able to have a frank, educated discussion with your doctor about what's best for *you.*

I am not recommending that you take hormones, nor am I advising you to avoid them. Only you and your doctor can arrive at a safe, reasonable approach that meets your individual needs.

When you discuss hormones with your doctor, or read about them on your own, you are likely to encounter the issue of bioidentical hormones as well as many different ways of taking hormones other than by mouth. Each of these is discussed in detail in the pages that follow. Making the right choice begins with being informed.

In the discussion of HT, it must be acknowledged that there has been no greater influence for women today than the Women's Health Initiative (WHI). The results of this important study have been so misconstrued that until you have a clear, full understanding of them you cannot make an informed decision about HT. That is why I begin this chapter with an examination of what the WHI has *really* taught us.

Making Sense of the Women's Health Initiative Study

The federally funded WHI was the largest, most compre-hensive examination of postmenopausal women's health ever under-taken. It is a pivotal study because so many women were included in it and because it was set up in the classic "randomized double-blind placebo-controlled" manner, which is the gold standard for scientific studies. Women were randomly assigned to receive either active hormone pills or sugar pills (placebo); neither they nor their doctors knew which they were getting. The hormones studied were Pre-marin (synthetic estrogen, synthesized from horse urine) and Prem-pro (synthetic estrogen combined with synthetic progesterone).

Women everywhere were distressed when, in July 2002, WHI in-vestigators reported halting research early on the Prempro group be-cause of the increased risk to the health of the women involved. The medical community was also disturbed by the report. WHI stated that the study was stopped because initial data showed that the women who were taking these hormones had higher rates of breast cancer, heart attacks, strokes, and blood clots than the women who were taking placebos. Although the study was supposed to run for eight years, it was halted after five because of these results.

In April 2004, the WHI also stopped its research on estrogen-only therapy because it appeared to increase the risk of strokes and blood clots without providing any added protection against heart disease.

These events had an enormous impact on medicine. Many women who were taking hormones stopped abruptly, and women who were not on hormones hesitated to start taking them. Prescriptions for hormone therapy plummeted. As recently as January 2009 the re-sults of the study were debated and reanalyzed.

The current interpretation of the WHI data on hormones and heart disease is in keeping with what researchers and clinicians have observed for the past 30 years: *healthy women* (those without established heart disease, strokes, or blood clots) between ages 50 and 59 do NOT have a higher risk of heart attack if they take estro-gen or an estrogen and progesterone combination within the first 10 years of entering postmenopause. *Healthy women* in this age group who have spent less than 10 years in postmenopause may consider taking hormones to control severe hot flashes. In fact, some studies looking at hormone use in this particular group of healthy postmenopausal women show that their risk of heart disease is lower with hormone use.

Initially, the WHI reported the outcomes for the majority of the women in the study, who were over 60 years old, as if they represented all of the women in the study, including those under age 59. They also combined outcomes of women more than 15 years out from their last menstrual period with those less than 10 years into postmenopause. They reported their results as a global finding—as if it applied to all of the age groups studied. In fact, these early published results were very different from the experience of women in the study who were younger than 59 and closer to their last menstrual period. But the data for the women under 59 was not interpreted separately or published until 2007.

Other differences have emerged as the information gathered from the WHI study has been reexamined. For instance, more of the older-than-60 women were obese than participants in the younger age group. The older groups of women also had established heart disease in the form of high blood pressure and high cholesterol. Their arteries had already begun to harden. Estrogen is *not* advised for women who already have heart disease. Estrogen can lower the risk of heart disease in a *younger* woman; if heart disease is not present, she is capable of benefiting from the estrogen, which may protect her from heart disease. Once heart disease is established, however, there is no role for estrogen—as a matter of fact, it worsens the heart disease.

The risk of stroke is low in younger-than-60, healthy postmenopausal women who are less than 10 years from their final menstrual period and have not had a stroke in the past. The risk of stroke in 50- to 59-year-old women is much lower than the risk for women in their sixties and seventies, so if hormone prescriptions increase the risk by a small amount, few additional women age 59 or younger are likely to experience a stroke (as long as they are healthy and have no predisposition to having a stroke before filling the prescription).

A more in-depth review of the WHI data confirms that starting, or restarting, hormones in women over age 60 (and who are more than 15 years away from their last menstrual period) is *not* beneficial. A very different circumstance exists for women age 59 or younger (and who have had their final menstrual period within the last 10 years) who need hormones to quell severe, debilitating hot flashes. The risks and benefits for each group of women are not the same.

The influence of taking hormones in postmenopause on the risk of breast cancer is being debated. It is so complicated that researchers and clinicians have not reached a consensus about the impact of hormones on breast cancer risk. There are some facts that all can agree contribute to this risk:

- The risk of breast cancer goes up each year until a woman turns 79 (and remains almost as high until age 85, when it begins to decline).
- Obese women have a higher risk of breast cancer.
- Estrogen affects breast tissue and cancer risk differently from the estrogen and progesterone combination (Prempro, discussed shortly).
- The risk of taking hormones affects the risk of different tissue types of breast cancer in different ways.
- The longer a postmenopausal woman over 50 takes estrogen and progesterone, the more likely it is to increase her risk of breast cancer.
- The higher the dose of hormones she takes, the higher her risk of breast cancer.
- After a woman stops taking hormones, her risk of breast cancer decreases over time until it is no longer elevated.

Since more of the women age 60 and older in the WHI study were obese than women in the younger group, they were already at higher risk of breast cancer (as well as heart disease) by virtue of their obesity as well as their age.

Who Participated in the Women's Health Initiative Study?

The study had some drawbacks, often overlooked, which prevent the results from applying to all women:

1. Only 10 percent of the women in the WHI study were younger than 55, so the early, general conclusions drawn from the study do not apply to all perimenopausal and postmenopausal women. They are helpful in learning about women who have spent more than 10 years in postmenopause, but they do not necessarily predict outcomes for perimenopausal women or for younger, newly postmenopausal women.
2. Seventy percent of the participants were over 60 years old. Most of the women were 15 or 20 years into postmenopause.
3. The women were not screened for heart disease at the beginning of the study. Some of them had already developed heart disease; most of them would have had an elevated risk of heart disease and stroke by virtue of their age and length of time in postmenopause.
4. Some of the participants were already taking estrogen before they enrolled in the study, although they were required to stop taking hormones for three months before the study. This confuses the data regarding the length of time participants took hormone therapy. The total length of time some participants took hormones is actually much longer than the study suggests.
5. The study excluded women with severe hot flashes. Women who wanted estrogen to relieve these symptoms could not participate in the study. This is unfortunate, since one of the principal reasons for prescribing hormones is to relieve hot flashes.

What Hormones Did the Women's Health Initiative Study?

Decades ago researchers found that women with a uterus who take estrogen alone have an increased risk of getting uterine cancer. Adding progesterone to the estrogen reduced this risk. This information was factored into the WHI study from the outset.

The women in the WHI study were divided into two groups to study both scenarios:

1. The first study started with 10,739 women who had all had hysterectomies. These women were divided into two groups:
   - Group A (5,310 women) took 0.625 milligrams a day of Premarin, a synthetic estrogen prepared from the urine of pregnant mares.
   - Group B (5,429 women) was given a placebo.
2. The second study started with 16,608 women aged 50–79 years who all had an intact uterus.
   - Group A (8,506 women) was given Prempro 2.5, which is a combination of 0.625 milligrams of Premarin and 2.5 milligrams of Provera (synthetic progesterone).
   - Group B (8,102 women) took a placebo.

What Were the Results of the Premarin Study?

When it became clear that the women in the WHI study taking Premarin (synthetic estrogen alone, without progesterone) had a higher risk of stroke, the study was halted. It is important to note, however, that for the duration they participated in the study, the women taking estrogen alone did not have a higher risk of heart attack or breast cancer than the women taking a placebo. They also had stronger bones and a lower risk of colorectal cancer than they would have had without Premarin. When the data for women ages 50 to 59 was reanalyzed, it showed that the women age 59 and younger who took Premarin alone had a lower risk of breast cancer. In addition, the Premarin group had more than twice the risk of certain types of benign breast disease (the Premarin group experienced 155 cases of benign breast disease, while the placebo group had 77 cases).

Now that the results have been reanalyzed and sorted out by age and menopause status, experts believe that the increased risk of stroke mainly affects women over age 60, as well as those who have spent more than 10 years in postmenopause. Women over 60 or women more than 10 years from their final menstrual period are discouraged from starting or restarting estrogen therapy.

What Were the Results of the Prempro Study?

Prempro, a synthetic version of estrogen and progesterone, was thought to prevent heart disease when the WHI study began. One purpose of the study was to determine whether or not this was true. Initially, the researchers reported that Prempro worsened the risk of heart disease. As of 2007, this applies to the study participants over 60 years old who were more than 10 years into postmenopause. Healthy women under 59 years old who were less than 10 years from their last menstrual period did *not* have a higher risk of heart attack in the WHI study. In fact, women age 59 and under who took Prempro had a lower risk of heart disease if they were less than 10 years into postmenopause.

Prempro did not prevent heart disease in the women over 60 because they already had it—it was too late for prevention. However, in women under 59 years old who have not been postmenopausal for more than 10 years, estrogen does prevent heart disease. This does not mean that you should take estrogen to prevent heart disease if you are younger than 59. What it does show is that healthy women who choose to do so to quell debilitating hot flashes, and who are in the low-risk group by virtue of being under 59 and early postmenopause of less than 10 years duration, will not increase their risk of heart disease.

A noteworthy effect of taking combination estrogen/progestin hormones was an increase in false alarms from mammograms and more benign breast disease. It is believed that the estrogen component increased the density of the women's breast tissue, which led to an abnormally high number of false positive readings from mammograms. Since hormone therapy may make it harder to detect breast cancer, women who use it will want to make sure they keep up with checkups, including annual breast exams and mammograms.

The vast majority of hormone studies have been done on the synthetic hormones Premarin, Provera, and Prempro. Since there are not large studies looking at other hormone preparations, for now experts advise that women and their doctors assume all types of hormones have the same risks regardless of the way they are taken or how they are made. This includes natural, bioidentical, or plant-derived hormones as well. These are discussed in more detail at the end of this chapter.

Since menopause experts are using synthetic hormones as studied in WHI as the standard for assessing the risks and benefits of hormones in general, I think it is helpful to review the safety concerns and precautions that the WHI research study showed in more detail

What Did Doctors Learn from the Women's Health Initiative Study and Its Reinterpretation?

The WHI findings were splashed across headlines in a blanket fashion: "Hormones are dangerous—do not take them!" We now know this is an oversimplification and does not represent the WHI findings in an accurate way. It cheated many women of the benefits of estrogen by implying that all women on hormones are in danger. From the alarming press reports, women got the idea that *all* hormones are bad for *all* women in *all* settings.

Hormone Therapy and Risk of Heart Disease

In early observational studies of younger postmenopausal women, estrogen lowered the risk of heart disease. The reanalysis of the WHI study results for women under age 59 has reaffirmed this fact. A 2006 study published in the *Journal of Women's Health*, based on data from the Nurses' Health Study, concluded that women who begin taking combination hormones while they are still perimenopausal have a 30 percent lower risk of heart disease than women who do not take hormones. Perimenopausal women and women in early postmenopause may benefit from estrogen to prevent heart disease before their arteries have hardened and lost their flexibility.

Hormone Therapy and Risk of Breast Cancer

Initially, the WHI results showed that women did not increase their risk of breast cancer if they took Prempro (the combined hormone used in the study) for five years or less. Those who took Premarin alone had a lower risk of breast cancer. These results are controversial and are being reevaluated.

Women who take estrogen or an estrogen/progesterone combination should commit to scheduled mammograms to detect early breast cancers and precancers before they can be felt on exam. Ways to decrease the risk of breast cancer are discussed in Chapter 13.

Hormone Therapy and Risk of Ovarian Cancer

In Denmark, a study of over 900,000 postmenopausal women was done from 1995 to 2005 to assess whether taking hormones increases the risk of ovarian cancer. Different types and dosages of hormones were studied, including bioidentical hormones. Women who took hormones were slightly more likely to develop ovarian cancer than those who did not take them. Two years after the hormones were stopped, there was no increase in risk. For every 8,300 women who took hormones for one year, there was one extra case of ovarian cancer. These results are similar to those of the Million Women Study.

Is this risk great or small? For an individual woman, the risk is not huge. Ovarian cancer is relatively rare, so even doubling the rate would still yield a low number. But any case of ovarian cancer is devastating, and when the effect is multiplied by hundreds of thousands of women, it becomes a public health issue. It is possible that this increase in ovarian cancer is due to greater vigilance and diagnosis, since women on hormones get close follow-up prior to refilling their prescriptions. More data are needed on the doses and types of hormones that influence these results.

Hormone Therapy and Alcohol

Alcohol increases the risk of breast cancer even without hormones. A Danish study that included more than 5,000 women found that women who took estrogen and other hormones increased their risk of breast cancer threefold by consuming one or two drinks a day. Drinking more than two drinks daily was associated with almost five times the risk. Women who know they are going to be drinking will want to factor this into their decisions about hormone therapy.

Who Should Avoid Starting Systemic Estrogen?

Systemic estrogen may be taken by mouth or by applying a patch to the skin, rubbing a lotion into the skin, or spraying the skin. It can also be taken by using Femring, a ring placed in the vagina that releases enough estrogen to alleviate hot flashes as well as vaginal dryness. These forms of estrogen are meant to be absorbed into the body and to raise the blood level of estrogen. In general, you should avoid starting or restarting systemic estrogen if:

- There is any possibility you are pregnant.
- You have not had a menstrual period for more than 10 years.
- You have any unusual vaginal bleeding that has not been checked by your doctor.
- You have liver disease.
- You have had a heart attack, stroke, or other heart disease.
- You are over 60 years old and have spent more than 10 years in postmenopause.
- You do not have severe hot flashes or night sweats.
- You have had a deep vein clot in your leg or a pulmonary embolus (lung clot).
- You were recently diagnosed with breast cancer, or you have already had breast cancer in the past, and have not discussed estrogen with your oncologist, breast surgeon, gynecologist, and internist or primary care physician.

Who May Safely Start Taking Estrogen?

If you find the quality of your life is compromised by severe, debilitating hot flashes or night sweats, you will benefit the most and incur the least risk from taking hormones if you exhibit the four characteristics below:

- You are under 60 years old.
- You are perimenopausal or in early postmenopause, having experienced a normal menstrual period within the past 10 years.
- You have no personal history of heart disease, stroke, or breast cancer.
- Your hot flashes or night sweats are not due to another medical condition such as a thyroid disorder.

Many women who cannot get adequate relief of their symptoms by other means will accept the risk associated with hormone therapy. With close monitoring, these individuals may benefit from taking low-dose hormone therapy.

Other Precautions When Considering Hormones

Ask your doctor about specific precautions for the particular type of estrogen or progesterone prescribed for you. For example, Prometrium, a plant-derived progesterone taken by mouth, is made from peanut oil, so do not take it if you are allergic to peanuts.

In general, if you are taking any type of estrogen, avoid direct sun. You will be more sun-sensitive. A discoloration may develop on your skin, even on your face. Use sunscreen, wear a visor or hat, and wear sunglasses. You may not metabolize alcohol as well. Both alcohol and estrogen taken by mouth are processed through the liver. If you drink on a regular basis, you may increase the amount of estrogen in your blood because your liver is busy processing alcohol instead of estrogen. So, its processing of estrogen is less efficient and effective. A consequence of this may be a higher risk of breast cancer, since higher levels of alcohol are associated with a higher risk of breast cancer. Also, higher levels of estrogen are associated with higher rates of breast cancer.

JANE'S STORY

How Old Is Too Old for Hormone Therapy?

"I'm 57 and I started taking Prempro to control severe hot flashes and night sweats eight years ago, when I was 49. At that time, I was healthy, and both my gynecologist as well as primary care physician were confident that the estrogen would also lower my risk of heart disease and keep my bones strong. I did well on the hormones but recently decided to stop taking them. While my mammograms have been normal, my doctors and I are concerned that my risk of breast cancer may increase if I stay on them. So we agreed that I would stop the hormones. I'm also going to decrease the amount of alcohol I drink, based on a discussion with my doctor, to lower my risk of breast cancer. I also know that alcohol can affect hot flashes and I want to keep those under control."

Hormones and Early Menopause

A woman's body is designed to release estradiol from her ovaries until about the age of 50. As you read in the first chapter, some women go into menopause prematurely. When this occurs, hormone therapy can help postpone the effects of postmenopause. The side effects of hormones for these women are low compared to the substantial benefit.

⚡ PATRICIA'S STORY ⚡

Early Menopause

"I had my last menstrual period when I was 33. My doctor put me on Prempro at age 34 and I have felt well since. Now that I'm 41 and have been on Prempro for seven years, the results of the WHI study have made me very anxious. I made an appointment with my gynecologist to talk about stopping the Prempro. She explained that I became estrogen-deficient prematurely and that, in general, a woman's body is meant to have estrogen until her late forties or early fifties. She also explained that because I'm much younger than the women in the WHI study, the study does not address my problem directly. She encouraged me to continue to take a hormone supplement until I'm 50 to 'imitate the biology of natural postmenopause' as if my unusually early menopause had not interrupted it. My doctor has convinced me that the benefits of the hormones, including maintaining stronger bones and preventing heart disease, outweigh the possible risks in my case."

Hormones and Hysterectomy

A *hysterectomy* is the surgical removal of the uterus, or womb. A *complete hysterectomy* means that the cervix was removed with the uterus. (There are separate terms for the removal of the fallopian tubes and ovaries.)

Taking estrogen alone is not appropriate for a woman with an intact uterus because it is associated with an increased risk of uterine cancer. However, women who have undergone a hysterectomy and no longer have a uterus may take estrogen alone to relieve hot flashes. They may take it in pill form, such as estradiol, Premarin, Menest, or Ogen. Or they may use estrogen in the form of a skin patch, such as Climara, Estraderm, or Vivelle. Another option is to apply estrogen to the skin as a cream, Estrasorb. More recently, a spray form of estrogen, Evamist, has become available.

It is possible to have a complete hysterectomy and still have fallopian tubes and ovaries. If you have had a hysterectomy but kept your ovaries, they will still cycle and continue to produce both eggs and estrogen. You may still experience PMS (premenstrual syndrome), if you had it prior to your hysterectomy. You will not get pregnant (the sperm have no way to reach the eggs), however, and you will not experience any more menstrual periods. Menopause will eventually occur on your body's natural schedule, when your ovaries stop releasing eggs and making estrogen. You may or may not experience hot flashes at that time.

Premenopausal or perimenopausal women who have both ovaries removed at the time of a hysterectomy (described as a *total abdominal hysterectomy with bilateral salpingo-oophorectomy*) usually experience severe hot flashes within three days of surgery due to the sudden loss of estrogen. This does not occur if the woman already completed her menopause and the ovaries already released their last eggs more than a year prior.

Severe hot flashes after surgical removal of the ovaries may be avoided in most cases with the use of an estrogen patch after surgery.

ℵ Susan's Story ℤ

Hysterectomy and Premarin

"When I was 43, I had my uterus and ovaries removed because of large, painful ovarian cysts, in addition to a large fibroid in my uterus that caused pelvic pressure and hemorrhaging. After surgery, my doctor started me on Climara, an estrogen patch, and I felt fine. When the WHI study results were publicized, I wondered if I should continue to use the *patch. My friends and co-workers were discouraging me from using the medication. But my gynecologist felt differently. First, she pointed out to me that since I had no uterus, I was not at risk of developing uterine cancer. Second, the data indicated I could continue taking Climara until age 51. And having surgical menopause at an early age meant I had started taking hormones while they could still lower my risk of heart disease. They also helped postpone bone thinning. My doctor explained that while the WHI study indicated a higher risk of blood clots and stroke for the women who took Premarin, a synthetic pill form of estrogen, I was much younger than the women in the study. I decided to continue taking Climara for a while longer. My doctor advised me that in my case the benefits at my age and stage of menopause outweigh the risks."*

Vaginal Estrogen

Vaginal estrogen was not studied in WHI. It is used to relieve vaginal dryness or pain with intercourse in perimenopausal and postmenopausal women of all ages. It can be used in the form of an estrogen cream, a tablet, or a vaginal ring that slowly releases small doses of estrogen into the vaginal walls (for more information, see Chapter 7).

Hormones and Oral Contraceptives

Estrogen and progesterone hormones are used in birth control pills, but in higher doses than the amounts for postmenopausal women. Oral contraceptives use hormones to block ovulation and thin the uterine lining to prevent pregnancy. Hormone therapy for menopause is designed to make up for an age-related decline in natural hormone levels. Oral contraceptives may be helpful in relieving hot flashes in perimenopausal women. They may also help regulate irregular menstrual cycles. If you are a nonsmoker who is still perimenopausal, your doctor may be able to prescribe a low-dose oral contraceptive for you (for more information, see Chapter 8).

Hot Flashes and the Pill

"I'm 43 and still have regular periods. My husband and I divorced recently, after 22 years of marriage, and I've been under a lot of stress. I had returned to work full time a year before the divorce, and I need the job now for health insurance as well as income. I used to be able to manage the occasional, mild hot flashes I get the week before my period by cutting back on coffee, wearing layers of clothing, and carrying a small paper fan. But for the past three months, the hot flashes have been occurring five times a day, and night sweats wake me up more than three times a night. My gynecologist explained that I'm still making a significant amount of estrogen in my ovaries, but it's erratic. Since I'm a nonsmoker without any risk factors for blood clots or stroke, my gynecologist recommended a low-dose birth control pill to control the hot flashes and night sweats. She said the low doses of estrogen and progesterone in the Pill will give me a steady, predictable hormone pattern and minimize or eliminate my hot flashes. Plus, I want to avoid an unplanned pregnancy."

Hormones for Hot Flashes

If approaches such as lifestyle modifications and non-hormone prescriptions described in Chapter 2 don't work for you, and your symptoms are debilitating, you and your doctor may conclude that the benefits of hormone therapy outweigh the risks.

ESTROGEN ALONE

Estrogen provides the best and most complete relief of hot flashes and night sweats. Because of the WHI study results, women are less likely to be offered a starter prescription for estrogen. Women with early or premature menopause under age 40 may benefit from taking estrogen much longer, or until they reach 51 years old. A healthy woman who is younger than 59 years old, has had her uterus surgically removed, and has spent less than 10 years in postmenopause may be a good candidate for low-dose estrogen if other options have failed to provide adequate relief. There are many types of estrogen available, as well as a range of doses and various routes of delivery. The decision about which type of estrogen is best for you should be thoroughly discussed with your gynecologist and primary care physician.

PROGESTERONE ALONE

Another option to decrease hot flashes is to take progesterone alone, such as Provera or Prometrium. Progesterone is available in different forms, including some that are plant-based.

Progesterone helps hot flashes and does not cause uterine cancer, but it is associated with other risks. The manufacturer of Provera (medroxyprogesterone) notes in its product information and on its website that the drug may cause difficulty controlling blood sugar levels, and you have read about the results of the WHI study for Prempro, which includes Provera. Progesterone may be associated with irregular bleeding as well as weight gain or bloating, and in some cases (less than one in 100), it is associated with depression. The manufacturer also cautions against the use of progesterone for women who have had breast cancer.

PROGESTERONE CREAM

Lay web sites and books emphasize the benefits of progesterone cream in menopause, particularly to ease hot flashes. Researchers are less certain. Progesterone in cream form is not absorbed by the uterus lining reliably or in a predictable way, so it should not be used to balance estrogen in hormone therapy.

ESTROGEN AND PROGESTERONE COMBINED IN OTHER PREPARATIONS

As you have already seen, the WHI study using Prempro helped clarify the risks of combination hormone therapy for postmenopausal women. Other preparations that include both estrogen and progesterone in a pill form are Activella and Ortho Prefest. The CombiPatch includes estrogen and progesterone in a skin patch worn daily and changed twice a week. There is also an estrogen and progesterone vaginal ring, Femring, which has systemic doses of hormones to help hot flashes and local estrogen for the vagina.

⚄ SERENA'S STORY ⚄

Estrogen and Progesterone for Hot Flashes

"I'm 51 and teach high school equivalency courses in the evenings. My last menstrual period was a year ago. My classroom is not air-conditioned and I frequently have to interrupt teaching to wipe the sweat off my face and neck. During the hot flashes, my face turns bright red and I know it distracts my students from focusing on the subject matter. My best friend, Janet, who is 52, is opposed to hormone use. Her hot flashes were very mild and have already passed. She encourages me to tough it out without taking hormones until the hot flashes resolve naturally. But my gynecologist encouraged me to try a low dose of estrogen and progesterone every evening. I was experiencing such discomfort and loss of sleep that I agreed to try it. Within three weeks, I was sleeping through the night and was comfortable teaching again. The doctor advised me that my increased risk of breast cancer is minimal if I stay on the low dose of hormones for less than five years. He also advised me to keep up with breast exams and annual mammograms."

WHEN ORAL ESTROGEN STOPS WORKING

Some women taking oral estrogen for more than a year may find that the same dose of estrogen pills is no longer effective in relieving their hot flashes. They may get relief by changing to an estrogen skin patch, lotion, ring, or spray. When taken in pill form, estrogen passes through the liver for processing. The liver processing changes how much estrogen is bound and how much is free in the blood. Estrogen in the form of a skin patch, cream, lotion, or gel avoids this step and can banish the hot flashes without the need to take a higher dose of estrogen to get relief.

From Estrogen Pills to Estrogen Patch

"I'm 41 and work as a librarian. At 33, I was diagnosed with severe endometriosis and had my uterus and both ovaries removed. My hot flashes have been controlled with 0.625 milligrams of Premarin I take by mouth once a day. However, for the past three months, I've been waking up with terrible night sweats. During the day I have hot flashes even though the library is air-conditioned. I spoke with my gynecologist and he advised changing to a patch form of estrogen in a comparable dose. He prescribed the Vivelle patch, from which my body absorbs 0.05 milligrams of estrogen per day. Although the doses sound different, he explained that they are bioequivalent. I apply a new estrogen patch to my lower abdomen at the same time each Sunday and Thursday. The patch remains in place even during baths, showers, and swimming. The relief I'm getting from hot flashes now is comparable to when I first took the Premarin. My doctor tells me I will be safely able to continue to use the patch for years."

STOPPING ESTROGEN

Many women have the misconception that if they start taking estrogen, they will never be able to get off it without suffering from severe hot flashes or night sweats all over again. In truth, most women are able to stop their hormones without the return of troublesome hot flashes or night sweats. That said, some women find that hot flashes or night sweats do return.

If you take hormones and have not tried any lifestyle modifications, I recommend you put the lifestyle modifications in place first, then try to stop the hormones. (Chapter 2 has tips.) For example, learn paced respiration and also slowly decrease the amount of coffee and alcohol you consume. These strategies will make it more likely you will feel comfortable off hormones.

The possibilities for stopping hormones include:

- stopping "cold turkey." While some women can do this with no ill effects, others cannot. If you miss a pill or two and do not experience hot flashes, you may be able to stop taking estrogen without tapering off.
- tapering off by taking a slightly lower dose for weeks or months at a time. So far, studies have not shown a benefit to tapering off hormones rather than just stopping them. However, many of my patients who want to stop their hormones feel more comfortable tapering off them rather than stopping abruptly. If you feel this way, your doctor may gradually lower the dose of hormones you take by giving you a prescription for a lower dose. Alternatively, you can cut your pills or patches in half, but discuss this with your doctor first. As soon as you adjust to the new hormone dose and have no hot flashes, you can take an even lower dose, until you have stopped hormones completely.
- tapering off by changing the intervals—that is, taking the same dose, but less often, such as every other day, then every third day. You move on to less frequent dosing when the hot flashes have subsided on the current dose schedule.
- adding another prescription medication that is not a hormone, for example, Effexor, Neurontin, or Clonidine. This approach relieves hot flashes by a different mechanism. It may supply enough relief when combined with lifestyle modifications after estrogen is stopped completely.

If possible, avoid stopping hormones during the summer (unless you live in a hot climate year round). If you are going to try tapering off slowly, allow time to get comfortable with a given dose or frequency before taking the next step. Exceptions include an urgent medical problem, such as being diagnosed with breast cancer. Women with newly diagnosed breast cancer are advised to stop their estrogen immediately. Some (but not all) breast cancers are sensitive to estrogen, and may grow faster if the estrogen is continued.

Quitting Hormones "Cold Turkey" Was Too Difficult

"I'm 69 years old and was on Prempro for 20 years when I read the newspaper reports of the WHI study. I stopped taking the pills immediately, but then couldn't sleep due to horrific night sweats. I suffered for weeks before seeing my gynecologist. I had no signs of breast cancer, so my doctor suggested that I taper off the hormones slowly to allow my body a chance to adjust. He understood I was not comfortable stopping the hormones 'cold turkey' after all these years. First, over the summer, I took Prempro every Monday, Wednesday, and Friday, instead of daily, and had only a few hot flashes. By September, I was able to reduce the Prempro to every Sunday and Thursday without waking up due to night sweats. By November, I was able to stop the Prempro altogether, and have had only a few night sweats since then, but I associate those with enjoying an occasional beer."

BIOIDENTICAL ("NATURAL") HORMONES

There is a lot of hype about bioidentical hormones being better for women than synthetic hormones, but at this time no proof is available to back this claim. The term "bioidentical" is not a medical term with a specific, standardized meaning. The term has been used to describe a wide variety of different hormones. It may refer specifically to hormones that an individual pharmacist compounds for an individual patient. Or, more generally, it may refer to any hormone derived from plants.

It is reasonable to request plant-based hormones if you prefer; just remember that so far there is no data to support that they are safer or work better. Doctors can prescribe hormones made from plants that are approved by the Food and Drug Administration (FDA-approved). But you should know that all hormones, even those that are compounded or bioidentical, are synthesized. Those that are not FDA-approved may not meet the same quality and purity standards and have not been extensively tested to see how well they work, or how safe they are for you. I recommend you strongly consider FDA-approved hormones that are plant-derived if you choose to avoid hormones synthesized from horse urine. Plant-derived hormones come in many forms, including skin patches, lotions, vaginal rings, and skin sprays as well as some oral forms such as Menest, Prometrium, Activella, and OrthoPrefest.

There are theories that hormones absorbed through a skin patch, lotion, or spray have fewer risks. They do not get processed through the liver before they reach the bloodstream, and this may decrease the risk of clots. Further proof is needed.

The FDA agrees with this determination and requires that a black box warning with the side effects of estrogen and progesterone hormones be placed on all types of hormones, regardless of the way they are processed. FDA-approved hormones derived from plants carry the black box warning. Hormones compounded by a pharmacist are not nationally standardized or FDA-approved, and do not receive the black box label. This is not because the black box label does not apply! It is because the pharmacist who compounds a hormone preparation, or a hormone preparation sold as a supplement, does not have the same labeling requirements for this type of preparation. In January 2008, the FDA stated it considers the claims made about bioidentical hormones false and misleading because they are not supported by medical evidence — a violation of federal law.

Most often, I prescribe bioidentical hormones that are derived from plants but are also FDA-approved because they have been more widely tested than the non-FDA-approved hormones. The medical community would welcome definitive proof that hormones made from plants are safer than synthetic hormones but the evidence is not there yet.

All hormones are powerful medications, regardless of their source. The Million Women Study, published in August 2003, showed that many types of estrogen, including estradiol, which is often referred to as a natural or bioidentical estrogen, contribute to an increased risk of breast cancer. If you and your doctor agree you will be taking hormones to control severe hot flashes, you will work together to find the lowest dose that keeps you comfortable.

Making the Decision

Hormone therapy is still the most effective treatment for certain symptoms of menopause, and today we are clearer about which menopausal women are most at risk from taking hormones, as well as which women can benefit the most, based on their age and stage of menopause.

If you have symptoms such as hot flashes and night sweats that don't respond to non-hormone interventions and they interfere with your quality of life, you may want to discuss hormones with your doctor, particularly if you are in the low-risk group. Making this decision is a very individual process.

Today, the decision you make about hormone use is less likely to be the same as your friend's, your co-worker's, or even your sister's. Your current circumstances and medical requirements are unique and change from year to year. These are an essential part of your decision process. Consult your gynecologist or health provider to ensure that you get up-to-date advice that is appropriate for you at each annual visit. The discussion with your doctor is the only way to integrate your personal medical history, family history, and individual circumstances, including how severe your symptoms are and where you are in menopause.

RESOURCES

The table of risks on page 51 in this chapter is modified from "Facts about Menopausal Hormone Therapy," an excellent general resource that can be found at "Facts about Menopausal Hormone Therapy," www.nhlbi .nih.gov/health/public/heart/other/pht_fact.htm, page 8, modified from Box 8, "Table of Increased Risk on Estrogen Plus Progestin." Last accessed on December 21, 2008.

Two other government websites for the Women's Health Initiative that provide helpful overviews as well as updates on new studies are Women's Health Initiative (www.nhlbi.nih.gov/whi) and Menopausal Hormone Therapy information (National Institutes of Health [NIH]) (www.nih .gov/PHTindex.htm).

Heart Disease:
The Risk of Doing Nothing

I find it troubling—and frustrating!—that many people distrust modern medicine. At the same time, it is understandable. Some people grew up with stoic parents who never went to the doctor, so they think that's normal. Others have read about the hazards of taking hormones and the perils of other prescription medications and have decided that medications are never to be trusted. And many women believe that since menopause is not a disease, all they have to do is let nature take its course—particularly if they feel well.

If you don't visit your doctor on a regular basis, you cannot expect to stay healthy and active in postmenopause. In most health settings, having a gynecologist as well as an internist or family doctor will serve you best at this time. Choosing to do nothing is risky. Your doctors are qualified to do more than just treat your occasional vaginal itch or bladder infection. They monitor changes in your health from year to year and are skilled at diagnosing all the hidden threats I've mentioned earlier—including cardiovascular disease (which causes heart attacks and strokes), diabetes, osteoporosis, and cancer. Even better, they can provide you with good preventive care so you do not develop these problems in the first place.

Now that women in North America have an average life span of 84 years, they are asking how they can stay as healthy and active as possible during their postmenopausal years. Preventive medicine is essential to reach that goal.

It's good to keep up with the news and be well informed about health matters, but it isn't a substitute for visiting your doctor, who understands what will help you personally. A prevention strategy that is beneficial for one woman may be ineffective or even harmful for another.

Many people attribute their aches and pains and fatigue to "just getting old." Some changes and deterioration are natural with aging, but others are not inevitable. Many of the changes women and their doctors formerly attributed to aging have now been shown to be due to factors that are well within your control, such as activity and diet.

Even if you feel fine, assess your risk for heart disease and stroke. Cardiovascular disease is women's largest silent killer. Fine-tune your prevention and treatment regimens every year with your doctor, who can help decide if your current approach is best or if it is time for you to incorporate the results of a new medical breakthrough or newly available natural remedy.

Why Prevention Is So Important

It's a lot easier to prevent heart disease than it is to treat it once it has developed. Moreover, although treatment is possible, you may never again be as healthy as you once were. Treatment may not be delivered in time to preserve your lifestyle and independence. If you have a stroke, for example, you could become debilitated and dependent upon friends, relatives, or nursing home care. You could even die. I encourage you to work with a doctor to prevent serious health problems.

Women are fearful of breast cancer and ovarian cancer. These fears are legitimate and deserve to be addressed, but cancer is much less likely to kill a perimenopausal or postmenopausal woman than heart disease. Breast cancer has a higher profile than heart disease, but it does not kill more women. While one out of every 25 women will die of breast cancer, one out of every two women over the age of 50 will die of cardiovascular disease. But heart disease is silent, so without your doctor's help, you won't even know you have it.

Here are some facts you need to know:

- Cardiovascular disease (CVD) is the number one killer of women in the United States.
- Heart disease is the leading cause of death for women over age 50.
- CVD kills more women every year than all types of cancer combined.
- Half a million women die from heart disease each year.
- More than half of American women will experience a heart attack in their lifetime, most with no warning.

Since most women will never be warned before their first heart attack, prevention is the best policy. Neglecting your risk of heart disease can be a fatal mistake.

What Are the Risk Factors for Cardiovascular Disease?

Cardiovascular disease progresses along a spectrum, from early risk factors that you can control, to the development of hardened arteries, to advanced or acute problems. The earlier you intercede in this progression, the more successful you will be at restoring your health.

Are you at risk for cardiovascular disease? Each of the following common risks is a red flag for CVD. If you have one or more risk factors, consult your doctor about detecting and preventing CVD. These guidelines are specific for women; they differ from men's guidelines.

SMOKING

Smoking increases your risk of cardiovascular disease dramatically. According to the American Heart Association, smoking increases your blood pressure, increases the tendency for blood to clot, lowers your "good" cholesterol, and decreases your tolerance for exercise. Women who smoke and use oral contraceptives increase their risk of CVD and stroke. To add perspective, the Women's Health Initiative study initially reported that Prempro increased the risk of breast cancer by 26 percent, increasing the number of breast cancer cases from 33 women out of 10,000 women in a year to 41 women out of 10,000 in a year (or 8 more women per year). Smoking increases the risk of heart disease by 2,400 percent, almost 100 times the risk!

POOR DIET

A high-fat diet with few fruits and vegetables but an abundance of processed foods makes it more likely that you will develop high cholesterol and hardening of the arteries. The typical American diet is high in calories but low in nutrients.

FAMILY HISTORY OF HEART DISEASE

If you have a family history of heart attacks or strokes, you may be genetically susceptible to heart disease.

INACTIVE LIFESTYLE

Although family history is important to help determine your risk of heart disease, it is not the only component. Your lifestyle is a large factor. A sedentary lifestyle increases the risk of both stroke and heart attack. Preventive measures to lower the risk of stroke include staying physically active. If you don't get much exercise, increasing your activity level will help alleviate nearly everything that is bothering you!

OBESITY

You are considered at risk for cardiovascular disease if your weight is more than 10 pounds higher than when you graduated from high school or your body mass index (BMI) is over 25. Another risk factor is body weight that is distributed in an apple shape. If you have more weight around your waist than your hips or thighs, you may have developed the apple shape. To find out, divide your waist measurement in inches by your hip measurement in inches. If the number is 0.8 or more, you are at high risk for CVD and diabetes. If your waist measures more than 35 inches, you are also at higher risk. Since women have different builds and different amounts of muscle, the waist measurement is growing in importance. If you have a lot of muscle, your BMI may be elevated out of the normal range, but your waist measurement would still be normal. The waist circumference reflects the amount of fat around the internal organs. Excess fat around the internal organs is a risk factor for diabetes as well as heart disease. To measure your waist, feel the top of your hip bones, and measure around the smallest part of your abdomen above the hips.

More than 60 percent of American women are overweight. Women who exceed their ideal body weight are at higher risk for heart attack, stroke, and diabetes. Guidelines for determining your ideal body weight and BMI are provided in Chapter 12. Although younger women don't always suffer the medical consequences of being overweight, perimenopausal and postmenopausal women cannot avoid them.

DIABETES

A family history of diabetes increases the odds that you will develop heart disease. If you have diabetes yourself, it is a risk factor for CVD. Even if you are younger, or still perimenopausal, you are at risk for a stroke if you have diabetes. If you don't modify your lifestyle and eating habits now, you may develop complications of diabetes, such as poor circulation, leg swelling, open leg ulcers, poor eyesight that cannot be corrected with glasses, or loss of sensation in your feet. When these late complications of diabetes occur, they are not reversible.

If you hear the alarms sound before you are diagnosed with diabetes, or soon thereafter, you may be able to stop the progress of the disease with more nutritious eating, exercise, and attaining a healthier body weight. (For more information on nutrition and attaining a healthy body weight, see Chapter 12.)

High Cholesterol

Your chance of developing cardiovascular disease is raised if you have high total cholesterol (over 200 milligrams per deciliter fasting), your triglycerides are high (over 150 milligrams per deciliter fasting), and your high-density lipoprotein (HDL) protective cholesterol level is low (under 50 milligrams per deciliter).

What Is Cardiovascular Disease?

"Cardiovascular disease" is a general term for diseases that affect the heart or blood vessels, including high blood pressure, coronary artery disease, heart failure, heart attack, and stroke. Some forms of CVD, such as congenital heart problems, are not due to risk factors we can control. Most often, CVD is brought on by a lifetime of habits that are not heart-healthy.

High Blood Pressure

High blood pressure means your blood is pumping through your blood vessels with excessive force. It is considered an early form of heart disease. If high blood pressure is not controlled, it can lead to hardening of the arteries, heart attack, or stroke. Your blood pressure is a cause for concern if it is borderline (includes prehypertension) or high—over 120 millimeters of mercury *systolic* (top number), or over 80 millimeters of mercury *diastolic* (bottom number). About one in four Americans has high blood pressure. A normal blood pressure reading is 120/80 or under. If you already have diabetes, your doctor may recommend a goal of even lower blood pressure numbers to stay healthy.

Arteriosclerosis

Hardening of the arteries can occur anywhere in your body. When the arteries carrying blood to your brain are affected, you could have a transient ischemic attack (TIA) or stroke. When the arteries of the heart are affected, you could have a heart attack. Sometimes arteriosclerosis is associated with an aneurysm, which is a dangerous bulge in the wall of an artery.

Coronary Artery Disease

The arteries of the heart—the coronary arteries—supply blood to the muscle wall of the heart. If they become narrow, either due to spasm of the vessel wall or due to hardened fatty deposits called plaque, or both, the likelihood of having a heart attack is increased. Coronary artery disease may be associated with angina (chest pain).

Congestive Heart Failure

Sometimes the heart becomes less effective and can't pump enough blood to meet the needs of your body's organs and tissues. This can cause shortness of breath, fluid retention, and fatigue. Technically, "congestive heart failure" means that heart failure has led to fluid buildup. Heart failure may occur after other cardiovascular conditions, such as coronary artery disease, have damaged or weakened the heart.

Stroke

Strokes are considered a form of CVD. An *ischemic* stroke occurs when blood flow to the brain is interrupted. This may be caused by a blood clot or by plaque in the blood vessels of the neck or the brain. A *hemorrhagic* stroke is when a blood vessel in the brain ruptures. Strokes vary in severity, and their consequences depend on the part of the brain that is affected. Loss of function may be temporary or permanent. Some individuals suffer partial paralysis after a stroke and cannot move an arm or leg. Stroke is also considered a neurological disorder because of the many complications it causes.

Heart Attack

When the blood supply to the heart is cut off—usually because a blood clot blocks the flow of blood through a coronary artery—the muscle of the heart can be injured. The medical term for heart attack is *myocardial infarction,* sometimes called MI by health care workers.

Bringing Down Cholesterol and High Blood Pressure without Prescription Medications

Lucy, 49 and perimenopausal, is a schoolteacher with two teenage children. "I have hot flashes that worsen with stress, but I usually sleep well. My menstrual periods are lighter than they used to be and occur once every two to six months. After my children were born, I gained 25 pounds. Most of the weight had gathered around my waist. My fasting cholesterol was over 270 and my blood pressure was 140/90 — both too high, according to my doctor. I prefer not to take prescription medications or hormones, so when my doctor told me I was at high risk for a heart attack and diabetes, I was very willing to listen to how I might be able to address these problems and avoid prescription medications.

"He told me I could lower my blood pressure and cholesterol if I exercised regularly and lost weight. If my blood pressure and cholesterol did not improve, I would need medication. After getting the green light to exercise from my doctor, I began walking every day during my lunch break and joined Weight Watchers. In three months, I lost 10 pounds. My blood pressure returned to normal, and my cholesterol came down 35 points. I have continued to exercise and keep a written food diary, and now my cholesterol is under 200. I'm glad I was able to avoid taking prescription medications, and another great benefit was losing two inches off my waist, I went from 36 to 34 inches. I've now been sticking to my exercise program for over a year."

Heart Disease Affects Men and Women Differently

CVD is the number one killer of American men and women. But CVD is even more lethal for women; it kills them more often than it kills men. It is more difficult to detect and treat in women. Although advances in medical research and treatment have lowered men's risk of dying from a heart attack, women have not yet benefited.

Until recently, medical research was done on white males. Researchers who studied heart disease in men thought their findings applied to both sexes as well as different ethnic groups. Now we know that is not the case. Further research is still needed to understand differences between ethnic groups and to learn more about how heart disease differs in women. So far, clinical experience and more sophisticated tests show us that female heart disease looks very different from male heart disease.

WOMEN HAVE DIFFERENT SYMPTOMS OF A HEART ATTACK THAN MEN

Many women who have heart attack symptoms experience them differently from men. The typical warning signals of a male heart attack are often completely absent in a female. The tests used to identify a man's heart attack may not identify a woman's heart attack. The variety of symptoms, and the fact that they are atypical and subtle, often causes fatal delays in diagnosis and treatment for women having a heart attack.

If a woman has a heart attack, she is more likely to die from that heart attack than a man. This is true even if she is in perimenopause.

Surviving a heart attack is only part of the battle. Of 100 women who have a heart attack, 38 will die within 12 months. Of those who survive (62), almost 50 percent will be disabled. That leaves only 31 of the original 100 women alive and unaffected by disability.

⚥ HARVEY'S STORY ⚥

Male Heart Attack Victim

"My dad had a heart attack when he was 45. When I was 49, I had one. I had cut back on cigarettes but hadn't quit. During a particularly stressful day at work, I felt a crushing pain on the left side of my chest. I was sweating and short of breath, and I told my co-workers that the pain was traveling to my jaw. Lucky for me, they recognized these as classic symptoms of a heart attack and called an ambulance.

The hospital confirmed I had had a heart attack and I was admitted for treatment and monitoring."

⚡ HARVEY'S SISTER, SANDRA ⚡

Female Heart Attack Victim

"One afternoon, when I was 59, I told my daughter I was feeling anxious and I noticed my heart was racing. My daughter brought me to the emergency room, but they said my heart rate was only mildly elevated. The EKG [electrocardiogram] did not show any changes indicating a heart attack. I was reassured that since my EKG was normal, I was probably having a panic attack. I was given a mild tranquilizer and told to rest and later follow up with my regular doctor. My regular doctor was concerned and ordered an echocardiogram, a sound wave test that images the heart as it is beating. He also scheduled a Cardiolite exercise stress test, a dye test that studies the heart as it is working. During the Cardiolite stress test, I walked on a treadmill, with monitoring. When my heart was stressed with exercise, the dye study showed areas of weakness in the heart muscle, pointing to a recent heart attack. So, I actually had had a heart attack but they didn't know it when I went to the emergency room."

⚡ ADRIANA ⚡

Female Heart Attack Victim

"By the time I was 46, I was through with my periods, I was diabetic, and I was overweight. My doctor said that although I was young, I was at high risk for having a heart attack, due to the diabetes, obesity, and being in postmenopause, even though I had no family history of heart disease. One night after dinner I felt nausea, indigestion, and discomfort in my upper middle abdomen, and I took antacids, but they didn't help. So, I went to my doctor, and she did a detailed cardiac workup. She said the tests indicated a recent heart attack."

A Woman's Risk of Heart Disease and Stroke Rises with Her Age

Due to the protective effect of estrogen made by the ovaries, young women who still have menstrual periods have a lower risk of heart disease than their male counterparts. Earlier in life, women suffer from fewer heart attacks than their male contemporaries. Perimenopausal women begin to lose that advantage as they begin to lose their estrogen. In postmenopause, when the ovaries have stopped making estrogen, the protective advantage is lost. A woman's risk of heart disease rises dramatically when she crosses the threshold into postmenopause. After entering postmenopause, the risk of CVD rises until, at age 65, CVD occurs as often in women as in men. Strokes commonly affect postmenopausal women.

Women with high blood pressure, a waist measurement thicker than 35 inches, high cholesterol, or diabetes are at even greater risk for heart disease when they lose their estrogen. Addressing these risk factors with lifestyle changes or medication during perimenopause can be lifesaving.

Once a woman reaches age 50, she has a 50 percent chance of dying from CVD. Although CVD usually affects women over 50, risk factors such as smoking, diabetes, and obesity can cause the development of CVD in younger women. Once a woman has heart disease, she is much less likely to live a long healthy life. Once she is diagnosed with heart disease, she has a 50 percent chance it will kill her before age 74. Put another way, half of the women who have heart disease will die before age 74, even though the average American woman lives to 84.

Becoming postmenopausal increases the risk of heart attack 8 to 10 times. Entering postmenopause younger than age 40 (premature menopause) increases the risk of heart disease 8 times; entering postmenopause between age 50 and 55 increases the risk of heart disease 10 times. Heart disease is the most common cause of death during perimenopause and postmenopause, not cancer.

A Warning in the Form of a Heart Attack

"Last year, when I was 57, I had high blood pressure and was 40 pounds over my ideal body weight. I had a prescription for blood pressure medication, but often forgot to take it. That was partly because I was so dedicated to my job and worked such long hours. The job was sedentary and involved lots of meetings. When my doctor advised me to lose weight and exercise more regularly, I rationalized that there was no need to be alarmed because no one in my family had heart disease. I also reassured myself that men were the ones who got heart disease. None of my female friends were worried about heart disease, although several of them had already had breast cancer.

"Although I tried different weight-loss diets, as soon as I stopped them, I'd revert to my old eating patterns and regain the weight. It was frustrating. I could never find time to exercise because of my busy professional schedule. Eventually, I had a heart attack and required open-heart surgery. I am now in cardiac rehabilitation and out on disability for three months. My perspective on things has changed. I have promised myself, and my doctor, that I will build time for exercise into my schedule when I return to work, and I can now see that's really doable. I am also committed now to reaching my target weight and following a maintenance program once I do."

How to Lower Your Risk of Heart Disease

- *Lose weight.* To attain a healthier body weight, consider a program with a suitable proportion of healthy fats. Heart-healthy programs include the South Beach Diet, Weight Watchers Core Program with filling foods, a Mediterranean diet, a low-fat vegetarian option, or a diabetic diet (for more nutrition information, see Chapter 12).

- *Lower your cholesterol and control your high blood pressure.* Although they are beyond the scope of this book, there are medications that can help with both of these risk factors. In some cases, a woman may attain a healthy body weight and exercise regularly, but still be frustrated by high blood pressure or high cholesterol. She may have an underlying cause of her high blood pressure, such as kidney disease or a hereditary tendency to have high cholesterol. In those cases, medication may be the best route to tame the high risk of CVD.

- *Exercise.* Find ways of increasing your physical activity on most days. If you are a healthy woman with no medical restrictions from your doctor, you may start with as little as five minutes daily and gradually increase the amount of time you spend each day. Eventually, work up to 30 minutes of activity four days a week or more. Exercising four days a week for a total of 40 minutes a day will decrease your risk of stroke by 60 percent, as well as decrease your risk of heart attack.

- *Stop smoking.* Smoking causes heart disease, stroke, peripheral vascular disease (PVD), and high blood pressure, not to mention cancer. It's never too late to stop smoking, and the benefit to your health begins as soon as you do. Your doctor can help you find a smoking cessation program that's right for you — hypnosis, prescription patch, and chewing gum are just a few of the choices available.

If you don't like taking medications, keep in mind they may be a temporary inconvenience. Some women who develop habits of regular, consistent exercise and maintain a healthy weight are able to stop some or all of their medications with their doctor's blessing.

With pharmaceutical companies' heavy direct-to-consumer advertising campaigns on television, the Internet, and in magazines, it is easy to conclude that we all need prescription medications to be healthy. This is simply not true. Not everyone needs to take a blood pressure medication or a cholesterol-lowering prescription to enjoy good health. However, some individuals may not be able to lower their risk of heart disease or stroke without them. Each perimenopausal and postmenopausal woman owes it to herself to learn what medications are available to her. Once you and your doctor review your personal risks and benefits for a specific medication, and the medical condition it treats or prevents, you can decide if that medication meets your needs.

⚔ HANNAH'S STORY ⚔

Reversing the Risk Factors for CVD

"Five years ago, at age 48, I decided to take steps to decrease my risk of heart disease. I work as a customer support representative at a software firm and am on the phone or at my computer all day long. At my last checkup, I had a high blood pressure reading (150/100) and high cholesterol (280). My doctor told me I had a high risk of CVD. She asked me about the rest of my health. I also have indigestion and occasional discomfort in my jaw. Even though I have no chest pain, she recommended I have an exercise stress test to be certain my heart would tolerate an increase in physical activity. Once the test results were back, she gave me the green light to begin moving more. I started a low-fat diet, which means I'm getting less than 20 percent of my total daily calories from fat. I've also switched from saturated fats to healthy oils, like olive oil. I exercise four times a week instead of once or twice. Even if I can't get in a 40-minute workout, I've found I can manage 10-minute mini-exercise routines on those days, which are just as effective in preventing heart disease. There are lots of easy ways to do that.

"I walk for 10 minutes at lunchtime whenever I can. I park at the edge of the company lot and walk five extra minutes to and from the corner of the lot to my office, morning and evening. I take the stairs at work and climb them more at home, rather than avoiding them. My cholesterol went down to normal (190) within a year of my lifestyle changes, but my blood pressure did not. Further evaluation showed that I had a kidney problem that caused the high blood pressure. With medication, I'm keeping the blood pressure normal, and that's helping me avoid a heart attack. I feel better now, five years later, than I have in years."

Aspirin and Heart Disease

Taking an aspirin daily has been shown to lower the risk of CVD, but it does not lower the risk of heart attack and stroke in women who are at average or lower risk of CVD. Aspirin therapy has only been shown to lower the risk of heart disease in those at higher than normal risk. A doctor can assess your CVD risk and advise you about personal prevention strategies that will be most helpful and beneficial for you.

⚜ Angelina's Story ⚜

Aspirin and High Risk of CVD

"My doctor has told me that I'm at high risk of heart disease. My mother died of a heart attack at age 52; I'm now 58. I've smoked cigarettes since I was 16. I have high blood pressure and a sedentary lifestyle. Based on my family history, blood pressure, lifestyle, and smoking, all of which contribute to increasing my personal risk for a heart attack or stroke, my doctor advised me to take one aspirin daily."

⚜ Janet's Story ⚜

Aspirin and Low Risk of CVD

"My friend Angelina suggested that I lower my risk of heart disease by taking aspirin daily. Her doctor had recently recommended it for her. I started, and developed a painful bleeding stomach ulcer. I needed ulcer medication for six months until the symptoms subsided. When I saw my doctor for the ulcer, he explained that those at low risk of heart disease — like me — do not benefit from taking aspirin and are more likely to experience side effects or problems. I'm a nonsmoker who exercises three times a week. I also have no family history of heart attack, stroke, or diabetes. So the aspirin therapy was not going to lower my risk of heart disease and it actually caused harm."

Why are people at high risk of CVD less likely to get ulcers from aspirin? They aren't. Anyone can get an ulcer from taking aspirin. If you are at medium or low risk of getting CVD, the aspirin will not lower your risk of CVD enough to make it worth the potential side effects. In contrast, if you have a high risk of heart attack, you will substantially reduce your risk of CVD by taking aspirin. This substantial reduction in your risk of CVD outweighs the lesser risk of side effects. This is an example of weighing the risks of taking a preventive measure against the benefits. Having a discussion with your doctor that weighs the relative risks and benefits allows you to reach the best strategy to optimize your health.

RESOURCES

American Heart Association (www.aha.org).

"Dietary Patterns and Risk of Mortality from Cardiovascular Disease, Cancer, and All Causes in a Prospective Cohort of Women" (www.american heart.org) (the full article citation can be found in the References at the end of this book). This review for patients was written July 7, 2008. I last accessed it December 13, 2008. The Nurses' Health Study is a large prospective study that surveyed more than 120,000 American female nurses in 11 different states and followed their health status over the next 18 years using questionnaires, blood samples, and toenail clippings from the participants. The subjects had no prior history of major heart or vascular disease, cancer, or diabetes. Those who ate more vegetables and fish lowered their risk for death from heart disease by 28 percent. They lowered their risk of death from other common diseases (not heart disease or cancer) by 30 percent. Those who ate more red meat, French fries, and sweets increased their risk of death. This site hails this study as "the largest and most definitive study ever that demonstrates a connection between a diet rich in vegetables, whole grains, legumes and fish and a longer, healthier life." The study, and the review, stress that the pattern of eating, not particular nutrients or supplements, is responsible for the risk reduction.

Hearthub.org (www.hearthub.org) includes tools for risk assessments and a BMI calculator as well as other features.

Goldberg, Nieca. *The Women's Healthy Heart Program: Lifesaving Strategies for Preventing and Healing Heart Disease.* Ballantine, 2006.

Understanding Unexpected Bleeding

Irregular bleeding patterns are the most common change noted by perimenopausal women. More than 80 percent of perimenopausal women experience some irregularity in their menstrual cycles. While some variations in menstrual bleeding pattern may be a sign of perimenopause itself, unusual or unexpected bleeding can be an ominous sign that something is wrong. Don't try to figure out the difference on your own. For example, some women in perimenopause have irregular menstrual periods. That may be normal. But bleeding every three to six months over time also can be associated with polyps, endometrial hyperplasia, or endometrial cancer. For conditions like these, you need a doctor's diagnosis.

Internet research and polling friends and relatives for their opinions cannot replicate a trained clinician's assessment. At times, even trained medical specialists find it difficult to determine which bleeding patterns are normal variants and which are abnormal and warrant further investigation.

There are a great many myths and misunderstandings about bleeding patterns among women over 35. These misconceptions can be very harmful to your health. Too often, abnormal bleeding patterns are ignored because women "feel fine" or they are waiting for the problem to "go away on its own." If there is an underlying problem, it will only get worse as time passes. I have treated women who kept thinking their bleeding was due to "one last period," when in fact it was a sign of something else.

Sometimes a woman won't visit the doctor because she is afraid that the only solution for her heavy bleeding will be a hysterectomy. In fact, there are several new and effective approaches to eliminate heavy bleeding without major surgery. There is usually no need for a woman to keep enduring heavy periods.

For perimenopausal women, bleeding is common, but not necessarily normal. For women in postmenopause, bleeding is *never* normal. Causes of postmenopausal bleeding range from the relatively ordinary to the life-threatening. For example, one in 10 women with postmenopausal bleeding may have endometrial cancer.

Possible explanations for abnormal bleeding include:

- thyroid disease
- a sexually transmitted infection of the cervix, such as Chlamydia or gonorrhea
- polyps (soft, fleshy tissue growths)
- fibroids (solid muscle wall tumors)
- adenomyosis ("back-bleeding")
- endometrial hyperplasia (precancer of the uterus)
- uterine cancer (cancer of the lining of the uterus, or endometrium)

Keep Track of Your Bleeding Patterns

The key to identifying abnormal bleeding is keeping an accurate menstrual chart or calendar. In Chapter 1, I mentioned the importance of monitoring your normal bleeding patterns so that you and your doctor can see at a glance if you experience a change that could be significant.

Heavy menstrual periods have a different significance in women over age 35. Under age 35, uterine cancer is rare. Other physical causes of heavy bleeding, such as fibroids and polyps, are also less common under age 35. As a woman ages past 35, endometrial cancer and other physical causes of abnormal bleeding become increasingly common over time. Heavy or irregular menstrual periods may be the only signal that a cancer or precancerous change is developing. This is why your record of your bleeding becomes an important part of your health history.

Gynecologists evaluate menstrual cycle length from the first day of any bleeding episode to the first day of the next bleeding episode, regardless of how many days the bleeding itself lasts. For example, a woman who begins a 7-day menstrual period on July 1, then re-bleeds on July 19, has a 19-day cycle. If her flow lasts 14 days instead of 7, her menstrual cycle length still remains the same at 19 days due to the same starting date for each bleeding episode. So the length of a menstrual period and the menstrual cycle length are two different aspects of the bleeding pattern. Each is important in its own way.

Different bleeding patterns suggest different possible causes. They also point to key tests that will pinpoint the cause of the bleeding. Further, they may help determine the most helpful order in which to do the tests. If I have a high suspicion that endometrial hyperplasia (a precancerous change of the lining of the uterus) is the cause of a woman's abnormal bleeding, I may do a biopsy of the uterine lining (the endometrium) early in the evaluation to check for cancer and precancerous changes.

Postmenopausal Bleeding Is Never OK

I've said it before, but it bears repeating: bleeding during postmenopause is not normal! Any amount or type of bleeding (after 12 consecutive months with no bleeding, which signals postmeno-pause) is abnormal and is called postmenopausal bleeding. A woman with postmenopausal bleeding should consult a gynecologist, even if the bleeding episode looks and feels exactly like all the menstrual periods she experienced in the past. Any postmenopausal bleeding warrants medical assessment — even if the bleeding is so scant that it covers an area smaller than a dime. The risk of cancer is as high as one in 10 for women with postmenopausal bleeding. Although 9 of 10 women will not have cancer, they often have other benign or noncancerous causes for their bleeding, including polyps, fibroids,

Keep Track of Your Bleeding Patterns

During perimenopause, the significance of different types of irregular bleeding varies. Women who track their bleeding patterns have a baseline for comparison. Begin jotting down your individual bleeding pattern, even if it does not seem unusual right now. If and when it starts to change, you'll have lots of information to share with your doctor.

Keep a chart or written record including:

- the day your menstrual period begins
- how many days the bleeding lasts
- whether or not it comes and goes (there are days with no bleeding)
- how heavy it is each day (in pads or tampons per hour)
- the size of the protection being used (for example, super tampon, a maxi thin pad, or an overnight pad)
- the date of any spotting or episode of irregular bleeding
- the presence of any blood clots, and their approximate size (for example, dime-sized, or the size of a silver dollar)
- if the bleeding is related to intercourse

The simplest way to record this information is on a menstrual calendar or chart. Make an "X" every day that you see any blood, circle it if the bleeding is heavy, and make a dot if there is only spotting. Doctors need to know the length of each bleeding cycle, the length of each bleeding episode, and changes in these patterns that may occur over time. If you produce a chart with this information, the doctor can glance at it and quickly get a lot of information that will improve your medical care.

Many women who have heavy or irregular bleeding attribute it to perimenopause but there may be other causes, including polyps, fibroids, or a precancerous condition of the uterus called endometrial hyperplasia. These problems are rare in 20-year-olds but are common in 40- and 50-year-old women.

endometrial hyperplasia, or even adenomyosis (discussed later in this chapter).

Abnormal Bleeding in Perimenopause

I strongly recommend that you record your bleeding patterns, even if you have not noticed any changes yet. Any deviation from a woman's normal pattern is considered "abnormal bleeding," and it is helpful to establish the baseline pattern early.

Abnormal bleeding can take many forms—too many to describe here. Do not assume that if the unusual bleeding is light, or merely spotting, or painless, that it is not important. The rules change for bleeding patterns during perimenopause and postmenopause. Light bleeding or spotting is significant. While a woman in her early thirties may not be concerned about light bleeding, a woman over 35 should not ignore it. Light bleeding that occurs too often or for a prolonged period of time is not normal. Even light bleeding that occurs infrequently or at irregular intervals such as every 3 or 13 months warrants investigation. Such bleeding, although light, could still be a sign of a polyp, endometrial hyperplasia, or even endometrial cancer.

Women who begin to bleed or spot every 21 days or less are bleeding too frequently. This is often erroneously attributed to perimenopause, but it is not a normal change. While an occasional menstrual cycle may start earlier than normal during perimenopause, persistent cycles that begin 21 days or fewer after the start of the last bleeding episode warrant investigation.

Here are some questions to help you evaluate whether or not your bleeding is abnormal:

- Is this pattern different from your usual pattern of menstrual bleeding?
- Have you noticed the change for more than three months?
- Does the duration or severity of the bleeding stop you from following your usual routine?
- Do you ever soak through a regular pad or tampon in one or two hours (three or four hours for a maxi pad or super tampon)?
- Do you bleed through your clothes without warning, or soak through your nightclothes or bedding?
- Do you ever re-bleed sooner than 21 days from the start of your last bleeding episode?
- Do any of your bleeding episodes last more than eight days—including any spotting immediately before or after?
- Do you bleed between periods or after sex?

- Have you skipped menstrual cycles for more than three months at a time? for more than a year?
- Have you bled or spotted blood after you have gone 12 consecutive months with no period?

If you answer "yes" to any of these questions, seek a medical evaluation. The doctor will use your medical history, stage of menopause, specific bleeding pattern, and pelvic examination findings to choose the most appropriate tests. Most often it will involve an endometrial biopsy or a dilatation and curettage (D&C).

The severity of the bleeding or the amount of blood lost is helpful to know, but difficult to estimate. Research shows that women's assessment of the amount of blood they actually lose during a menstrual period is seldom accurate. The reasons are unclear. One reason may be that blood dissolving into the toilet may give the appearance of a larger loss. Another reason may be that a super tampon, a maxi pad, or an overnight pad can absorb a large amount of blood while giving the appearance of minimal blood loss. Some women are accustomed to losing large amounts of blood with their menstrual periods and do not consider a heavy flow abnormal. For others, there is an element of denial. They do not want to deal with the bleeding problem.

Some women lose a lot of blood with their menstrual periods, but the blood loss does not occur through the vagina. Some of the menstrual blood never passes out through the cervix to the vagina. Instead, it pushes back into the wall of the uterus, where it is reabsorbed into the abdominal cavity. This is called adenomyosis, or back-bleeding (see below).

Bleeding after Intercourse

Bleeding after intercourse has many possible causes, from sexually transmitted diseases like Chlamydia or gonorrhea, to a precancerous or cancerous change in the cervix, to a soft growth such as a polyp in the cervix or uterine lining. It may also be due to a vaginal infection, such as yeast or bacterial vaginosis. Bacterial infections are readily treated with antibiotics (see Chapter 6).

Changes in the cervix can be diagnosed with a microscope exam and a biopsy; polyps can be removed with a biopsy or a D&C.

Bleeding during or after intercourse is not normal and warrants a medical evaluation.

Diagnosing the Problem: Helpful Tests

Gynecologists use a woman's medical history, pelvic examination findings, and laboratory results to determine whether her current bleeding pattern is a normal variant for her or a sign of a problem. By taking a detailed medical history and performing a careful pelvic exam, a gynecologist can determine which additional tests will help pinpoint the most likely causes of the bleeding.

This area of women's health has become increasingly complex in the past 10 years. Now we have diagnostic tools such as pelvic and transvaginal ultrasounds, hysteroscopy, and saline sonohysterograms. New treatment options include endometrial ablations and uterine artery embolizations (described later in this chapter). These advances in the diagnosis and treatment of abnormal bleeding are a double-edged sword. They offer excellent relief for women with certain medical needs, but are hazardous to others.

A woman's doctor will guide her as to which tests are most helpful in her circumstances and which are not applicable. Transvaginal ultrasound and sonohysterograms (also known as saline-infusion sonography exams) are playing a more critical role in helping clinicians determine which individuals need a lining biopsy and which biopsy technique is best for that individual. The definitive diagnosis of endometrial cancer or pre-cancer is made by examining lining tissue under the microscope.

Pap Smear

A Pap smear checks for precancer and cancer of the cervix.

Swab Test

A swab test of the cervix can check for Chlamydia and gonorrhea.

Specialized Blood Tests

In some cases, specialized blood tests may help identify the cause of the abnormal bleeding or persistent anemia. Blood tests can identify forms of anemia that are hereditary, such as Thalassemia. Another hereditary condition, Von Willebrand's, impairs the ability of blood to clot in a timely fashion.

Hematocrit and Ferritin

A hematocrit blood test checks current blood levels for adequate iron and oxygen-carrying ability. This helps determine the severity of the bleeding and whether it is affecting a woman's energy level. It checks for current, recent anemia—a low red blood cell count. Hematocrit is the blood test that is done to see if you are anemic or whether you can donate blood. However, it is not the only way to check for anemia. Low iron reserves that are depleted over time may not show up as a low hematocrit. Sometimes only a ferritin level will reflect this type of anemia.

A ferritin level is a blood test that helps check the iron reserves over a period of time. If a woman has just become anemic recently, her ferritin may be normal and her anemia is reflected only in her low hematocrit level. A ferritin blood test checks iron reserves that accumulate over time and can detect chronic anemia that is more subtle but long-lasting. When abnormal bleeding has persisted over a long period of time, iron reserves will likely be low.

A woman may feel fatigued with a low ferritin, even if her hematocrit is normal. A low ferritin is like a gas tank that is just reading empty. If your gas tank reads empty, you may have enough gas to get to the gas station, but you cannot go anywhere else. You cannot do errands, go to work, go shopping, or go home; you can only go directly to the gas station. Those women with a low ferritin *and* a low hematocrit are experiencing a situation analogous to having an empty gas tank. They have no reserves and cannot make it to the gas station. A low hematocrit or a low ferritin is a common cause of fatigue and may indicate the need for iron supplements as well as further testing and treatment for anemia.

On the other hand, if a woman has been anemic for a long time but she has had successful treatment of her heavy menstrual bleeding and has been taking iron, her hematocrit level may have reached the normal range, but her ferritin may show that her iron reserves are still low.

In women who smoke, the hematocrit is often abnormally high. A smoker needs more red blood cells to carry oxygen to her body. If a smoker is hemorrhaging, her hematocrit could still be well in the normal range, and her anemia may only show with a low ferritin.

Thyroid Tests

Blood tests for thyroid function can reveal a hormone imbalance. This can be treated with medication that corrects the thyroid hormone imbalance and restores a normal bleeding pattern.

ENDOMETRIAL BIOPSY

An endometrial biopsy is a procedure for collecting a sample of the tissue lining the uterus (endometrium). It can be done in a gynecologist's office. Numbing may or may not be offered. One technique is to insert a slender device into the uterine cavity, then attach a syringe that can be used to create negative pressure. The negative pressure allows a small tissue sample to be withdrawn and sent for analysis to help evaluate the contents of the uterine lining. The tissue analysis may reveal infection, endometrial hyperplasia, a precancerous change, a hormone imbalance from irregular cycles (all of the tissue in the sample is not in the same phase of the menstrual cycle), or endometrial cancer.

An endometrial biopsy is not a reliable method to remove a polyp, if there is one, because there is no direct visualization.

HYSTEROSCOPY

A hysteroscope is a slender microscope that is inserted into the uterine cavity. It allows direct visualization of the cavity and provides a view of any blood vessel changes, polyps, or fibroids that may protrude into the lining. A hysteroscopy, a visualization process using this special microscope, can be done in a doctor's office or in the operating room. Hysteroscopy may be performed alone or as the prelude to another procedure, such as a D&C or an ablation. Hysteroscopy is not a substitute for a biopsy sample of the lining as not every type of change can be visualized with it.

Sonohysterogram or Saline-Infusion Sonography

During a sonohysterogram, sterile salt water is infused into the uterine cavity through a small tube. The inside of the cavity is then examined with ultrasound as the salt water separates the walls of the uterine lining. Some gynecologists use this method to visualize a polyp or fibroid protruding into the lining. It gives an indirect image much like a fuzzy old-fashioned black-and-white television image. Sonohysterogram may be used to pinpoint areas that should be biopsied that might otherwise be missed.

Pelvic and Transvaginal Ultrasound

A pelvic ultrasound is an examination that uses a probe over the pelvis, above the pubic bone, to get an image of the uterus and ovaries using sound waves. This creates a "sketch" of the organs and their dimensions. It is not the same as direct visualization. The pelvic organs are imaged by looking through the full bladder as a window. A transvaginal ultrasound involves a trained technician. For the vaginal portion of the examination, the technician or the patient herself inserts a slender sterile probe into the vagina (much like inserting a tampon) that allows imaging of the uterine lining, the uterine wall, and the ovaries. While measuring the thickness of the uterine lining is not a substitute for a tissue sample obtained from an endometrial biopsy or a D&C, in some cases, a thin lining measuring under 4 millimeters (1/6 of an inch) in a postmenopausal woman may preclude the need for a tissue sample.

Dilatation and Curettage

A dilatation and curettage, or D&C, is a sampling of uterine tissue involving dilation of the cervix. The opening of the cervix is gently widened with dilators to allow other instruments to be introduced into the uterine cavity, permitting removal of a tissue sample. The lining is not scraped away entirely (the goal is not to remove the lining), nor is the goal to "clean out" the uterine cavity. A D&C is not a cure; it is a diagnostic procedure used most often to determine the cause of abnormal bleeding.

At one time, women thought of a D&C as a "dusting and cleaning." Unfortunately, that misnomer persists. A D&C also samples the cervical lining tissue, which is traditionally sent in a separate container for analysis. Some gynecologists offer a modified office D&C using softer instruments and minimal dilatation. This procedure is more thorough than an endometrial biopsy because the instruments used for the D&C are capable of removing a polyp if there is one present, whereas the endometrial biopsy is likely to leave a uterine polyp unscathed. Also, more tissue is obtained for evaluation during an office D&C than during an endometrial biopsy.

Bonnie's Story

Modified D&C

"I'm 57, and because I still buy sanitary pads for an occasional period, my friends tease me—even my younger friends have long since stopped buying them. I usually bleed once a month for two or three months, and then have no period for four months in a row. After that the monthly bleeding begins again, followed by another stretch of four months with no bleeding, and the cycle repeats itself. This pattern has persisted for five years. I've had a history of uterine lining polyps in the past, which were removed with a D&C. My longtime gynecologist has retired and I've recently established with a new doctor. She informed me that I am at risk for endometrial hyperplasia and explained how my lining was building up without shedding for four months straight. Even though the bleeding I experienced was not heavy at any time, I did become concerned. I had simply assumed the four months of missed periods was a sign that I was getting closer to menopause. Although this is true, my doctor explained how my bleeding history could put me at higher risk for endometrial hyperplasia. My doctor suggested a modified D&C, which would allow her to remove polyps if they were present

in the upper endometrium. This was performed in her office, and the pathology results showed simple endometrial hyperplasia. I was treated with progesterone by mouth for three months. After I finished the medication I had another biopsy, which showed the hyperplasia had resolved. I was glad not to have a higher risk of cancer."

Some Causes of Abnormal Bleeding

Some of the following problems are easier to pinpoint than others. Some are easier to treat than others. But none of them should scare you away from the doctor's office. Every day many women face—and conquer—these problems.

UTERINE CANCER

The results of your Pap smear are not related to the condition of your uterus and cannot be routinely used to detect uterine cancer. A Pap smear detects abnormal cells on the cervix, the tissue at the opening of the uterus. The Pap smear is designed to detect only cervical cancer, not uterine cancer. Uterine cancer is much more common in perimenopause and postmenopause than cervical cancer.

In some cases, a clue that there may be a precancer or cancer of the uterine lining *may* be found on a Pap smear. The Pap smear "clue" may be a report of gland cells from the upper lining with a reading of "atypical glandular cells of uncertain significance" (commonly abbreviated AGCUS or AGUS). That reading may suggest trouble in the upper uterine lining and indicates that a biopsy of the uterine lining is needed. But that clue can often be absent.

Remember, women under age 35 seldom get uterine cancer or precancer. These conditions become much more common after age 35, as do polyps, fibroids, and adenomyosis. Uterine cancer should be identified and treated before it spreads.

ADENOMYOSIS

Adenomyosis is a form of local endometriosis where the tissue lining of the uterus does not stay where it belongs but migrates into the uterine muscle wall. There it may cause pain and swelling of the uterus, bloating, or severe menstrual cramps. The lining of the uterus acts as if it is leaky. Blood may push back across the lining into the uterine wall instead of passing out into the vagina as normal menstrual blood. The term "back-bleeding" captures what happens to the menstrual blood in women with adenomyosis. This back-bleeding forces blood into the uterine muscle wall, where some of it slowly reabsorbs back into the abdominal cavity instead of exiting the body through the vagina.

Adenomyosis is difficult to diagnose, except at the time of hysterectomy, when the uterus is cut open and analyzed for changes deep in the muscle wall. If other causes of abnormal uterine bleeding are not detected, adenomyosis may be the cause. It can also be present in women who have other causes for their abnormal bleeding, such as fibroids or polyps.

Women with back-bleeding do not see all of the blood they are losing because some of it is lost through the abdominal cavity and does not exit from the vagina. These women suffer from bloating as the uterus swells from the extra blood pushed back into the wall. They may also spot between menstrual periods as some of the blood may eventually leak back out into the vagina at a later date, well after the end of the regular menstrual period. They may feel extra pelvic pressure from the swollen, engorged uterus since the extra blood is trapped in the uterine wall and is absorbed more slowly than normal. If the pelvic examination shows the uterus is enlarged at times, but other times it is not, or the ultrasound does not show uterine enlargement when the pelvic examination does, adenomyosis may be the cause.

Adenomyosis is difficult to identify with the common tests used to check causes of heavy bleeding, a large uterus, and/or anemia. An ultrasound usually cannot identify adenomyosis because it is a dynamic process of back-bleeding and does not leave telltale signs visible on a sound wave test.

A biopsy of the uterine lining, an endometrial biopsy, or a D&C may not directly reveal that adenomyosis is the prime suspect causing the abnormal bleeding. And biopsies of the uterine muscle wall are not practical.

Hysterectomy (surgical removal of the uterus) allows definitive identification of adenomyosis. After the uterus is removed, the uterine wall is cut open, examined carefully under a microscope, and sent to the pathology laboratory. For women who have their uterus and wish to keep it, magnetic resonance imaging (MRI) may reveal changes that suggest adenomyosis. In some cases all the signs of adenomyosis are present, and nothing else can explain the changes.

⚡ ANNETTE'S STORY ⚡

Adenomyosis

"When I was 46, I started experiencing changes in my menstrual cycles that weren't normal for me. For 30 years, my periods always started every 28 days and lasted 6 days. The bleeding was heavy for two of those days. Even when it was heavy, I never needed more than a pad or a tampon in two hours, although at times I noticed blood clots. When my periods started changing, I began having periods every 23 days and they lasted longer—10 days, with heavy bleeding for the first 4 days. When I talked with my gynecologist about this, she updated my medical history, performed a pelvic examination, and ordered blood tests, including a hematocrit and a ferritin, as well as thyroid tests. The blood test results showed I had borderline anemia, but my thyroid was normal. She found my uterus was slightly enlarged on pelvic examination. She scheduled an endometrial biopsy, which, thankfully, showed no cancer or precancerous changes. Since I'm a nonsmoker, she prescribed a low-dose oral contraceptive to control my periods and make them shorter, lighter, and regular, once every four weeks.

"After six months using the pills, my doctor and I agreed I would stop them. I was fine for a year, but after that, the periods became heavier again. I was bleeding through a large pad in less than two hours, and the heavy bleeding lasted for more than five days. This time, blood tests showed my hematocrit was low, indicating anemia, so my doctor had me start taking iron. During the pelvic examination, she found my uterus was even larger, but an ultrasound did not reveal any fibroids. She suspected adenomyosis, since the ultrasound did not show any fibroids and no masses were felt in the physical exam. I had a D&C with hysteros-

copy, which confirmed there was still no cancer or endometrial hyperplasia, and no polyps or fibroids were found.

"My doctor and I discussed the choices. She recommended an endometrial ablation. Even though ablations are not always effective for adenomyosis, and the only 'sure thing' is to have my uterus removed with surgery, she advised I consider having a type of ablation that had a better track record in providing relief for women who may have 'back-bleeding,' or adenomyosis. If the ablation did not provide relief, then a hysterectomy would stop the heavy periods. I had an ablation and have been pleased to have short, light menstrual periods since then, for the past three years."

ENDOMETRIAL HYPERPLASIA

Endometrial hyperplasia is a form of precancer characterized by a microscopic change in the uterine lining. Precancers are not cancers: they behave differently. The path of a cancer is set; it will not improve without surgical removal, chemotherapy, radiation, or a combination of these three. The path for a precancer is very different; it may have any number of unexpected twists and turns. A precancer may turn into a cancer over time, or it may remain unchanged, or it may resolve on its own. The timeframe a precancer takes to go away or become cancerous depends upon the type of precancer and how severe the changes are.

Examining a biopsy sample of the uterine lining under the microscope shows glands growing too close together and forming abnormal clusters. There are different types of endometrial hyperplasia, some more ominous than others. Simple hyperplasia is a more innocent (least worrisome) type and is the most common. It is the least likely type of hyperplasia to turn into endometrial (uterine lining) cancer over time (a less than 5 percent chance). It is most likely to be completely cured with medication alone, which prevents it from progressing to endometrial cancer.

Hyperplasia is identified by an endometrial biopsy of the uterine lining or a D&C. If simple hyperplasia is identified, it can be treated with a medication such as Provera or Megace, which are types of progesterone. Progesterone corrects the hormonal imbalance caused by too much estrogen influencing the uterine lining. The progesterone is usually taken by mouth for three months.

After treatment, it is crucial to resample the uterine lining with another biopsy. This ensures that the hyperplasia has responded to the medication and has resolved. If the hyperplasia persists but has not progressed to a more severe type, the doctor may retry the medication and then resample the lining to see if the condition was cured; after reviewing the results, she or he may suggest other options.

If simple hyperplasia worsens despite medication, the uterus may have to be removed to decrease the risk of cancer. If a biopsy shows severe hyperplasia or complex hyperplasia or hyperplasia with atypia, it indicates the features are more worrisome and are more likely to progress to cancer. Atypia describes nuclei in the cells that are angry and more aggressive than normal. They may influence the cells to grow erratically and become cancerous rather than follow a normal growth pattern. Those with hyperplasia that has both complex and atypical features are more likely to have actual uterine cancer present next to the hyperplasia in the uterine lining. Women with severe hyperplasia or complex or atypical hyperplasia may be best served by a hysterectomy (surgical removal of the uterus) to prevent uterine cancer or remove early uterine cancer.

Hyperplasia of the uterine lining is more common in women over 35. It is also more common in women who are overweight. You may recall from Chapter 1 that women make an estrogen in their fatty tissues called estrone. Women who are overweight make more estrone. This excess estrogen stimulates the uterine lining to get too thick and promotes cancer and precancerous changes. Exercising and removing excess weight can decrease the risk of forming endometrial hyperplasia and endometrial cancer by decreasing the amount of estrone made in the fatty tissues.

The clinical clues suggesting that endometrial hyperplasia may be present are confusing. On the one hand, endometrial hyperplasia is associated with heavy or prolonged bleeding in women in their mid-thirties and older. On the other hand, it is also found in women who bleed too seldom. A woman who bleeds every three to six months, or even less frequently, does not shed her lining every month. The resulting buildup of tissue can promote hyperplasia. This is common in perimenopause as a woman's cycles become irregular. It can also occur in postmenopausal women who have not bled for 12 consecutive months and then re-bleed.

Endometrial hyperplasia causes the lining to become thick microscopically. While a transvaginal ultrasound can measure the thickness of the uterine lining, it is not sensitive enough to detect endometrial hyperplasia in its early stages. Therefore, an ultrasound measurement of the uterine lining thickness should *not* take the place of an endometrial biopsy or D&C to detect endometrial hyperplasia.

Endometrial hyperplasia can also form inside of a soft tissue growth called a polyp. However, removal of the polyp does not always ensure that the endometrial hyperplasia is gone for good.

⚜ BERYL'S STORY ⚜

Postmenopausal Bleeding

"I'm 55, and my periods stopped a year ago, when I was 54. I went through the menopause transition smoothly. But after 13 months with no bleeding, one day I noticed some pink spotting. The amount was so small that I was tempted to ignore it, but I recalled my gynecologist emphasizing that I should be seen if I bled at all after 12 consecutive months of no bleeding. My neighbor, whom I mentioned this to, thought I was overreacting since the amount of bleeding was so small. 'Why don't you wait and see if the bleeding happens again and then call your doctor? You don't want to be an alarmist.' I thought about waiting but then decided to see my doctor. He advised an endometrial biopsy.

"The biopsy showed endometrial hyperplasia, a mild precancer. He prescribed medication to treat the hyperplasia, and I took progesterone daily for three months. I then had another endometrial biopsy, which showed the hyperplasia had not responded and still persisted, although it had not progressed to a more severe type. My gynecologist offered me two choices: I could undergo a hysterectomy or I could take a stronger medication to try to eradicate the hyperplasia. I chose to try a stronger

medication, Megace, which I took twice a day for three months. I con-
tinued to have mild, irregular bleeding while on the medication. After
three months of Megace, I had a D&C with hysteroscopy. It showed that
the hyperplasia was completely gone and the Megace worked well. My
doctor explained that if I could increase my daily activity by walking
more or exercising, and if I could lose weight, I'd decrease my chances of
getting hyperplasia again and decrease the amount of estrone my body
was making in the excess fatty tissue I was carrying."

Polyps

Polyps are mushroom-shaped soft tissue growths. They may occur in the cervix or in the lining of the uterus (womb). Sometimes they are attached to the uterus or cervical lining without a stalk and are called sessile polyps. They may be benign (innocent), precancerous, or cancerous. Precancerous polyps have the ability to turn into cancer over time. Polyps are removed to be certain they are not cancerous and to prevent them from turning into cancer.

Polyps can cause bleeding or spotting between menstrual cycles after a few days or weeks with no bleeding. They can also cause bleeding after intercourse. They are common in perimenopause as well as postmenopause. They may cause heavy or light bleeding or a combination. The key is the timing of the bleeding.

The spotting from polyps may occur in the middle of the menstrual cycle when no bleeding is expected, or they may cause spotting before or after a regular menstrual period, prolonging it beyond the normal timeframe. Polyps may cause anemia due to prolonged and/or frequent spotting over time.

If there is a polyp in the uterus, it may not be visible by speculum exam in the office, especially if it is attached high in the uterine cavity. Unless they happen to protrude from the cervical opening, much like the center of an old-fashioned bell, polyps are not visible on a routine pelvic exam. An ultrasound study might not be able to identify polyps either. At times, polyps can cause the uterine lining to appear thicker when measured by ultrasound, but this is not always the case.

Polyps can be seen with a hysteroscope or identified using a sonohysterogram. Regardless of how they are seen, they can be removed with a D&C.

Polyps should be removed because they cause abnormal bleeding and because they can turn into cancer, although they usually do not. Even though uterine polyps are rarely cancerous, they should be tested for cancer when they are removed.

⚘ JASMINE'S STORY ⚘

Irregular Spotting Due to a Polyp

"At 39, I'd been having heavy menstrual bleeding for five years. My doctor knew about it, and I managed the periods pretty well. My co-workers gave me extra breaks during my period and told me it was a sign of early menopause. Over time, I developed fatigue, to the extent that my doctor checked my blood count. I was not anemic, but I had low iron reserves. My ferritin was only 4. I learned that although low normal is 20, most healthy women have a value over 50! In addition, my thyroid blood test was abnormal. My doctor treated that and the bleeding became normal.

"When I was 40, I started having unusual spotting every month for about five days before my period. After three months of this I saw my doctor, and she had the thyroid test redone; everything was normal. My pelvic exam was normal. She put me on a three-month course of progesterone to rebalance the uterine lining, which did eliminate the spotting, but then it recurred. At that point, my gynecologist suspected a polyp or hyperplasia. She performed a D&C in her office and found and removed a benign endometrial polyp. Now, three years later, my periods have been normal ever since. I keep track of my monthly bleeding pattern so that if anything becomes abnormal again, I will have a history that will help my doctor determine what's going on."

FIBROIDS

Fibroids are common, firm muscle wall tumors. One out of five women in their thirties has them. Studies show that all women develop fibroids by the time they reach old age. Fibroids can grow slowly or increase in size very rapidly. Rapidly enlarging fibroids may represent sarcoma, a cancerous form, although that's not common; only one in 10,000 fibroids are cancerous. Fibroids that are very large or increase in size rapidly should be assessed for a possible sarcoma.

Fibroids result from mutations. The development of fibroids in the uterine muscle wall over time is analogous to the changes in one's skin over a lifetime. A baby's skin is smooth and clear. As the baby grows, her skin stays smooth and clear into her twenties. At age 40 her skin no longer "duplicates" as accurately or as well. Mutations begin to form, and genetic "mistakes" occur during skin growth. Brown or red dots and areas of discoloration may appear with age.

Similarly, the uterine muscle wall cells do not replicate as well by the time a woman is in her thirties. Over the next decade the mistakes include the formation of fibroids, firm muscle tumors that look like whorls or gnarls on an old tree. They begin in the muscle wall of the uterus as small nodules, smaller than a raisin. The fibroids may expand or push into the uterine lining, or push outward to the surface of the uterus. Fibroids that are not too numerous and not too large may be inconsequential. At times fibroids may get as large as a small watermelon. The fibroids are stimulated by estrogen. In Chapter 1, you read about the saw-tooth patterns of estrogen during perimenopause with erratic peaks of excessive estrogen levels. These high levels are particularly conducive to fibroid growth.

Large fibroids or too many fibroids may cause pressure and bloating from an enlarged uterus, as well as heavy bleeding. A very large uterus may silently press on the ureters, the tubes that carry the urine from the kidney to the bladder. In some cases, over time this pressure can even cause silent kidney failure. More than 20 years ago, women were commonly offered a hysterectomy to remove the uterus with the fibroids and cure the problem of pressure and/or heavy bleeding. Now there are many other alternatives to treat the problems resulting from a large uterus or heavy bleeding due to fibroids.

Medical Procedures to Stop Bleeding

Treatment options vary by the type of bleeding, its cause, and the phase of menopause a woman is in. Sometimes the options include observation. Other times it is imperative to treat a woman with medication or a surgical procedure to avoid the need for a blood transfusion or taxing the heart from severe anemia, or to prevent the development of uterine cancer.

Endometrial Ablation

Twenty years ago, women over 35 with heavy or prolonged bleeding were advised to have a hysterectomy. Today there are other options. One is an endometrial ablation. Endometrial ablations involve treating the endometrium (uterine lining) to prevent excess bleeding.

Endometrial ablations have evolved over the past 17 years or so since they were first introduced. The original ablation techniques to reduce heavy bleeding involved surgically removing the entire endometrium. A resectoscope was used with a loop to scoop out lining tissue. Cautery or a laser was used to seal the blood vessels and minimize blood loss. The woman kept her uterus.

Another early technique involved cauterizing the entire surface of the endometrium using a "roller-ball." A miniature metal steam roller no wider than a thumbnail was passed over the lining surface, cauterizing the lining tissue down to the base. The procedure was done painstakingly in rows, much like mowing a lawn.

There were hazards associated with these early techniques. The principal one was that a large amount of fluid was needed to keep the walls of the uterine lining apart to maintain visualization during the procedure. As the lining was removed and blood vessels were exposed, fluid went into the blood vessels. During longer or more difficult procedures a substantial amount of fluid caused imbalances in the body, sometimes causing brain swelling.

Another concern raised was whether cancer could form but escape detection after the lining was cauterized. To date, the few isolated cases of endometrial cancer that have been reported after endometrial ablations occurred in women who did not have a timely biopsy of the endometrium prior to the ablation. The uterine cancer was present but not identified before the ablation was performed.

Safer techniques have been developed. Today, if the traditional methods of ablation are used, the amount of fluid is carefully measured during the procedure. And now there are a variety of newer ways to safely perform an endometrial ablation that do not involve using fluid at all. In some cases, the cavity may be visualized directly with hysteroscope prior to the procedure, but the actual ablation is performed without direct observation. Each method has different pros and cons, risks and benefits. Some techniques are better suited than others to a particular woman's history, physical examination, and uterine anatomy.

For example, if the uterine lining cavity is less than 12 centimeters (4.8 inches) in length, the NovaSure method is one option. A fan-shaped mesh device is introduced into the endometrial cavity to distribute energy from radio waves across the endometrial surface. After the surface is sealed, the device is withdrawn from the uterine cavity. One advantage of the NovaSure method is that no hormonal preparation is required before the procedure, and it can be performed during any part of the menstrual cycle, even during active bleeding. A disadvantage is that it may not be possible to use the technique in a uterus where the endometrial cavity has a very irregular shape.

The satisfaction rate for this technique is very high. For every 100 women who have a NovaSure endometrial ablation, 95 are satisfied with it and would recommend it to others. Of the satisfied women, some have a short, light menstrual flow after their endometrial ablation. Others no longer have any menstrual bleeding after the ablation.

Doctors cannot predict who will no longer have any menstrual bleeding and who will still get a light flow. Even those who no longer have any bleeding are still premenopausal and fertile and may feel cyclic changes such as mild PMS (premenstrual syndrome), if they had them prior to the procedure. Their hormonal balance is unchanged. A NovaSure ablation, unlike many other types of ablation, also helps many women with adenomyosis.

The Thermachoice balloon was the first ablation technique to cauterize the whole endometrial lining at once. A balloon is introduced into the uterine cavity and then filled with hot water. The hot water heats the lining touching the balloon. After the lining is heated, the water is removed and the balloon is deflated and withdrawn. One disadvantage is that the endometrial lining must be prepared with hormones ahead of time. Another is that the balloon will not fit into endometrial cavities distorted by protruding fibroids or those without a smooth or regular shape.

Yet another technique is hydrothermal ablation, or HTA. This technique involves monitoring the endometrial cavity with a hysteroscope and filling it with sterile salt water (saline) under direct observation. After the cavity is filled, the base of the cavity is sealed off and the sterile water in the uterine cavity is heated for 10 minutes until the lining is thinned. Then the water is cooled and removed, and the instruments are withdrawn. Advantages include the ability to treat any cavity, regardless of size or shape, as the saline can go into all of the crevices. One disadvantage is that the seal between the cervix and the device may loosen during the procedure. This may increase the chance of the hot saline leaking into the vagina, causing a burn.

Finally, cryoablation (commercial name, HerOption) involves freezing the uterine lining with an ice ball that extends into the myometrium, or muscle wall. The process is monitored with ultrasound to ensure that the freezing is done for the desired length of time and in the most strategic locations.

Endometrial ablations do not affect the timing of postmenopause, and they do not change a woman's hormone balance. They are designed exclusively to eliminate heavy and/or prolonged abnormal bleeding while allowing a woman to keep her uterus. The procedures have helped many women to avoid hysterectomies and other surgical procedures. In some cases, the results are not permanent. Other women are fortunate enough to reach postmenopause on their own before the ablation wears off. A few but not all of these procedures are also effective for adenomyosis.

Endometrial ablations are not recommended for women who wish to conceive. An ablation decreases the blood supply to the uterine lining. It also alters the contours and qualities of the uterine cavity so it is no longer hospitable to a fetus. An ablation may make the uterine lining unsuitable for healthy fetal growth, but does not prevent pregnancy. So women who have an ablation should use reliable contraception throughout perimenopause.

Endometrial ablations are not suitable for women with postmenopausal bleeding. They are only FDA-approved for perimenopausal bleeding or for younger women with heavy or prolonged abnormal bleeding that are premenopausal and have not yet reached perimenopause.

Those with endometrial hyperplasia should not consider an endometrial ablation unless they have simple hyperplasia that has been completely treated and resolved on a follow-up biopsy or D&C. Some experts advise a hysteroscope prior to the ablation as well as a recent endometrial sampling to ensure that the lining being treated is free of cancerous and precancerous changes.

◢ POLLY'S STORY ◣

Endometrial Ablation with NovaSure Technique

"I'm 49 and have smoked two packs of cigarettes a day since I was 17. I did stop once successfully, but took up smoking again after my divorce. About a year ago, I went to my gynecologist because I'd been having unusually heavy periods for a little over a year. My doctor found, during the pelvic exam, that my uterus was enlarged. Blood work showed my thyroid was normal. But even though my hematocrit was 42, which she told me was high-normal for a woman, I was exhausted. My blood level of ferritin was 5. The doctor said this substantial reduction in my iron reserves explained my fatigue. The diagnosis was a severe chronic anemia. First, I sought several opinions about how to manage the bleeding and considered a vaginal hysterectomy to remove my uterus. But then, after giving it more thought, I decided to undergo an endometrial ablation. The procedure was successful, and within three months, I was having short, light periods lasting only two days. I was

actually able to wear a panty liner for half a day. For an entire year I took an iron supplement once a day, until tests showed my iron reserves were restored to a normal level. I was less fatigued within three months of the ablation, but returned to my normal energy level completely only after my iron reserves returned to normal."

ANTI-ESTROGEN INJECTIONS

One option for temporary relief of bleeding due to large or numerous fibroids is a medication called Lupron, given as an injection. Lupron works, within two weeks, to turn off the ovaries as if they were in postmenopause. This stops the ovaries' production of estrogen and halts estrogen stimulation of fibroid growth. The benefit of the injection wears off in one to three months, depending upon the strength of the injection. Side effects include hot flashes. With long-term use beyond six months, osteoporosis becomes a concern. Unfortunately, as soon as the injection wears off, the ovaries become active in releasing estrogen again and the fibroids regrow. So Lupron is not a long-term or permanent solution.

⚥ JUANITA'S STORY ⚥

Treating Adenomyosis with Lupron Injections

"I've had worsening cramping and heavier bleeding during my menstrual periods for the past three years, since I was 41. Now, it has become so severe I have to leave work on the first day of my period. I've kept a menstrual calendar and it shows my periods are longer and heavier. Between menstrual periods, I spot for more than a week. My gynecologist has noted that my uterus is more swollen and enlarged. He ordered an ultrasound, which did not show any fibroids or growths in the uterine wall. A biopsy of the uterine lining showed no cancer, polyps, or infection. He said this was typical of adenomyosis. He explained that even though menstrual periods commonly get more irregular during perimenopause, they should not get heavier. My doctor found that my blood count was low, which explained my fatigue. He prescribed an injection of Lupron, which he said contains a hormone that 'turns off' the ovaries

temporarily and simulates postmenopause. I had two injections of Lu-
pron, one month apart. The uterus swelling went down and my cramps
vanished. I continued to take iron once a day and I continued to feel less
tired. However, after two months of Lupron shots, the effects wore off.
My doctor suggested an endometrial ablation or a hysterectomy. Since I
wanted to keep my options open to maybe have one more child, I chose
the option of going back on a low-dose oral contraceptive pill until my
anemia was completely cured."

HORMONES FOR BLEEDING, INCLUDING PILLS OR A MEDICATED INTRAUTERINE DEVICE

Perimenopausal women may have the option to try progesterone to rebalance their uterine lining and diminish their bleeding. Nonsmoking perimenopausal women may benefit from the use
of a low-dose oral contraceptive to regulate their menstrual periods
if they are too heavy, prolonged, or too frequent. This is safest after
the lining has been biopsied, especially in women over 40.

Another option to control heavy bleeding in both smokers and
nonsmokers is the Levonorgestrel Intrauterine Device, or IUD, available by prescription. This device is placed in the uterus during
an office visit to the gynecologist and slowly releases small doses
of progesterone into the uterine cavity continuously over time. It
serves as contraception as well as playing a role in decreasing heavy
bleeding. If a woman wishes to conceive, the IUD can usually be
removed in the doctor's office.

MYOMECTOMY

Another strategy especially suited to one or two large
fibroids causing pressure or excessive bleeding is to perform a myomectomy. This surgery removes fibroids from the uterine muscle
wall. Traditionally, this was performed through an open incision, or
cut. More recently, it has become possible to remove some fibroids
using a laparoscope (a microscope introduced through the navel).
Depending upon the size and location of the fibroids, it may be possible to remove them through an operation using a hysteroscope.

The downside of a myomectomy to remove troublesome fibroids is that they regrow in three to five years. As a result, myomectomy is more often used in cases where women want to preserve their fertility. Myomectomies may be offered to other women as well, as long as the women are aware that their fibroids may regrow after the surgical removal.

Not all fibroids can be treated with these methods. Newer methods are being explored, such as treating larger individual fibroids with ultrasound as a treatment modality to decrease their size.

Uterine Artery Embolization

Uterine artery embolization (UAE) is a newer technique to decrease the blood flow to the uterus. If fibroids are present, they will shrink as a result of the diminished blood supply. Dye is injected to identify the arteries that supply the uterus. Tiny synthetic particles are passed through a small tube inserted in the groin. These particles create a road block in the major arteries that supply the uterine wall and the fibroids. Specialists called interventional radiologists are trained to perform UAE. Local numbing is used at the groin site where the particles are injected, but no general anesthesia is needed. The woman may go home after a period of observation, or remain in the hospital overnight for pain management. Since the blood supply is cut off suddenly, an enlarged uterus will shrink quickly, in some cases causing severe cramping. Some fibroids may even pass out through the vagina. Some radiologists perform a nerve block at the time of the embolization, reducing the discomfort considerably.

One risk of the procedure is that the blood supply to the ovaries may be affected and compromised, but this is rare. In most cases the blockage does not affect the blood supply to the ovaries at all. It is designed to block only the blood supply to the uterus, and that does not change a woman's menopause status. Perimenopausal women who undergo a successful UAE procedure usually remain perimenopausal (even if they stop bleeding afterward), because their ovaries continue to function normally.

Another disadvantage is that the procedure is not permanent.

The relief from fibroids and heavy bleeding lasts from one to three years. After that, the blood supply may reestablish and the fibroids may regrow.

HYSTERECTOMY

A hysterectomy with removal of the uterus removes the uterine wall, so fibroids cannot re-form. If a supracervical hysterectomy is performed, where the body of the uterus is removed but the cervix nubbin remains, fibroids may regrow from the inner stump of the cervix and residual bleeding may occur from a menstrual period generated by a small amount of remaining uterine lining tissue attached to the cervix.

Occasionally a hysterectomy is needed to solve a woman's abnormal bleeding problem.

❧ MARNI'S STORY ❧

Blood Loss, Anemia, and Hysterectomy

"I've always been someone who is wary of taking any medication if I'm not desperately ill. Shortly after I turned 50, I started having much heavier periods, but they remained regular and appeared every 25 days. Eventually, about a year and a half ago, when I was 53, the periods got even heavier, and then became irregular. I was also passing large clots, wider than a silver dollar. The bleeding became so unexpected that I would soak through my clothes with no warning, even wearing overnight pads. These accidents became more frequent and were terribly embarrassing. When I visited my gynecologist, he did a blood count that showed I had severe anemia and had lost the equivalent of at least four units of blood over time! My iron reserves were close to zero. Taking iron was not going to help me fast enough; he said I was in danger of needing a blood transfusion.

"The blood test to check my thyroid hormone was normal. I had a modified D&C in my gynecologist's office, during which a polyp was removed from the upper uterine lining. It was sent to a pathology laboratory for analysis, and the report showed complex endometrial hyperplasia, a severe form of precancer. I took iron for six months, but the

bleeding continued and the anemia persisted. My doctor discussed the alternatives. I could take Megace, strong progesterone, for three months and then have another endometrial sample to see if the hyperplasia responded. If it persisted or worsened, he recommended a vaginal hysterectomy. Or, if I chose, I could have a vaginal hysterectomy sooner and not take the medication or have another biopsy. I had experienced headaches in the past when I tried a low-dose birth control pill and so was reluctant to try a hormonal medication even though it was a progesterone and not estrogen. One day, I passed out due to severe blood loss. I also developed an elevated heart rate from the anemia and required a blood transfusion. That's when I decided to have a vaginal hysterectomy.

"After the surgery, when the uterus was examined in the lab, a small endometrial cancer was found next to the complex hyperplasia. My doctor assured me that the hysterectomy 'cured' me and I didn't require any chemotherapy or radiation. After I recovered from the surgery, I didn't have any further bleeding. Since the hysterectomy was done through the vagina, I had no incision and healed well. It took a year of taking iron to completely replenish my iron reserves."

How Anemia Affects Your Health

If you reassure yourself that your bleeding pattern is normal when it is not, you may become anemic. Anemia (low iron in the blood) leads to fatigue and extra stress on the heart. A woman who has bled heavily since her teens may be complacent in her mid-thirties. She is accustomed to bleeding heavily. However, heavy bleeding not only has a different significance in terms of abnormalities of the uterine lining, it can affect the function of the heart, especially after age 40. Women over 40 already face a higher risk of heart disease over the next two decades of their lives as a result of age. Becoming anemic over age 40 may result in more than fatigue; women who become anemic after age 40 may not only feel tired but also tax their heart at an age when the risk of heart disease is already rising quickly. The heart is taxed because the blood is carrying less oxygen than normal. The heart must therefore pump harder to send more blood to the tissues and organs to deliver the same amount of oxygen.

Sometimes I am asked if taking iron alone will solve the problem and correct the anemia. Taking iron alone is like trying to fill a sink without plugging the drain. If too much blood continues to be lost on a regular basis, taking iron may not be enough to correct the anemia and replenish the iron reserves. Taking iron will not fix the problem until the cause of the heavy bleeding is identified and treated and the amount of blood loss is reduced. Taking iron is important, but doing so is not enough to correct a more severe problem. Severe anemia and excess blood loss over time can even lead to a blood transfusion or emergency surgery to correct the problem.

⚘ LILA'S STORY ⚘

Blood Loss and Anemia

"I'm 46 and have always had heavy menstrual periods. My doctor encouraged me to keep a menstrual calendar, which I've been doing faithfully. It shows that I bleed for 10 days at a time, and I change an overnight pad every three hours for the first 3 days of my cycle. My doctor was concerned by this heavy bleeding and ordered tests, which determined that I'm anemic. Once my doctor knew that, she recommended further testing to check the causes of the heavy bleeding. But I declined, since I had been bleeding this heavily for more than 25 years. I told her, 'This is just me; I can live with it.'

"My doctor was persistent. She explained that at my age, 46, I was at higher risk for cancer and precancer of the uterus than I had been at age 26. Plus, I have a greater chance of having a physical, curable cause for the heavy periods, such as fibroids, adenomyosis, or polyps. She also said that a healthy woman my age with no other reasons for her anemia is probably anemic due to heavy menstrual bleeding. She advised me to have tests done to detect the causes of the heavy bleeding and anemia; it shouldn't be written off. I wanted to address the problem by continuing to take iron daily, and nothing else. We discussed my options over several months at different visits. I eventually agreed to have additional blood tests. One of the tests revealed a thyroid disorder. Two months after the *thyroid disorder had first been treated with daily medication I took by mouth, my periods lightened and became more regular."*

Blood Thinners

Women taking aspirin regularly may have prolonged or excessive bleeding and anemia. Aspirin will increase the severity and duration of the bleeding, but aspirin alone is not likely to start abnormal bleeding.

Some over-the-counter supplements are known to increase the amount of bleeding or prolong the duration of the bleeding. Examples of such supplements include St. John's wort, ginkgo or ginkgo biloba, ginseng, and dong quai (more details on these are included in Chapter 2).

Common Concerns

E ven if a woman enjoys robust health in her younger years, she may experience numerous discomforts as she ages. Sometimes it's hard to tell if a problem is vaginal or urinary, gastrointestinal or reproductive. This chapter is designed to clarify some of the common concerns of women over 40, and to give you a framework for approaching your doctor with any further questions you may have. The sooner you visit your doctor, the sooner he or she will be able to diagnose and treat your problem. In many cases, this can prevent a small incident from becoming a big nuisance.

Urinary Problems

Postmenopausal women may develop problems with urination. They may urinate too often, or lose urine when they cough or sneeze. Sometimes the problem is due to dryness of the vagina associated with the lack of estrogen. Other times the bladder sits lower in the vagina due to weakening of the supporting tissue. Or there may be malfunctions of the muscles or nerves of the bladder or urethra (the narrow outlet through which urine exits the bladder). It is possible to have one or more of these problems at the same time. Fortunately, there are prevention strategies that lower your chances of having these problems, as well as a range of treatment options available for each.

A gynecologist or urologist (a specialist in the urinary system) can do a specialized evaluation. In some medical centers a urogynecologist, a gynecologist with additional training in women's urinary problems, will be available.

URINARY TRACT INFECTION OR BLADDER INFECTION

Postmenopausal women are more prone to getting a urinary tract infection (UTI) or a bladder infection (cystitis). Once the vaginal tissues become thinner and less well lubricated with the loss of estrogen, they are more vulnerable to infection.

Symptoms of a bladder infection can include:

- pain while urinating
- bladder pain
- blood in the urine
- odd-smelling urine
- a sudden, urgent need to go to the bathroom
- inability to completely empty the bladder
- needing to void again immediately after voiding

Causes of a bladder infection, in addition to thinning vaginal tissues, comprise:

- not drinking enough water/dehydration
- intercourse without adequate lubrication
- wiping from back to front after a bowel movement (allowing fecal bacteria to get in)
- a polyp or growth in the bladder or urethra
- kidney stones

Preventive measures include:

- getting adequate hydration
- wiping from front to back after urination or a bowel movement
- urinating immediately before and after sex

- avoiding the use of soap and washcloths in the vagina and around the urethra
- using cranberry juice, cranberry supplements, and whole cranberries (to help prevent bacteria from sticking to the bladder walls)

While these measures are effective prevention strategies, they are not adequate treatment once a UTI has begun. At that point, antibiotics are needed to eradicate the bacteria. The urinary tract is normally sterile, and bacteria in the bladder or urethra are not normal.

⚡ CHARLOTTE'S STORY ⚡

Urinary Tract Infections

"When I was 44, I began experiencing a burning sensation when urinating. I had trouble getting to the bathroom on time and noticed an unfamiliar odor in my urine. Urination was extremely painful, and the color of my urine was darker than usual. When it continued for a week, I made an appointment to see my gynecologist. I couldn't imagine what was going on since I had never had a urinary tract infection. While I waited the three days to see my doctor, I tried drinking cranberry juice, but it didn't help. During the pelvic exam, my bladder was tender. My doctor suspected a urinary tract infection. I left a urine sample, which she said would be used to identify the specific type of bacteria causing the infection. But the doctor said I needed an antibiotic right away to treat my infection quickly and thoroughly. She prescribed an antibiotic, to take twice a day for three days. After three doses, which was only half of my prescription, the burning stopped and I felt better. So, I didn't finish the prescription.

"One week later, the burning sensation during urination returned. When I told my doctor that I had stopped taking the antibiotic after only three doses, she told me that was a mistake. If I had taken the full course of antibiotic, my urinary tract infection would have been gone. She explained that even though the original urine culture showed that I was on the correct medication to kick the infection, I would now need a different antibiotic. What most likely occurred is that the first three *doses of the antibiotic wiped out most but not all of the bacteria, which was why I felt so much better. But the remaining bacteria had an opportunity to adapt and become resistant to the antibiotic. My UTI was completely gone after a full course of the second antibiotic. Then, three weeks later, the burning with urination returned.*

"My doctor was concerned because I had had two urinary tract infections in one month with no history of prior infections. The pelvic examination showed that I had developed a urethrocele, a small out-pouching of lining tissue that looks like a skin tag, protruding from the opening of the urethra (the urine tube leading out of the bladder). My doctor sent me to a urologist, who performed a cystoscopy to examine the inside of my urethra and bladder with a microscope. He found a polyp, a soft tissue growth, protruding from the lining of the bladder. He removed it through the scope and also removed a growth from the urethral opening. I have not had any further urinary tract infections since then."

Incontinence/Unexpected Leakage

You will undoubtedly be surprised the first time some urine leaks out when you are not near a bathroom. You have lots of company. This is a common occurrence in perimenopause and postmenopause.

Stress Incontinence

This term describes urine loss that occurs when a woman puts extra stress or strain on her bladder. The urine may leak out when you sneeze, cough, laugh, or lift something heavy. In the past, stress incontinence was attributed solely to changes in anatomy resulting from childbirth. More recently collagen has been implicated. Collagen is a protein-based fibrous support tissue that holds the body together. It provides strength and flexibility in a variety of tissues, including bones and teeth as well as soft tissues such as those lining the vagina and supporting the bladder. Collagen degrades slowly with age.

The quality of collagen varies with each individual. Just as one woman may inherit collagen under the skin of her face that weakens at an early age and forms premature wrinkles, another woman may inherit collagen beneath the surface of her vagina that is less supportive of her vaginal tissues and bladder. In addition, there are lifestyle choices that can influence bladder support. Women who are overweight have more pressure on their bladder supports and are more prone to incontinence. Fortunately, with weight loss, the incontinence symptoms often improve or even disappear completely.

Treatment options for stress incontinence include losing weight if you are overweight and learning Kegel exercises (described later in this chapter). Another option is to have a pessary fit by your gynecologist. A pessary is a rubber or plastic device that comes in different shapes, such as a ring, cube, or miniature hammock. First, the doctor determines what size and shape will fit you. Then the doctor inserts the pessary in the vagina, under the pubic bone, to support the bladder. It can stay in the vagina for months at a time and then be removed, cleaned, and replaced. Periodic examination of the vaginal tissues in the doctor's office ensures there are no ulcers or sores on the vaginal walls behind the pessary. Finally, there are a variety of surgical procedures, many of which are performed through the vaginal opening, which re-create the original support of the vaginal tissues and reposition the bladder back at the apex of the vagina.

Urge Incontinence

This term describes a bladder that develops "a mind of its own." It may contract and empty at random times whether or not it is full, independent of whether you have chosen to make a trip to the bathroom or not. Bladder irritants can make urge incontinence worse. Avoiding smoking, coffee, alcohol, and soda can help decrease irritation of the bladder. Hydration is also important. Drinking too little water can cause the bladder to spasm. Urge incontinence can also result from problems with the muscles or the nerves that control urination. Treatment approaches include a variety of medications that act on different nerve receptors in the bladder and urethra, either facilitating or inhibiting their function as needed.

Another approach is cognitive behavioral therapy (CBT). After you keep a voiding diary, a trained clinician retrains your bladder with you so that you are able to urinate at reasonable intervals, when you would normally want to make a trip to the bathroom, as opposed to battling a feeling of urgency every 20 minutes or so. In addition, a newer type of therapy involves using electrical stimulation to control the bladder impulses. Initially, the device to control the electrical stimulation is worn next to the body. Once it is adjusted and proven to be helpful, it can be implanted under the skin to control the bladder contractions long term, much as a pacemaker is implanted under the skin to control an irregular heart rhythm.

Mixed Incontinence

This encompasses both types of incontinence, stress and urge. In this case, a combination of treatments may be needed to return to a normal pattern of urination.

⚘ CELINE's STORY ⚘

Urge Incontinence

"By the time I turned 60, I'd been having difficulty getting to the bathroom 'on time' for a while. I have very little warning before I need to go, and often leak a little urine before I get to the toilet. The urgency I feel before urinating sometimes involves brief but painful spasms. During my annual exam, I discussed this with my doctor and she said I have a chronic problem of urge incontinence. She had a urine test done to check for bacteria or a bladder infection, but that and my exam were normal. So, she recommended that I try eliminating coffee, which is a bladder irritant, and that helped. But the problem did not go away completely, so she prescribed a medication to counteract the untimely bladder contractions and spasms. This still was not enough to resolve the symptoms. I also spoke with the nurse practitioner at my urologist's office who helped me with a program of behavior modification and feedback to 'retrain' my bladder so I could go to the bathroom at normal intervals without discomfort. I've done well since."

Medications That Can Cause Urinary Symptoms

If you are having bladder symptoms, the doctor will review the list of medications you are taking, looking for those that can cause urinary problems. For example, some medications for glaucoma (an eye condition) influence bladder function and urination because they work through the same part of the nervous system. Some allergy pills or over-the-counter decongestants also work through the nervous system and affect the nerves in the bladder that influence urination patterns and even cause vaginal dryness.

When Internal Support Weakens

Earlier, you read that weakened collagen may cause the support of the bladder to weaken. Weak collagen, surgery, childbirth, and other factors may result in the supports of the uterus, bladder, rectum, or even the vaginal walls themselves weakening and bulging into the vaginal canal. At times the weak tissue may extend outside the vagina, where it may be seen as well as felt.

Cystocele

A bladder that is no longer well supported high in the vagina, or that has "dropped," may be another cause of problems with urination. The bladder can be repositioned; this can be achieved with a pessary (a ring or other device placed in the vagina to hold up the tissue). Alternatively, surgery may be used to restore bladder support and return the bladder to its normal position in the vagina. This is a common problem that probably has a hereditary component. Some women have weaker connective tissue than others. The connective tissue helps keep the bladder and pelvic organs suspended in place at the top of the vagina. Over time, if the connective tissue weakens, the uterus, vagina, or bladder can drop lower into the vagina.

Kegel exercises help strengthen the tissue and muscles supporting the bladder. To see results, Kegels must be done at least three times a day on a regular basis. It may take three to six months to notice an improvement. The technique for doing Kegel exercises is to identify the muscles by stopping the flow of urine while you are on the toilet. Then, when you are not urinating, squeeze the muscles 10 times, 3 times a day. Hold the squeeze for three seconds. You can do the Kegel exercises standing, sitting, or lying down, and no one can tell you're doing them. I suggest you pick triggers to remind you to do them: for example, waiting in line at the bank, while on hold on the telephone, while downloading email, at red lights, and so forth. Avoiding weight gain also helps prevent pressure on the pelvic organs and bladder.

⚑ JENNIFER'S STORY ⚑

Helping Urine Loss with Kegels

"I considered myself to be a youthful 47, so when I started noticing that I accidentally leaked a little urine when I laughed, coughed, or exercised, I was distressed. When I had my annual exam, I told my doctor about the problem and that it had worsened over the past 10 months, to the point where I experienced chronic urine loss. I did not have any burning sensation or trouble getting to the bathroom on time. During the pelvic exam, my doctor noted that my bladder was positioned lower in the vagina. She said it was sinking slightly into the top of my vagina and was sitting lower in the vaginal canal than it had three years ago. The vaginal roof, instead of being flat, was shaped more like a hammock. If the bladder drop worsened, or if I experienced uncomfortable pressure, my doctor said I could try a pessary or surgical repair of the problem. My doctor taught me how to do Kegel exercises, and after doing them three times a day for three months, urine loss is extremely rare for me. I was glad not to have to consider additional treatment."

RECTOCELE

The roof of the rectum borders the floor of the vagina. When the support tissue weakens, the rectum bulges into the weakened vaginal floor, forming a rectocele. Some women develop this over time and need to press down on the floor of the vagina with their fingers to help a bowel movement to pass. Problems passing stool due to a bulging rectocele may be eased with over-the-counter stool softeners, adequate hydration with water, increased fiber consumption, and increased daily physical activity as well as achieving a healthy body weight. Constipation and inactivity aggravate rectocele symptoms. Also, excess body weight puts pressure on the supporting tissue that can aggravate a cystocele or rectocele. If the conservative measures just mentioned do not provide adequate relief, or the rectocele worsens or interferes with intercourse, it can be corrected with a surgical procedure in the operating room called a posterior repair or rectocele repair.

UTERINE AND VAGINAL PROLAPSE

The attachments or ligaments that hold the uterus in place can loosen over time and weaken. They may be affected by inherited weaker collagen, collagen weakened by age, smoking or poor nutrition, childbirth, surgery, excess weight gain, chronic cough, or long-term heavy lifting. This can be alleviated with a pessary or corrected surgically. Protrusion of vaginal tissues may also occur for similar reasons. The loosened vaginal walls may be associated with the loss of other support for the uterus, bladder, or rectum. A gynecologic exam can help determine which organs have lost their natural support. While a pessary may help in some cases, others require a surgical repair to restore the normal anatomy.

Problems That Cause Vulvar and Vaginal Discomfort

If you have itching or discomfort in the genital area, you owe it to yourself to have a gynecologic exam to determine the cause. Self-diagnosing an itch as "just a yeast infection" may mean missing a bacterial infection, a sexually transmitted disease, a skin condition, or even a precancerous change. Even prolonged scratching can cause problems with the skin outside the vagina. And choosing to live with discomfort may make the problem harder to diagnose or treat over time.

At times it can be difficult to pinpoint where the problem of itch or discomfort originates. Some infections affect the skin outside the vagina either inside the pubic hair or the smoother tissue closer to the vaginal opening. Or, the itching may be only in the vagina itself. At times, the infection may affect both the outer skin and the vagina.

Vaginal dryness occurs when your estrogen levels drop. Your vagina is usually very elastic, able to easily stretch for sex and childbirth. It is also a self-cleaning organ, providing its own lubrication for sex as well as for cleansing purposes. But as estrogen levels go down, your vaginal walls get thinner and lose some of their elasticity. Your vagina also becomes drier and takes longer to become lubricated (for more on vaginal dryness, see Chapter 7).

Atrophic vaginitis can be caused by lower estrogen levels after menopause. Symptoms include dryness and irritation. There may even be a dark yellow or mustard-colored discharge.

VAGINAL SYMPTOMS THAT INDICATE A VISIT TO THE DOCTOR IS IN ORDER

The symptoms of very different problems may be similar. Only a doctor can correctly identify the underlying problem and prescribe appropriate medications. Schedule a visit to your doctor if you have any of these symptoms:

- odor
- irritation
- itching
- discharge

A fishy or ammonia-like odor may be a sign of a bacterial infection. Irritation or burning also may indicate bacterial infection, or atrophic vaginitis, or both.

Vaginal infections may produce initial pain or irritation with sex. Although yeast is the most well-known vaginal infection, it is not the most common type. Different types of vaginal infections include:

- yeast infections
- bacterial infections
- sexually transmitted diseases

It is also possible to have a combined type of vaginal infection such as yeast and bacterial vaginosis. Each of these infections is discussed separately in the pages that follow.

YEAST INFECTIONS

A yeast infection inside the vagina is called Candida vaginitis. If it occurs on the skin outside the vagina, on the vulva, it is called Candida vulvitis. Often, both the vagina and the vulva are involved, and that is called Candida vulvovaginitis.

Yeast infections in either or both locations are common after taking antibiotics. The antibiotics alter the normal complement of bacteria that are supposed to live in the vagina. When healthy, the vagina is acidic. That is one reason that using soap to clean the vagina goes against your body's natural way of keeping the vagina clean and healthy. Soap is basic—it has a higher pH than the vagina's low acidic pH. The soap actually disturbs the natural pH balance of the vagina. Basically, soap cleans out the bacteria that are *supposed* to stay. As a result, the vagina's natural barriers are compromised, allowing bacteria that do not belong there to enter.

Many women are brought up to believe that their vulvas and vaginas are "dirty" and therefore must be thoroughly scrubbed and cleaned. This is unfortunate, since the vagina is a self-cleaning organ, just like the eyeballs. Your eyeballs do not require scrubbing or the application of soap and neither does your vagina. Similarly, the mouth has bacteria that normally live there, and the saliva keeps the sides of the mouth lubricated and clean (although not the teeth and gums).

There are different kinds of yeast that can cause vulvovaginitis. Usually the most common kinds respond well to over-the-counter anti-yeast preparations. If you use them frequently, however, or when you actually have another type of infection, you can become resistant to these medications. Other types of yeast may grow, requiring a different treatment approach.

I think it is reasonable to use an over-the-counter preparation to treat yeast if you have taken an antibiotic in the past six weeks or so, but if you do not get completely better, see your doctor. Also, be aware that if you have itching on the vulvar skin outside the vagina, using a vaginal yeast cream or suppository inside the vagina will not cure the vulvar yeast infection. You will need to apply the yeast cream directly to the skin outside the vulva to get relief.

BACTERIAL INFECTIONS

Bacterial vaginosis is the most common vaginal infection in women. It can occur at any age, from the teen years to the nineties. It is usually not contracted from a sexual partner.

Bacteria from the rectum may settle in the vagina and cause a fishy or ammonia-like odor. There also may be irritation or burning at times, and dryness or discomfort with sex. Examination and evaluation of the discharge will reveal the type of infection to be bacterial vaginosis, not yeast. Over-the-counter yeast medications or douching will *not* clear this infection and should be avoided. Bacterial vaginosis requires an antibiotic to correct the problem.

One common way to acquire bacterial vaginosis is to wipe the wrong way and bring bacteria from the rectum into the vagina. Wipe from front to back to avoid this risk. Also avoid introducing soap or a washcloth into the vagina, which can sweep in the wrong kind of bacteria (see Vaginal Health, below).

While yeast will respond to over-the-counter treatment, a bacterial infection requires prescription antibiotics to resolve. Bacterial vaginosis is only relieved by taking antibiotics by mouth or placing them directly in the vagina. Both the oral and topical antibiotics are obtained by prescription. If the bacterial infection persists, or recurs after treatment with antibiotics, the woman's sexual partner should also be treated with antibiotics to prevent passing the infection back and forth.

Every year I see many women like Valerie.

🙏 VALERIE'S STORY 🙏

Same Symptom, Different Cause

"I'm 54 and have been married for 30 years. I made an appointment to see my gynecologist between annual exams because I was experiencing pain with intercourse and had vaginal burning at other times. I had tried an over-the-counter yeast medication, but the symptoms did not improve. At my annual exam four months earlier, I was fine. I thought it must be part of postmenopause. I told my doctor I was concerned about vaginal dryness. As it turned out, that wasn't my problem. The pelvic exam revealed vaginal discharge with an atypical color and odor. The discharge was analyzed under a microscope and revealed bacterial vaginosis. My doctor explained the importance of wiping from front to back, which may have been the source of my problem. She prescribed an antibiotic, Flagyl, and gave me some information about vaginal care to prevent further episodes.

"Six months later, I was back because of burning inside the vagina, which I'd been experiencing for three weeks. I was concerned that the bacterial infection had returned. During the exam, I told my doctor that I had taken antibiotics for bronchitis a month before. The pelvic examination and laboratory tests showed that I had a yeast infection, and my doctor advised me to buy an over-the-counter antifungal treatment that included a suppository or cream for the vagina. She said the yeast infection was unrelated to my bacterial vaginal infection, but rather was related to the antibiotic I had taken for bronchitis. Instead of buying the preparation she suggested, I used an over-the-counter medication I already had in my medicine cabinet: Vagisil, a product that I was to learn is not a true antifungal. The itch and burn lessened but never completely disappeared. Because my symptoms felt somewhat better, I didn't call my doctor. But the infection persisted, and then worsened.

"I developed burning and itching of the skin outside the vagina. At that point, although I didn't know it, I had an even more extensive yeast infection, affecting not only the vaginal canal, but also the vulva. Now I would need to use an antifungal treatment with an insert for the vagina and cream for the skin. My doctor explained that treating a vaginal yeast infection does not treat a vulvar yeast infection. Even though these in-

fections felt similar to me, they required different treatment. Neglecting the first yeast infection led to a more extensive problem."

Sexually Transmitted Diseases

Postmenopausal women can still acquire sexually transmitted diseases even though they are no longer fertile or having periods. Many of these sexually transmitted diseases will also cause pain or discomfort. The sexually transmitted diseases that can plague any woman earlier in her life may still descend on the menopausal woman.

HERPES

Women who have intercourse are at risk for herpes, a virus that produces painful genital ulcers. Herpes pain may be alleviated with antiviral medication to shorten the duration of symptoms.

GENITAL WARTS

The human papilloma virus (HPV) causes genital warts, or condylomata. One out of three young women (in their late teens and early twenties) now carries this virus. There are more than 100 DNA types of HPV. Once infected with this virus, you can harbor it for the rest of your life. It is not known how many postmenopausal women have been exposed to HPV. You can acquire the virus earlier in life, or from a partner, and not know. For example, you may have had a wart on your hand or foot as a child. This means you were exposed to HPV then. The virus may remain dormant for decades.

The virus may produce raised white cauliflower-like lesions, which may occur on the hands, on the feet, or inside or outside the genital area in men or women. If you contract the wart virus, it may result in an abnormal Pap smear of your cervix. If you had a wart on your hand, and then wiped or cleaned your genital area, you could acquire genital warts without having them sexually transmitted. Wart virus is acquired and spread by skin-to-skin contact.

Women of any age may show signs of wart virus on their Pap smear, even if they have not been sexually active for years. They should be examined by a gynecologist and treated for the virus if it produces abnormal precancerous changes on their Pap smear. At this point, if wart lesions are found, they are treated. Or, if the HPV causes a change on the cervix, such as a dysplasia or precancer, that may be treated to prevent progression to cancer (see Chapter 13).

If you have ever had warts, inform your doctor and be certain to have regular Pap smears. The wart virus may produce precancers or dysplasias of the cervix, which may be found on a Pap smear. Treating the precancer of the cervix will prevent it from progressing to cervical cancer in the future. Once precancers are signaled on the Pap smear, a microscope exam and a biopsy may identify abnormalities of the cervix that require treatment. It is possible to test for HPV with a swab test or during a Pap test (for more information, see Chapter 13).

At present, researchers are looking for a vaccine to treat wart virus. Your doctor will keep you posted.

HIV/AIDS

Menopausal women may also contract human immunodeficiency virus (HIV/AIDS). Using condoms will help prevent this possibility.

Chlamydia

This is an infection of the cervix that can spread to other pelvic organs and cause pain with intercourse, abnormal bleeding, or vaginal discharge. It is diagnosed using pelvic examinations and cultures or microscope analysis and is treated with antibiotics.

⚜ Sonya's Story ⚜

Chlamydia

"As a 54-year-old woman in postmenopause, I was not concerned about getting pregnant and did not use a condom with my new sexual partner. Unfortunately, I began to experience bleeding and deep

pain during intercourse. My gynecologist performed a history and com-
plete physical examination. A test for Chlamydia came back positive. I
took antibiotics, and my partner was tested for Chlamydia by his doctor.
Although his test came back negative, he also took antibiotics. I was
retested after treatment, and the bleeding and pain stopped."

GONORRHEA

Gonorrhea can infect the cervix and must be treated with antibiotics. It is diagnosed using pelvic examinations and cultures or by microscope analysis. While postmenopausal women with new partners need not be concerned with contraception, they may consider using condoms to help protect against gonorrhea, Chlamydia, and HIV.

TRICHOMONAS

Trichomonas infections produce a characteristic foul odor with an irritating discharge and red swollen surfaces inside the vagina. It is usually sexually transmitted. It may cause burning or odor and a green watery vaginal discharge. Analyzing the discharge under the microscope and identifying the organism that causes the infection (a protozoan, or type of microorganism related to algae) clinches the diagnosis. Treatment consists of a prescription antibiotic. The sexual partner should also receive treatment.

Vulvar Changes

Postmenopausal women are more vulnerable to vulvar problems. Itching and burning may be chalked up to a yeast infection but not be caused by yeast at all, nor are they always associated with an infection. There are a wide variety of problems that may be causing the itch and warrant a different approach to treatment.

Skin problems elsewhere on the body, such as psoriasis or eczema, can also occur on the vulva. Sometimes psoriasis or eczema shows up on the vulva before it appears anywhere else. Treatment includes prescription-strength creams prescribed by a dermatologist, gynecologist, internist, or family doctor familiar with this condition.

There are other skin disorders unique to the vulva that can cause swelling, pain, itching, burning, and pain with intercourse. If neglected, the swelling can be severe enough to make sitting or walking difficult. There are distinct features of the three common vulvar skin conditions that can be diagnosed by medical history and physical exam.

Contact Dermatitis

Contact dermatitis is an irritation of the skin that results from exposure to a particular substance such as a scented product. Soap, fabric softener, detergent, dryer sheets, douches, wipes, pads, lotions, creams containing alcohol, and panty liners are all possible offenders. Even Vagisil, an over-the-counter product sold to help vulvovaginal symptoms, is itself a common cause of dermatitis. It contains Benzocaine, an allergen. Other products contain preservatives or perfume that may not agree with you.

Treatment includes stopping contact with the offending product or additive. It also involves stopping the vicious cycle of itching that produces more scratching. Infections need to be treated, but the inflammation resulting from the irritation and scratching often points to the need for a mild steroid cream such as Triamcinolone. Why not treat this yourself, using over-the-counter steroid cream? If you use steroid cream and you have a yeast infection, the infection will get worse. It is important to get a doctor's evaluation, including a careful history and physical examination, to prescribe the most helpful treatment and not worsen the condition. If contact dermatitis occurs in the setting of incontinence, topical estrogen may help as well.

Lichen Simplex Chronicus

This condition occurs when chronic itching leads to more scratching and more itching over a period of time. It gets worse with hot, humid conditions as well as stress and irritants. It is common in women who also have conditions such as psoriasis or contact dermatitis. The itching that results is difficult to tolerate. On physical examination the skin is actually thickened from repeated scratching. One or both sides of the vulva may show differences in color as the pigment in the skin evaporates. There may be scratch marks or hair loss. The doctor will check to be certain that the only cause is prolonged scratching and to ensure there are no precancerous areas present. They can look similar. At times, a biopsy is needed to identify the cause of the changes.

LICHEN SCLEROSIS

Lichen sclerosis (LS) is a chronic condition that occurs only on the vulva; it does not involve the vagina. It is caused by an immune response that produces changes in the vulvar skin that include white areas, tissue thinning, and scarring. It can also cause red areas near the white patches or white areas as well as fissures. The white areas, red changes, and fissures characteristic of LS may be mistaken for changes associated with vulvar yeast or Candida vulvitis. Lichen sclerosis can cause burning or itching, pain with urination, and pain with sex.

But sometimes, lichen sclerosis is asymptomatic and silent, causing the vulva to shrink, thin, scar, or even fade away without a warning pain, burn, or itch. I have seen vulvar scarring in women who did not know that they had the changes of lichen sclerosis. Those not familiar with this condition may attribute the vulvar thinning and scarring to old age. While there is some loss of the fat pad under the vulvar skin with age, the tissues of the vulva, including the covering of the clitoris, are not designed to vanish or scar over with age. Even in the absence of itching or burning, vulvar scarring may result if you have lichen sclerosis that is neglected. To me, LS alone makes a strong case for having regular pelvic exams during postmenopause.

Pelvic exams that identify asymptomatic LS early allow for treatment before the vulva shrinks, thins, scars, or fades away, especially if there are no warning symptoms. For those who do get them, it is important to get a pelvic exam to avoid falsely attributing these symptoms to a yeast infection. Once the type of vulvar dystrophy is identified, special creams may be applied to the area to reverse the changes and treat the symptoms. Many months of treatment are usually needed to treat these types of skin changes. Hygiene changes are also advised.

While there isn't proof that lichen sclerosis causes vulvar cancer, LS is more common in women with squamous cell cancer of the vulva. There is a genetic predisposition, such as thyroid disease or lupus; almost half of the women with lichen sclerosis have auto-antibodies, and many have an actual autoimmune disease, such as thyroid and lupus.

Vaginal Health

Proper care of the genital area can prevent many common problems. In my experience, women have many misconceptions about vaginal care. Sometimes their efforts to stay clean and fresh actually do more harm than good. Here are up-to-date guidelines that will help minimize any episodes of vaginal discomfort.

- Wipe from front to back—all the time, whether you have urinated or moved your bowels. Wiping from front to back will prevent the bacteria in the rectal area from getting into the vagina. This will also help prevent urinary tract infections. Healthy urine is sterile and contains no bacteria.
- Use unscented, plain white toilet paper.
- If you use pads or tampons, avoid the type with deodorant.
- Avoid dryer sheets and fabric softeners. They have strong chemicals in them that are harsh for menopausal skin. Many women get rashes and itching from using these products.
- Wear all-cotton panties (not nylon with a cotton crotch). Avoid thong underwear; they track bacteria from the rectum forward into the vagina.
- Avoid wearing tight jeans or slacks.
- Avoid wearing pantyhose under slacks. Even though they are called "pantyhose," wear all-cotton panties underneath.
- Put your underwear through an extra rinse cycle in your wash to avoid detergent residues that may irritate your skin, or use half the amount of liquid detergent recommended so there is

Despite the many products available online and at your local drugstore, do not douche. The vagina has a delicate balance of acidity (pH). The normal vaginal pH encourages healthy bacteria to live in the vagina and discourages foreign bacteria from inhabiting it. Commercial products or douches cannot mimic or improve nature's own balance. Douching is now suspected of causing serious infections of the fallopian tubes and ovaries, as well as abnormal Pap smears. The lining tissue of the vagina is similar to the lining tissue of the mouth. You wouldn't use soap to clean out the inside of your mouth. It isn't necessary to douche or use soap inside your vagina, either.

less soap residue. Use liquid rather than powder; it will dissolve more thoroughly. When you do the laundry, dissolve the detergent in the machine water before adding your clothes.

- Do not clean the vagina with a washcloth. It will disturb the protective function of the vulvar and vaginal surfaces. No matter how carefully you use the washcloth, it will also spread bacteria from the rectum into the vagina since they are often less than an inch apart.
- Avoid deodorant or antiperspirant soaps in this area. They have harsh, irritating chemicals. Try using mild glycerin soap for the hip, lower stomach, and groin area.
- If you have a hand-held shower head, do not point the nozzle into your vagina when showering. Use a sitz bath to clean the genital area (see below).
- If you are traveling and cannot use a sitz bath, carry the over-the-counter product Balneol, a perineal lubricant and cleanser. Put a dime size dab of the lotion on clean toilet paper, wipe front to back, then continue to wipe with clean pieces of toilet paper until they are no longer soiled. This also helps clean around hemorrhoids.

Hᴏᴡ ᴛᴏ Usᴇ ᴀ Sɪᴛᴢ Bᴀᴛʜ

Sitz baths are plastic basins that look like bedpans. They may be purchased at your pharmacy without a prescription. Raise the toilet seat the way men do. Put very warm water in the sitz bath and place it on the base of the toilet bowl. It will not touch the toilet water. Sit in the sitz bath for a few minutes. (You do not need to use the plastic tubing that comes with the sitz.) Spread the folds of the vulva apart and cleanse the area.

A sitz bath cleanses the skin outside the vagina without moving bacteria in the wrong direction. It rinses away sweat and secretions without harming the body's natural balance. A sitz bath with warm water will not irritate any dry areas or aggravate other skin conditions. It is also effective for soothing and preventing hemorrhoids.

RESOURCES

The American College of Obstetricians and Gynecologists (ACOG) has a patient information pamphlet on urinary incontinence available at www .acog.org/publications/patient. It may also be available at your gynecologist's office.

Stewart, Elizabeth Gunther, and Paula Spencer. *The V Book: A Doctor's Guide to Complete Vulvovaginal Health.* Bantam Books, 2002.

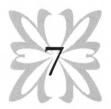

Smoother Sex

Many women assume that sex will become painful and less pleasurable with age. In fact, for many women, sex becomes *more* pleasurable. The worries about an unplanned pregnancy are behind you. You have fewer responsibilities for young children or less pressure on the job—which translates into less anxiety and more opportunities for fun. Part of this increased enjoyment of sex may stem from the fact that some women simply become more comfortable with themselves over time.

This chapter should reassure you that menopausal women do not all "dry up" and have pain with intercourse. Many women enjoy intercourse in their postmenopausal years without pain or dryness. Although some women experience temporary decreases in their libido, overall the research in this area is encouraging. In fact, we are finding that women report more satisfaction with their sex lives after postmenopause than before.

The good news from researchers is that the sexual response in postmenopausal women is healthy and intact. Women are responsive. They can still enjoy orgasms if they were orgasmic before. They can learn to be more responsive if they so desire. Your actual enjoyment of intercourse or being intimate need not diminish with postmenopause. Women in their fifties, sixties, seventies, and beyond can (and do) enjoy a healthy sex life. This chapter is not intended to encourage self-diagnosis or treatment. It is an introduction to a complex topic and provides an overview of issues and questions that you may wish to discuss with your physician.

Age-related Physical Changes That Can Affect Sex

A long-term lack of estrogen can cause physical changes that might affect your sex life. With age and lower levels of estrogen, there is less blood flow to the vagina. With less estrogen, the vagina becomes less acidic. Less acidity makes the vaginal tissues more susceptible to infection. Vaginal wall thickness and elasticity are also lost. There is also less lubrication, and lubrication during sexual activity takes longer to achieve. In addition, the vagina may atrophy, becoming somewhat smaller in width and length. More stimulation may be required to achieve arousal. Spending more time on foreplay is helpful. Different positions may be more comfortable or pleasurable. These include the woman positioning herself on top, next to, or in front of her partner so she can control the depth of penetration. Women's genital anatomy is not structured for maximum sexual stimulation with penile-vaginal intercourse, especially in the missionary position with the woman on the bottom and the man on the top. For most women, orgasm is most easily reached through direct vulvar stimulation, not by intercourse (in contrast, the neuroanatomy of men's genitals results in intercourse providing a very efficient way to stimulate the nerves around the tip of the penis).

Long-term lack of estrogen may also have an effect on the central and peripheral nervous systems, affecting sensation, touch, and vibration. This compromise in nerve function is more commonly seen in diabetics, whose nerves are affected by their condition.

Other physical changes in postmenopause include thinner skin over the clitoris. This offers less protection and can result in increased sensitivity of the clitoris. Loss of fat in the thickness of the vulva, or folds of skin outside of the vagina, occurs over decades. Pubic hair loss also occurs. Remaining pubic hair usually turns gray. The degree of these changes varies with each individual.

A woman's physical health and well-being impacts her sexuality.

Fatigue, chronic pain, depression, limited mobility, and incontinence of urine or stool may impact sexual health. Diabetes may affect autonomic nerve conduction and compromise genital sex response. Body image can be affected after a mastectomy or a hysterectomy. And women's sex responses are negatively affected by a male partner's sexual dysfunction, such as premature ejaculation or inability to have an erection.

Age-related Physical Changes in Men and Their Impact on Female Partners

As men age, they experience an increase in erectile dysfunction. Fortunately, there is no corresponding sexual dysfunction in women as they age, although there is a subtle decrease in desire with age and menopause. Despite the changes in women's genitalia with age—less volume of clitoral tissue and less vascularity in the vulva and vaginal areas—these changes don't usually correlate with sexual symptoms. The increase in congestion around the vagina in response to an erotic stimulation is similar in women with and without estrogen.

Erectile dysfunction in men affects both partners. There are now prescription medications to address this problem, including Viagra and Cialis. However, women's increased sexual enjoyment and satisfaction is not an automatic consequence of these therapies because using them can result in less foreplay. Surveys questioning women in healthy marriages report foreplay as the most satisfying component of partner sex. A woman whose partner requires Viagra may have some genital atrophy and she may need longer foreplay and stimulation prior to intercourse. Men who use Viagra to attain an erection can adjust the timing of taking the Viagra to match the needs of their partners. Viagra produces a rapid erection without allowing a woman to have the time she needs to lubricate. One strategy for such couples is to encourage foreplay prior to the male partner taking Viagra. Couples should try to be intimate together first and allow time for the woman to "warm up" prior to the man taking Viagra. This puts less pressure on the woman to have intercourse before she is well lubricated and ready. Otherwise, the woman is not likely to be satisfied with the sexual outcome.

The same strategy is advised for couples where the man has a penile implant to treat erectile dysfunction. Some men have erectile problems due to the medication they take to control high blood pressure. They may benefit from a new blood pressure medication that does not affect sexual function. A medical evaluation will define which options have the best chance of working.

Medications That Can Affect Sex

ANTIBIOTICS

One common side effect of taking antibiotics is developing a yeast infection inside the vagina, outside the vagina, or both. If a woman has taken antibiotics in the past two months, she may develop a yeast infection. Yeast infections can produce itching, burning, or irritation. The discomfort may occur days or even weeks after taking the medication. Yeast infections that are not detected or treated may cause vaginal dryness or discomfort with sex.

ANTIHISTAMINES

Prescription or over-the-counter antihistamines may cause dryness of the vaginal tissues as well as a dry mouth. Lubrication is reduced, causing pain with intercourse. Drying effects from antihistamines may also cause constipation, resulting in deep pain with intercourse.

BLOOD PRESSURE MEDICATIONS

Diuretics push fluid out of the blood vessels. Beta-blockers (such as Atenolol) work by slowing the blood flow and reducing the pressure in the blood vessels. Both types of blood pressure medication may reduce blood flow to the pelvic organs enough to reduce sensation during sex or to suppress orgasms. Changing to a different type of blood pressure medication may result in a return to normal sexual arousal and orgasms.

Depression is tied to impaired sexual desire in most studies. Those women with impaired desire are twice as likely to have a history of a major depression. Chronic anxiety is also linked to impaired sexual function and low desire. Unfortunately, some antidepressants are associated with sexual dysfunction and lack of sex drive. This paradox is frustrating. Fortunately, certain antidepressant medications will not disturb a healthy sex drive. Some women will find their sex drive dampened by one antidepressant but not by a sister medication in the same class. If changing to another antidepressant is not an option, some doctors recommend a "drug holiday" where the antidepressant medication that's effective for treating the depression but is causing a dampened sex drive is stopped for the weekend and then resumed. This strategy must be used with a knowledgeable doctor since stopping certain antidepressants without medical supervision can produce severe side effects.

Medical Conditions That Can Affect Sex

Sex may be different due to other changes in your health or personal situation. Medical conditions affect the amount of energy you have for sex, your physical response during sex, and your physical comfort during sex. Problems with sexual intercourse are varied and complex. Sometimes a problem, such as a vaginal infection, can be diagnosed and treated during an office visit. Survivors of child abuse, rape, post-traumatic stress disorder, or chronic pelvic pain require longer-term treatment.

Rectocele, Cystocele, Uterine and Vaginal Prolapse

Protrusion of vaginal tissues, the uterus, or the bladder is common in postmenopausal women and may influence their experience during sex. A gynecologic exam can help determine which organs have lost their natural support. Options to correct the problem include using a pessary to support the loose tissue or a surgical repair to restore the anatomy.

Ovarian Cysts

Another cause of deep pain with sex is ovarian cysts. Ovarian cysts form regularly during the years that you menstruate. A small cyst forms during the middle of the menstrual cycle at the time of ovulation, or egg formation. Another cyst forms just prior to the menstrual period itself. These types of cysts are referred to as physiologic, or cycle, cysts. These small cysts usually do not enlarge and are considered a variation of normal. They dissolve in a short time while they are still small.

When a cyst gets too large or persists too long it may cause pain. Some cysts develop abnormal features and no longer look clear and simple inside as a physiologic cyst would. These cysts may persist as tumors or even become cancerous. These must be watched carefully by a gynecologist or, in some cases, surgically removed.

In addition to the medical history, a pelvic examination can raise the possibility of a cyst. Pain, tenderness, or fullness may be detected on exam. An ultrasound can provide more information about the specific features of the cyst, including its size. In some cases, a cyst may be harmless. A small cyst, under an inch, with no alarming features on ultrasound may be observed over time. Your gynecologist will advise you whether your cyst needs to be watched or biopsied or removed. A larger cyst, or one with worrisome features on ultrasound, may warrant analysis or even removal for biopsy. Whether or not the ovarian cyst causes pain with intercourse or any other pain, you should work closely with your gynecologist until the cyst is resolved.

While postmenopausal women are not expected to bleed or cycle, they may still form ovarian cysts. More information about ovarian cysts is provided in Chapter 13.

Bartholin Gland Cyst

Another cause of initial pain or discomfort with sex is a Bartholin gland cyst. This is a swelling of the lower vulva, the skin just outside the vaginal opening. The gland deep in this skin may get blocked off. When a cyst forms, it may fill with fluid, become painful, and cause a partial blockage. The cyst may cause pain when sex is initiated as well as at other times. If it enlarges enough, it can even make walking or sitting uncomfortable. A Bartholin gland cyst can become infected, requiring antibiotics and, at times, drainage in a doctor's office or emergency room. A gynecologist can tell if it needs to be drained to release the fluid or to control the infection. A doctor can prevent the cyst and infection from recurring by using a simple surgical technique called marsupialization.

Skin Changes of the Vulva

Another common cause of pain or discomfort with sex in women over 40 is skin changes of the vulva. Thinning of the skin, raised or thick areas, or white or red color changes may be found on exam. Types of discomfort that may be attributed to these changes include dryness, itching, or burning. Many of these types of skin changes will be diagnosed as vulvar dystrophies. Other changes of the vulva skin may echo changes elsewhere on the body such as eczema or psoriasis. Yeast infections will also produce red itchy changes of the vulva in many women, not just vaginal discharge as is commonly believed. (For more on these conditions, see Chapter 6.)

Diabetes

Diabetes often goes undiagnosed in women who do not metabolize sugar normally. Women with diabetes may be slender, of average weight, or over their ideal weight. Diabetics are predisposed to getting yeast infections inside and outside the vagina. Dryness, burning, itching, and actual pain during sex may result. Women with long-term diabetes may have less blood flow to the pelvic organs. Your doctor can diagnose diabetes by checking your blood sugar level or testing your urine for sugar. Diabetes runs in families but also occurs in those who do not have a family history of diabetes.

Thyroid Problems

As you read in Chapter 2, thyroid problems are more common in women than in men, and thyroid disease is more common with increasing age. When thyroid function becomes overactive or underactive, it affects metabolism and sex drive as well as lubrication. Once the thyroid gland abnormality is diagnosed and treated, the related problems usually resolve. Body weight can normalize over time, sex drive may return to normal, and the rest of the body rebalances.

Urinary Problems

A urinary tract infection can cause pain with sex. Once treated, the problem resolves. Women who leak urine when they laugh or cough may also leak urine during sex. The approaches to this problem are discussed in Chapter 6.

Vaginal Infection

As you read in Chapter 6, there are different kinds of infections that can cause vaginal discomfort and pain with sex. It is important to have a doctor check for a vaginal infection and treat it before assuming that you have pain with sex due to vaginal dryness.

Constipation

The most common cause of deep pain with sex is constipation. The intestines surround the pelvic organs. Stool can back up and cause pressure and pain in the area of the pelvic organs. Even if you move your bowels every one to three days, you may still suffer from a large amount of backed-up stool pressing in your pelvis, especially if your colon or intestinal tract is large.

Sufficient water intake on a daily basis is more important than ever. I find many women avoid drinking water so they do not have to run to the bathroom too frequently or at an inconvenient time. There are ways to work around this. If you have trouble with urination, either urinating too frequently or not being able to make it to the bathroom on time, you can train your bladder to work more efficiently (see Chapter 6). Try drinking 48 to 64 ounces of water a day. Additional water might be needed if you exercise or live in a warm climate.

Coffee and sodas are bladder irritants and may force the bladder to empty prematurely or more often. Try to get most of your fluids as water. If you like carbonated drinks, look for seltzer with no sugar, salt, or artificial sweetener.

Exercise can provide dramatic relief from constipation or backed-up stool. Be certain to drink adequate fluids daily to get the full benefit in eliminating the bulk of the stool.

A high-fiber diet is helpful. Many Western diets have less than 10 grams of fiber a day, while an ideal amount is 20 to 30 grams. Most processed foods have very little fiber. Fruits and vegetables eaten raw or cooked have good fiber content. Fruit juice does not have fiber (it is removed during processing). Brown rice and whole grain products and beans have a healthy amount of fiber. You may also use a product like Konsyl, Per Diem, Metamucil, or Citrucel. Use these as directed and make sure to drink extra water or they will not be effective. Try them for six weeks or more and then continue if you have relief.

Laxatives should not be used. They are not a healthy long-term alternative and can cause problems when they are stopped. The bulk agents in dietary fiber and the over-the-counter products listed above draw water into the colon to move the stool in a healthy way. Do not be concerned that these agents will cause diarrhea; they seldom do. Even those with irritable bowel syndrome, or who alternate between having diarrhea and being constipated, are usually able to use these bulk agents without problems. Consult your doctor if you are unsure.

Vaginal Dryness

The first thing that comes to a woman's mind when she experiences vaginal dryness is, "I'm drying up; it must be menopause." Fortunately, that's not always the case. Even if it is, it can be addressed. Vaginal dryness due to old age and menopause is not inevitable.

There are many causes of dryness that are not related to age or menopause that are treatable. Estrogen may provide relief to those women who do not have other causes for their discomfort, but not every woman must take estrogen to continue to have enjoyable sex in her menopausal years.

The first step is to have a gynecologic history and exam performed to identify the reasons for the dryness. This is not an area for self-diagnosis. There are many causes of vaginal dryness and many effective treatments to choose from are available once the specific cause is identified. An expert examination will go a long way to helping you address the problem that you *actually* have, not the problem you *think* you have.

If it is a vaginal infection or a reaction to a scented hygiene product, a woman can expect to return to her normal level of lubrication after the infection is treated or the hygiene routine is modified. You can become sensitive to certain products even if you used them without problems when you were younger. Eliminating the use of scented soaps, dryer sheets, and fabric softener may reduce irritation and dryness outside the vagina and at the vaginal opening. On the other hand, if the dryness is due to perimenopause or postmenopausal estrogen deficiency, there are many safe options for you to consider.

Vaginal dryness or discomfort with intercourse is a problem that may begin during perimenopause, but more commonly surfaces in postmenopause, especially if months or years go by without intercourse. Intercourse twice a week or masturbation maintains vaginal lubrication and vaginal health without supplemental estrogen. This has led some menopause experts to advise women to "use it or lose it." Women who have intercourse on a regular basis do not tend to notice dramatic changes that produce dryness or discomfort, even if they do not take estrogen. Long periods of abstinence may make the changes more pronounced, but they are still correctable.

Vaginal Lubricants

If no other cause of vaginal discomfort is identified, over-the-counter preparations to lubricate the vaginal walls during intercourse may be used. A water-soluble lubricant that contains no additives is the best choice to reduce friction during intercourse. Vitamin E may also be used as a lubricant. Examples of vaginal lubricants sold over the counter are Astroglide, Lubrin, and K-Y Jelly. If used at the time of intercourse, they will often decrease pain or discomfort. Avoid Vaseline or oil-based products. Do not use hand cream or other products containing perfume or alcohol; they may damage the vaginal wall tissues. Vaginal lubricants may be used even if you are using other products to moisturize, such as estrogen cream, but do not apply them at the same time. Estrogen cream is not a vaginal lubricant and should not be used during intercourse.

Vaginal Moisturizers

There are products that restore the thickness, elasticity, and moisture of the vaginal wall tissues. Moisturizers are not designed for use during sex. They work at other times to promote healthy vaginal wall tissues. Examples of over-the-counter moisturizers include Replens, Rephresh, and K-Y Long-Lasting Vaginal Moisturizer. You may find adequate relief with the use of a vaginal moisturizer, or you may find that you require prescription estrogen to get adequate relief and comfort.

Hormones for Vaginal Dryness

Women who take estrogen in pill form, as a skin patch, or as a lotion may or may not also require vaginal estrogen, lubricants, or moisturizers. Alternatively, those who do not take estrogen systemically may benefit from vaginal estrogen alone. Some women who take estrogen by mouth or in the form of a skin patch find that they have healthy vaginal wall tissue that is not too dry or fragile. Others may find that they only get adequate relief with topical or local estrogen cream or tablets in addition to what they take by mouth or by patch. Your gynecologist can detect the degree of vaginal dryness or elasticity of the vagina by doing a simple speculum exam in the office and correlate this with your medical history and comfort during sex and at other times.

If vaginal thinning has taken place, local estrogen restores the elasticity, strength, and moisture of the vaginal walls. Estrogen for this purpose is now available in a tablet form, a cream, and a ring. Once the vaginal walls are healthier, some women can maintain their own vaginal health over time, even without continuing to use estrogen, while others continue to benefit from vaginal estrogen use. Vaginal estrogen has fewer side effects than estrogen taken by mouth or other routes.

Estrogen Tablets

The tablet form may be inserted in the vagina intermittently and provide improvement in the vaginal wall tissue. Vagifem is a prescription estrogen tablet that is inserted in the vagina every night at bedtime for two weeks, followed by a maintenance regimen of inserting the tablet at bedtime every Monday and Thursday (only twice a week). If you have intercourse in the evening, plan to insert the Vagifem tablet after intercourse. Vagifem is not designed as a lubricant for intercourse. The Vagifem tablet is a very low dose of estrogen that is delivered locally to the vaginal tissues. It does not produce a high level of estrogen in the blood, nor does it expose the uterus lining to excess estrogen. At this time, it is not necessary to balance this low dose of vaginal estrogen with progesterone as it has not been associated with a thick uterine lining or uterine cancer.

Estrogen Cream

Estrogen cream is available by prescription. It is placed in the vagina with an applicator. It will usually restore elasticity to the vaginal lining tissue and eliminate vaginal dryness over time. If it has been many years since your vagina received the benefit of estrogen from your ovaries or from hormone replacement therapy, it will take longer to restore the vaginal lubrication.

Various types of prescription-strength estrogen creams are available. Your doctor will advise you how much to use based on your history and examination. He or she will also tell you how often to use the cream. At times you may bleed or get irritated from the tip of the plastic applicator. If this happens, see if your doctor recommends applying the cream with clean fingers until the vaginal walls get stronger and the applicator may be used without discomfort.

If you use estrogen cream in the vagina for an extended period of time, work closely with your gynecologist and get regular checkups. If you still have your uterus (you have not had a hysterectomy), you may need to have a biopsy of your uterine lining to make sure you do not develop a cancer or precancer from the unopposed estrogen. If you have a uterus, you should not take estrogen alone in any form without close supervision by your gynecologist to monitor you for endometrial hyperplasia or uterine cancer. Estrogen cream is more difficult to dose. If you use too much over time, you could expose your uterine lining to excess estrogen. Regular checkups with your gynecologist will help monitor for this possibility. Be certain to report any vaginal bleeding to your gynecologist, especially if you take estrogen.

Vaginal Ring

Vaginal estrogen may be prescribed in the form of Estring, a silastic ring that releases small doses of estrogen slowly over 24 hours, 7 days a week, for 3 months while the ring is left in place in the vagina. This soft plastic ring sits inside the vagina away from the opening. It slowly releases a small amount of estrogen into the vaginal wall tissues. The amount of estrogen is so small that it does not get into your bloodstream. For most women, the Estring vaginal ring is a safe alternative, even if they have had breast cancer or have other reasons not to take estrogen in other forms. The estrogen ring is available through your gynecologist by prescription. After you have a medical exam and the ring is inserted, it should be rechecked by your doctor within the first two weeks of use to be certain no ulcers or sores have developed under or behind it. Once this initial check has taken place, you can insert a new ring yourself every three months, or your doctor or other health provider can change it for you. The Estring ring stays in place during intercourse. This may be used as your only form of estrogen, or it may be used in conjunction with estrogen by mouth or in patch form. Many women prefer the estrogen vaginal ring to vaginal creams because they find the creams messy and more time-consuming than the ring.

The estrogen ring is a breakthrough for women who have survived breast cancer or other cancers where estrogen is to be avoided. The estrogen ring offers local delivery of the estrogen while protecting the rest of the body from receiving any significant amounts of estrogen. Postmenopausal women who do not take estrogen often have a blood level of 20 picograms per milliliter of estrogen. Studies of women using Estring show blood levels are also 20 picograms per milliliter, and are not elevated due to Estring usage. In view of this, some gynecologists, surgeons, and oncologists are comfortable prescribing Estring for breast cancer survivors who suffer from vaginal dryness and pain with intercourse because their blood levels of estrogen remain low with this dose and form of estrogen use.

Lifestyle Factors That Affect Sex

Ask a friend or partner: What is the most important female sex organ? Even medical professionals often answer this question incorrectly. The most important female sex organ is the brain. What a woman thinks and how she feels about herself and her partner, if she has one, influences her sexual experience. There are many aspects of her life that will affect her attitude toward sex, her motivation to have sex, and her physical experience when she does have sex. Analyzing these factors is a complex process. Our understanding of what contributes to sexual experience is still developing. This is a very difficult subject to research, as women vary widely in their experiences and expectations.

Currently there is a great emphasis placed on hormone levels, including estrogen and testosterone, but the key to sex in postmenopause goes beyond achieving an optimal balance of hormone levels. These are other important areas that influence female sexuality:

- *Stress level.* Many women have schedules so packed, they give up all of their down time. Those who have no unscheduled time away from life's stresses may not be able to maintain or restore their libido. Keeping a diary or logging how you spend your time each day may be an eye-opener and is often helpful. You may find time you currently commit to projects or other people that you can reclaim for yourself.

- *"Personal time."* Do you have any? A hectic schedule with no private time or couple time is not conducive to a healthy and pleasurable sexual experience, particularly in perimenopause and postmenopause. Changes in your routine can affect your sex drive or motivation to have sex.
- *Alcohol.* Alcohol loosens inhibitions, relaxes us, and makes it easier to enjoy sex. Ironically, alcohol chemically dampens sex drive and decreases sexual responsiveness. Finally, alcohol disturbs deep sleep. Less quality rest leads to a lower libido and compromised sex drive.
- *Physical exercise.* Exercise enhances blood flow throughout the body, including the pelvic area. Exercise also decreases stress by releasing endorphins, the "feel-good" hormones. If exercise came in pill form, doctors would prescribe it for every patient in postmenopause, including those with decreased libido. Exercising regularly will enhance your sex drive as well as your sexual experience. The exercise program does not have to be a formal one. Gardening, walking, and even housework can be part of your exercise routine (for more information about exercise, see Chapter 12).

Seeking Medical Care with Concerns about Sex

When seeking medical care with concerns about sex, it is helpful to organize your thoughts beforehand. List any medications that you take, including the dosages, and note how long you have been on each medication. Also, think about these questions:

- How long have you been noticing a change in your sex life?
- Can you pinpoint the change?

- Do you have physical discomfort or pain in your abdomen, pelvis, or joints?
- If so, is it during foreplay, initial penetration, or deep penetration?
- Do you notice a difference in your sex drive?
- Do you not feel like having sex?
- Do you enjoy it when you have it, but feel like you no longer want to initiate sex with your partner?
- Is it your desire or motivation to have sex that is waning?
- Is there pain or discomfort during sex?
- Is the pain triggered by certain positions and not others?
- Are you experiencing muscle spasms due to fear, anxiety, or anticipation of pain?

These questions may be embarrassing or difficult to consider. But your doctor needs to have this information to help pinpoint what is causing your problem and address your concerns. Consider writing down your questions or concerns prior to your doctor visit so you don't forget them. That way, you can hand the doctor the written questions at the start of your visit, or you can refer to them during your visit.

If your doctor feels he or she is not the best person to evaluate these problems, you may be referred to another specialist. Depending on your doctor's specialty and training, he or she may use a formal questionnaire or clinical judgment to assess your concerns while trying to pinpoint which areas of sexual function are relevant.

Different areas of concern suggest different medical approaches. Is desire or motivation for sex affected, or has arousal or the physical response to stimulation changed? Ability to achieve orgasm and satisfaction is another key area in addition to physical comfort during sex. Issues of pain or lubrication are fully evaluated using findings on pelvic examination as well as history taking.

Even though pain during sex is a separate issue from sex drive, they are intertwined. If your sex drive is initially intact, but you experience pain rather than pleasure with sex, your sex drive will suffer. Expect a time delay even after the cause of the pain is treated. It takes time for the brain to process that there is no longer going to be pain with sex. After the brain has reprogrammed, and there is consistently no more pain with sex, pleasurable sex can return.

Whether your concern is how to maintain your sex drive and sexual function or how to enhance or improve your sexual function, it is important to return for regular gynecologic exams. This will enable you and your gynecologist to be certain that you are physically healthy. If changes do occur in your body, your doctor can help you to address them early before the changes become more severe. And as new information is available, you and your physician can talk about what is best for you to maintain a healthy body that functions well for you.

How Interested Are You in Sex?

Libido, or sex drive, does not necessarily diminish with age. As the North American Menopause Study showed, the majority of women are delighted or at least satisfied with their sex drive and sexual function in their fifties, sixties, and seventies.

A British researcher recently found that for women, libido decreases after the first two years of a relationship regardless of a woman's age. A 60-year-old woman in a new relationship will have an intact sex drive for the first two years of that relationship, just as she would if she were 30. Despite this, there are women with long-term partners who remain delighted or satisfied with their sex drive and sexual function in their fifties and well beyond.

Be ready to adjust your expectations of your spontaneous sex drive during the perimenopausal years. New research tells us that women should adjust their expectations of what a normal female sex drive looks and feels like before, during, and after menopause. One author suggests that women should not expect to "get horny" as frequently as they might have in their twenties or early thirties.

Women often retain the ability to enjoy sex once it is initiated. Those women who were orgasmic prior to postmenopause continue to be orgasmic. For this group of women, the enjoyment of sex remains the same once they get going. The difference is that their motivation lags and they are less likely to initiate sex. Experts suggest that you plan to have sex. Waiting to "feel" motivated in your mature years may leave you without sexual experiences.

Are you always hungry when you make reservations to go out for dinner? Not necessarily. During perimenopause and postmenopause, you may want to "schedule" sex with your partner just as you would make dinner reservations in advance. If sex has been a welcome part of your relationship, do not wait for spontaneous opportunities to arise or until you are in the mood. While it is still terrific to have spontaneous sex if you are in the mood, don't count on that alone. Scheduling sex with your partner, even if the biologic urge is dormant, may help you weather perimenopause and early postmenopause.

If you experience pain or discomfort, be certain to see your gynecologist to pinpoint physical changes that may be diagnosed and treated. If you have a partner with a medical or physical condition that imposes limitations on your sexual activity, be open to other forms of sexual experience that do not include intercourse itself, for a short time or as a long-term approach.

Lower Libido

For women, feelings for their partner at the time of the sexual interaction as well as their emotional well-being predict whether sex will be a satisfying experience. Men don't operate the same way and may have a wider disconnect between their feelings, emotional well-being, and sexual function at times. For women, lack of sexual responsiveness in a problem setting is a normal, adaptive response. This does not mean that a woman does not function well sexually. In the past, clinicians and researchers tried to pinpoint a biologic or psychological cause of "sexual dysfunction." It is important to look at the environment and its stresses and how they impact a woman's physiology to see if it is conducive to a positive sexual encounter.

Especially during perimenopause and postmenopause, women may not engage in sex for reasons of desire. It is not clear whether changing hormone levels are the cause of this temporary dampening. Lack of desire may be a consequence of stress, lack of private time with a partner, lack of exercise, or lack of personal time / down time. Family pressures or illness of a parent, relative, or friend may influence sex drive or experiences. Financial pressures, "empty nest syndrome," or caring for grandchildren may dampen sexual desire or enjoyment. Still other menopausal women are inhibited by the presence of teenagers or adult children in the house. The good news is that the stimuli and context of the occasion can change a woman's neutral sexual stance to a responsive one. Do you feel old or undesirable? Do you have unrealistic expectations of what is sexually appealing to your partner, and do you therefore judge yourself to be falling short? You may be more critical of your appearance than your partner is. And physical changes that bother you may not be important to your partner.

Do you have a critical or unsupportive partner? Is your partner verbally or physically abusive? Are you bored? Do you lack stimulation or variety in your routine?

These are questions to consider and discuss with your doctor or a therapist. The doctor may suggest other resources to help address these areas.

Remain open to the other aspects of your health that impact your sex drive and sexual function, such as regular exercise, adequate hydration with water, and enough rest and relaxation with reprieves from stress. Allow more time for vaginal lubrication to take place. Monitor your overall health. Sleep deprivation, common with hot flashes or night sweats, will make you more irritable and may affect your sex drive.

Are you more concerned about changes in your sex drive or about discomfort during sex? The more specifically you can pinpoint your concerns, the more readily your doctor can determine the questions to ask, which portions of the physical exam to perform, and the most helpful tests to order. If the doctor you see does not address all of your questions, he or she will refer you to colleagues who do.

Enhancing the quality of sex in a relationship cannot be separated from enhancing the quality of the relationship itself. This becomes even more important in the menopausal years. The physical and psychological changes that men and women experience in their forties, fifties, and sixties are different from those they had in their twenties and thirties. Some women do not sleep in the same room as their partners at this time. Their relationship is not intimate and their ties with the partner or spouse are not close physically or emotionally. In the past, these women would be labeled as having a problem with sex. Now, with a broader understanding, it would be interpreted as a problem with the relationship and intimacy, not just a problem with sex.

In the menopausal years, there are several aspects to the relationship that become more important. The quality of the emotional intimacy is more critical. There may be fewer work and family distractions than there are for younger couples. Each partner must be able to maintain some independence while still staying connected as a couple and each needs the ability to manage stress.

For example, a stay-at-home wife with a husband who works outside the home may enjoy the support of her friends and her volunteer activities. When the husband retires and is home full time, away from his network of work associates, he may demand more of her time and the wife may not be able to access her friends. This can tax the relationship and unbalance it as each person in the couple no longer has the same routine with colleagues and friends.

Some couples enjoy being "empty nesters" and find that adult children and/or grandchildren returning to live at home cramp their style. Each of these factors contributes to the quality of the sexual relationship. A woman's expectations of herself as well as her partner may not be realistic. Studies have shown that having a youthful body is not required to have enjoyable sex. Pressuring oneself about attaining a "normal" frequency of sexual intercourse is also damaging. Such norms do not exist. Furthermore, they should be irrelevant to you. Although sex continues to be a part of many mature couples' relationships, it is not a part of every healthy relationship. If a woman and her partner are content without having sex, that is fine. Having sex once a month or once a year is fine if that works for you and your partner.

Some women are motivated to have sex but do not have a partner.

They may choose to masturbate. Still other women are in a relationship with a man who has medical problems or a disability that precludes him from having penile-vaginal sex. They may be open to different forms of intimacy and adjust by expanding their sexual repertoire. Options to consider include massages, caressing, mutual masturbation, oral sex, and taking baths or showers together. This reduces the pressure on both individuals to have penile-vaginal sex and maintains closeness and intimacy.

For women, feelings about their partner and pleasure are paramount. Concern about the physical sexual response has less influence on a woman's views on sex than her perception of the relationship she is in and the pleasure she gets from it in a multitude of areas. Brain studies can now image women during sexual arousal and show that areas in the brain responsible for emotional response and cognitive appraisal are activated separately from areas that perceive genital responses. Women's physical response does not necessarily correlate with their subjective arousal. This differs from similar studies in men.

For most women, sexual desire itself is not a frequent reason to agree to partnered sexual activity. Reasons women cite frequently include increasing emotional closeness to their partner and enhancing their sense of well-being. Women will also act to avoid negative consequences to a lack of sexual activity in a relationship. Women can enter into a sexual experience feeling neutral but willing to become aroused. Well into the experience, they may then feel sexual desire. If the experience is enjoyable and the outcome is rewarding, women will find it satisfactory.

Motivation to have sex and the mental processing of sexual stimuli are influenced by the larger context of a woman's life and the immediate potential sexual experience. Longer-term menopausal studies emphasize the importance of a woman's feelings for her partner in influencing her sexual appetite and responsiveness. Relationships with others and the demands of those relationships as well as her feelings about them also influence her sexual experience and frequency, as do society's standards.

Acquiring a new sexual partner has been proven to increase a woman's sexual desire and responsiveness; effort is being put into emotional closeness, and romantic, erotic contacts are more plentiful. Going out and getting a new partner, however, is not advised as a solution to a low sex drive!

If your emotional well-being is compromised, it is a strong predictor that you will have sexual stress. Worrying, experiencing anxiety, low self-esteem, and guilt are all emotions and experiences that dampen sexual response and desire. Addressing these areas may enhance your sex life.

Your sexual pleasure is also influenced by the expectations you have of your relationship and having the relationship be sexually exclusive. A sexually exclusive relationship has been found to be important to both men and women in a long-term relationship. It is tied to their emotional satisfaction and their physical pleasure from sex. A woman who expects her relationship to last indefinitely has more emotional satisfaction with sex.

MEDICATIONS TO IMPROVE LOW SEX DRIVE

Many women seek a "magic pill" that will restore their sex drive. Wouldn't it be wonderful if there truly were such a pill? In fact, most women do not need to resort to this. New research has shown that women who have intercourse regularly maintain vaginal health after perimenopause. They do not necessarily need hormones or other medications to enjoy sex. There are circumstances, however, where hormones may be helpful.

Testosterone

This male hormone is made in every woman's ovaries. It continues to be made by the ovaries in postmenopause, even after the ovaries stop making estrogen. In addition to the ovaries, another source of testosterone in healthy women is the adrenal glands; one sits on top of each kidney. The production of testosterone by the adrenal glands is not affected by the ovaries' production of testosterone. Enzymes in the skin also convert other hormones into testosterone.

Testosterone influences sex drive and motivation, but as described earlier, it is not the only influence. Circumstances, relationship issues, comfort during sex, stress levels, outlook, and many other forces influence sex drive besides testosterone.

Testosterone can be measured in the saliva or in the blood. Methods for measuring testosterone vary greatly and cannot be reliably compared to each other. Testosterone is difficult to measure accurately, regardless of testing method. As a result, normal levels of testosterone in healthy perimenopausal and postmenopausal women are not well established. We do know that there is a great degree of variation between individual women's testosterone levels.

Adding testosterone improves sex drive in some women. Side effects of excess testosterone include painful enlargement of the clitoris, weight gain, an increase in hair growth on the face, chest, or belly, and male-pattern balding. A woman's voice may become permanently lower from using testosterone, making it an unacceptable choice for some.

Although testosterone is touted for its ability to revive one's sex drive, the Food and Drug Administration (FDA) has not approved it for this purpose. Testosterone is only approved for treating severe hot flashes that do not respond to estrogen replacement. Therefore, if your doctor prescribes testosterone in a pill, patch, or cream form to enhance your sex drive, she or he is prescribing it "off label."

It's important that a woman have enough estrogen in her system when she is taking testosterone. Testosterone is not effective if a woman is lacking estrogen.

Women with elevated cholesterol or abnormal liver function should avoid taking testosterone by mouth. It can cause liver damage and worsen lipid levels (driving the cholesterol abnormally high). Doctors can check liver function and cholesterol blood tests prior to prescribing oral testosterone.

Women with normal cholesterol levels and liver tests who elect to try testosterone can have these levels monitored to be certain that they are not adversely affected. Those who develop abnormal blood levels of cholesterol will be advised to stop testosterone. At present there is not much research on long-term use of oral testosterone beyond three years; more information about safety is needed.

Dr. Jan Shifren, a clinical researcher and menopause specialist, published her findings about testosterone patches in the *New England Journal of Medicine*. First, she studied women who had complete hysterectomies and removal of both ovaries with the uterus. These women reported improved sex drive, improved sexual response, and a better sense of well-being after using testosterone patches. Subsequently, she published her study of the testosterone patch improving sex drive for women who still have their own uteruses and at least one ovary. The women ranged from age 40 to 70 and were distressed about their lack of desire. They reported improved sexual function, frequency, and drive after using a testosterone patch.

The testosterone patch has been reviewed by the FDA but has not been approved for use in treating low libido in women. Although women benefit from much lower doses of testosterone than their male counterparts, testosterone patches at low strengths suitable for women are not yet available.

Topical testosterone creams can be applied to the outer genital area to increase sex drive. Specialized pharmacists can compound these creams with a doctor's prescription. Well-controlled medical studies have not been done and there is no proof as yet that this cream is effective. In small amounts, the cream is unlikely to affect your voice, your cholesterol levels, or your blood liver tests. One known side effect of testosterone cream is painful clitoral enlargement.

Testosterone can be compounded with petrolatum (like petroleum jelly) to produce an ointment that can be rubbed into the clitoris and vulva to enhance sexual response. We do not have studies on large numbers of women to assess how well this works and what doses are most helpful.

In Europe and Canada a more specialized form of testosterone is available called Andriol, which may have fewer side effects for many women. It is not yet available in the United States.

EstraTest was the only FDA-approved oral testosterone preparation available in the United States. This pill contained both estrogen and testosterone and required a woman to take progesterone if she still had her uterus (had not had a hysterectomy). It was recently taken off the market and has not been replaced.

For years women have been asking for testosterone to reverse their lagging sex drives. But it is unwise to use testosterone supplementation as a starting point. A thorough history and physical examination with targeted testing sets the stage.

Remember, testosterone will not help a woman whose relationship with her partner is not working. The other components of a healthy relationship need to be in place for the testosterone to be successful. The relationship does not have to be perfect, but there has to be more potential than two people who are not even glad to spend time together in nonsexual settings.

✄ ANDREA'S STORY ✄

Distancing and Hostility in a Long-term Relationship

"At 59, after 30 years of marriage, I went to my doctor to request testosterone to help improve my sex drive. Before writing the prescription, my doctor asked about my relationship. I admitted that my husband and I did not sleep in the same bedroom and we no longer enjoyed each other's company. My husband has a prescription for Viagra. My doctor advised me that a prescription for testosterone would not be likely to help my sex drive if I didn't want to be in the same room as my husband. He made a referral to a marriage counselor."

Dehydroepiandrosterone

Dehydroepiandrosterone (DHEA) is a hormone made by the adrenal glands. DHEA does not drop suddenly during postmenopause; rather, it diminishes gradually over decades in both men and women. Its role in sexual function is not yet well defined.

Despite the lack of thorough research studies, DHEA has been touted as a cure for low sex drive. There are no large well-controlled studies that show DHEA is safe or effective in improving sex drive. As a result, at this time, most physicians believe it's unlikely to make a difference.

Estrogen

Estrogen, as you read in Chapter 1, is still produced by the ovaries in perimenopause. During this time its production becomes very erratic before essentially shutting down in postmenopause. Estrone, the principal form of estrogen produced in postmenopause, is synthesized in fatty tissue. Estrone is a weaker estrogen than estradiol. Even though estrone is a weaker estrogen, it may influence bleeding patterns in perimenopause and affect the uterine lining after menopause. The role of estrone in maintaining libido or vaginal health or controlling hot flashes has not been well studied.

Viagra for Women

Viagra is being studied to determine if it will help women with intercourse. Viagra and other similar medications, such as Cialis, help some men who have otherwise lost the ability to attain an erection. The preliminary data for women suggests that very few women will actually have more satisfying sex using Viagra. At present, studies show that the women who will benefit from Viagra are those who have suffered spinal cord injuries and therefore have compromised blood supply to the pelvis. Additional studies are under way.

Progesterone

Progesterone may help to revive a suppressed sex drive. Progesterone comes in pill form, a skin cream, and a vaginal cream. There are different types of progesterone hormone available. In a woman's body, some progesterone made by the ovaries is naturally converted into testosterone. If your doctor feels that progesterone is safe for you and you are not enthusiastic about trying testosterone, it provides another option.

Although concerns have been raised about Provera (medroxyprogesterone) regarding undesirable effects on the heart or the breast tissue, Prometrium, a plant-based progesterone, is better tolerated by some women. Women who are allergic to peanuts cannot take Prometrium because it is made from peanut oil.

Oral Estrogen

Indirectly, estrogen replacement may help with sex drive. If your sex drive is low due to poor sleep from hot flashes or night sweats, estrogen may improve the quantity and quality of your sleep, increase your sense of well-being, and allow your sex drive to return. Estrogen replacement will also help sex drive if the cause is related to vaginal dryness and poor lubrication. Discomfort is not conducive to pleasurable sex and will affect sex drive.

Oral estrogen is processed in the liver. There, it increases sex hormone binding globulin (SHBG). Oral estrogen also produces changes that result in less testosterone availability; because more testosterone is bound to receptors, there is less free testosterone in the blood for the body to access.

Over time, women who take estrogen by mouth increase the amount of SHBG in their bodies, making estrogen less available to the body, and less effective. In these cases, some women get better results by changing to a form of estrogen that is not taken by mouth, such as a patch, cream, lotion, or vaginal ring.

RESOURCES

Altman, Alan. Patient Information: Sexual problems in women. www.UpTo Date.com. Online Version 16.3. Last accessed December 10, 2008.

Altman, Alan, and Laurie Ashner. *Making Love the Way We Used To—Or Better: Secrets to Satisfying Midlife Sexuality*. Chicago: Contemporary Books, 2001. Dr. Alan Altman is a practicing gynecologist and assistant clinical professor of obstetrics, gynecology, and reproductive biology at Harvard Medical School. He focuses on menopausal issues and sexuality. His book is a practical approach to many common concerns in this area.

The Association of Reproductive Health Professionals and the National Women's Health Resource Center have combined their efforts in the joint website www.NurtureYourNature.org. Last accessed August 5, 2009, it provides information on sexuality to women and their health care providers.

Barbach, Lonnie, editor. *For Yourself: The Fulfillment of Female Sexuality.* Garden City, NY: Anchor Press, 1976, rev. 2000. Lonnie Barbach, Ph.D., is a sex therapist and leading authority on sexuality. She is on the clinical faculty at the University of California at San Francisco School of Medicine.

Minkin, Mary Jane, and Carol Wright. *A Woman's Guide to Sexual Health.* New Haven, CT: Yale University Press, 2005. Dr. Mary Jane Minkin is a clinical professor of obstetrics and gynecology at Yale Medical School and an internationally recognized menopause expert. Her book is an excellent resource written in question-and-answer format.

Westheimer, Ruth, with Pierre A. Lehu. *Dr. Ruth's Sex after 50: Revving up the Romance, Passion, and Excitement!* Sanger, CA: Quill Driver Books / Word Dancer Press, 2005. "Dr. Ruth" is the first expert who comes to mind, both within medical circles and outside them, when discussing women's sexuality.

Compatible Contraception

This chapter is for those women who are sexually active, perimenopausal, and not interested in becoming pregnant. If you and your doctor have confirmed that you are definitely postmenopausal, you no longer need to worry about becoming pregnant.

Perimenopausal women are still at risk for unplanned pregnancy. Nearly half of all pregnancies in the United States are unplanned, and the rate of unintended pregnancies in perimenopausal women is high. The pregnancy termination rate for women over 40 is 35 percent and even higher for women over 45. The only group with a higher rate of abortions is preteens. Just because you do not get a period does not mean that you cannot get pregnant; you can be ovulating, not see a period, and get pregnant. Younger perimenopausal women may find that their menstrual periods start up on their own again after a gap of 10 or 12 months. Your doctor can advise you when you can safely stop using contraception.

Contraception options for you to consider are discussed below. They are included because they are effective and/or user-friendly for women over age 40 and readily available. I have also included options that are available or appealing but are not well suited to perimenopausal women. Whether you are considering these options or others, you will want to discuss your choices with your doctor.

The Rhythm Method

Even if you successfully used the rhythm method of birth control during your twenties or thirties, and were meticulous about following your cervical mucus and determining your fertile time, this method will *not* serve you well in your forties. Your cycle can change with no warning at this age. You might not experience the expected mucus changes, but ovulate anyway and be able to conceive. This is one reason that the rhythm method of birth control is not considered reliable in the perimenopausal years. Irregular cycles and absent or disguised signs of ovulation make the failure rate of the rhythm method of birth control high, even for women who are experienced practitioners of this method.

The Withdrawal Method

Withdrawal is not a reliable method for preventing pregnancy at *any* age. Sperm can be produced in small amounts before ejaculation, which is why withdrawal has a 50 percent failure rate.

Over-the-counter Spermicides

The use of over-the-counter spermicides alone has a high failure rate, although spermicides used *with* condoms or a diaphragm are effective methods for preventing pregnancy.

Barrier Methods

You may elect to use a barrier method of contraception. The advantage is that there is nothing to take by mouth, and you can use it only when you need it, at the time of intercourse. Barrier methods are effective regardless of where you are in your menstrual cycle, and they do not affect your bleeding pattern. You only use this method when you actually have sex, and there are no hormones involved.

The two most common barrier methods are condoms (for men)

and the diaphragm (for women). Both also offer varying degrees of protection against sexually transmitted diseases (STDs) such as HIV/AIDS as well as others.

FEMALE CONDOM

A female condom is available, which has also been shown to protect against sexually transmitted disease. The condom has a pouch that rests inside the vagina and a wide rim that presses against the outside of the vagina and covers much of the vulva (outer lips). It has been tested extensively in Africa and Mexico.

CONDOMS

Condoms for men are 98 percent effective in preventing pregnancy if they are used correctly and reliably. During perimenopause, do not decide on whether to use a condom according to your cycle. During perimenopause your cycle can become irregular with no warning. If condoms are your birth control method of choice, use them at *all* times. Use a lubricant that is compatible with the type of condom you are using, and select one with as few additives as possible. If you are sensitive to latex products, be certain to select a non-latex condom. Also avoid scented products. Some women are sensitive to the additives included in some spermicides and lubricants. Allow extra space at the tip of the condom so that it is less likely to break. Condoms should not be reused.

In addition to preventing pregnancy, condoms help prevent the spread of STDs.

THE DIAPHRAGM

Prior to intercourse, the diaphragm (coated with spermicidal cream or gel) is inserted into the vagina by the woman or her partner. It must remain in place six to eight hours after intercourse. When properly fitted, it will cover the cervix and the upper vagina, preventing sperm from entering the cervix. It should always be used with spermicide, which forms a seal around the inside rim of the diaphragm. The diaphragm is fit in a doctor's office; a prescription is written for the size and type that fits you best. Have your diaphragm refit if you gain or lose more than 15 pounds, as the fit may change and you may need a new size. The diaphragm protects the cervix from sexually transmitted diseases, but not the vaginal cavity or the vulva outside the vagina. The diaphragm should be cleaned after each use and checked for holes by holding it up to the light for a visual check and by testing that water does not leak through it.

The "Morning-after" Pill

"Plan B," also known as "The Morning-after Pill," reduces the chance of pregnancy after unprotected sex. It is available as a backup method only. It is not suitable for regular, frequent, or routine use. Common circumstances where Plan B may be a helpful option include after a condom breaks or tears, or in the devastating instance of a rape.

Plan B may be purchased at a pharmacy without a prescription, or "over the counter." The Plan B kit includes two progesterone pills that are taken by mouth 12 hours apart. Side effects do not always occur, but may include nausea or vomiting, stomach pain, breast pain, headache, dizziness, diarrhea, fatigue, or menstrual changes. Taking Plan B within 72 hours after unprotected intercourse will prevent pregnancy more than 90 percent of the time. It works best if taken within the first 24 hours after unprotected sex. Plan B should not be used if you are pregnant. However, it is not likely to harm an existing pregnancy that may not yet be evident. Plan B is not the same as the "abortion pill" (RU486). Plan B does not cause an abortion to take place; it does substantially reduce the chance that a pregnancy will be successful in the next three weeks or so.

If you are unable to purchase Plan B, your doctor may recommend that you take a certain number of pills from a regular birth control pill pack in a particular way to achieve the same result of preventing ovulation. The dosage will differ depending upon the type of pill being used, so do not compare your instructions to those of a friend's.

The Intrauterine Device

The intrauterine device (IUD) acquired a bad reputation among baby boomers. But since the 1960s, the IUD has been upgraded and revamped and is safer today. The newer IUDs can be effective for 5 or even up to 10 years. If you decide you want to conceive, you can have the IUD removed. In the past, some women bled more heavily or had more prolonged or irregular bleeding with an IUD in place. Now, the Mirena IUD has progesterone in it. The progesterone is slowly released into the uterine cavity and can help to reduce heavy or prolonged bleeding.

The IUD is not recommended for women who have a history of an ectopic, or tubal, pregnancy. In a tubal pregnancy the embryo accidentally implants in the tube instead of the uterus. The IUD increases the risk of ectopic pregnancies even in those women who have not had one. Those with a history of pelvic infection such as PID (pelvic inflammatory disease) should also avoid IUDs because they can increase the risk of a pelvic infection. Women who have multiple partners are not ideal candidates for IUDs because multiple partners increase the risk of pelvic infection.

The IUD is inserted into the uterus in a doctor's office. This procedure is mildly uncomfortable, but the brief cramps may be relieved with an over-the-counter anti-inflammatory medication. An IUD can usually be removed in the office, especially if the string is still visible in the vagina.

Depo Provera

Depo Provera is a long-acting birth control method that is reversible. It involves getting an injection of progesterone every three months. There is no estrogen in the preparation. Depo Provera injections may produce light or irregular periods, or result in no menstrual periods at all. Depo Provera is not a suitable long-term choice for a perimenopausal woman because it is associated with bone thinning when used for more than a year.

Oral Contraceptives

Birth control pills are a helpful option for the perimeno-pausal woman. The newer low-dose birth control pills may be taken safely by the vast majority of them. The pills available today are safer than ever, due to newer formulations that contain even lower doses of hormones. Most of the low-dose birth control pills contain small amounts of estrogen and progesterone. A few oral contraceptives contain progesterone only.

Oral contraceptives are not appropriate for women in postmeno-pause or women who smoke. Even low-dose oral contraceptives have too much estrogen in them for a postmenopausal woman. In addition, the oral contraceptives deliver hormones in a cyclic fashion that does not match the biology of the postmenopausal woman.

Smokers over the age of 35 should not take the estrogen-progesterone birth control pill. For them, the risk of strokes, heart attacks, and deep blood clots in the veins is significantly higher. Some doctors are comfortable prescribing birth control pills to women with high blood pressure as long as the blood pressure is being treated and has been brought into the normal range with medication. These women should be closely monitored by their medical doctors. Some women have hereditary high cholesterol or triglycerides and may experience a further increase in cholesterol or triglycerides while taking an oral contraceptive. Your doctor will guide you on these more complex issues based upon your personal and family history and laboratory results. While these medical issues are certainly of concern, many experts conclude that pregnancy in a woman with high blood pressure is much riskier than taking a low-dose birth control pill.

For most nonsmokers, the birth control pill is an appealing option. It may help to regulate irregular or heavy menstrual periods. The estrogen in the pill may alleviate hot flashes. It produces regular, light cycles that many women appreciate.

It is important to take folate, a B vitamin, while you are on oral contraceptives. If you were to conceive, it is important to have adequate levels of folate in your system to lower the risk of birth defects in the brain and spine of the developing fetus.

In the past, there was a concern that birth control pills caused breast cancer, and a number of studies supported this concern. Large reviews of multiple studies have not produced a clear conclusion, so many experts in gynecology conclude that oral contraceptives do not cause a significant increase in breast cancer risk. That said, if you have a personal history of breast cancer, you should not take oral contraceptives. Those with a family history of breast cancer should not have an increased risk, but the decision is best made with a doctor's input to weigh the pros and cons, risks and benefits, for you as an individual.

Taking oral contraceptives can mask the exact timing of menopause. Sometimes, taking oral contraceptives during perimenopause can spur bleeding cycles when a woman may otherwise have stopped bleeding on her own. There is no one agreed-upon strategy to determine the onset of postmenopause in a woman taking oral contraceptives. Your doctor will advise you of the best strategy for your individual situation. It is not safe to assume that if you stop bleeding you are postmenopausal, since some women on oral contraceptives stop bleeding due to a thin uterine lining. On the other hand, it is not accurate to assume that you are still perimenopausal if you continue to bleed on oral contraceptives, as they can induce cyclic bleeding after postmenopause due to the way the hormones are sequenced.

The Pill does not prevent sexually transmitted diseases. If you have more than one sexual partner or are not in a stable relationship, condoms will lower your risk of getting a sexually transmitted disease. The birth control pill lowers your risk of ovarian cancer by 50 percent. The Pill also lowers the risk of uterine (endometrial) cancer.

♏ Melissa's Story ♏

Hot Flashes and the Pill

"I began having irregular menstrual periods three years ago, when I was 46. I would skip a period every three or four months. I was also experiencing debilitating hot flashes, which were extremely difficult to cope with in my job as a flight attendant, especially during long flights. I'd always had an erratic sleep routine with my unpredictable work schedule and layovers in different time zones. Once I began having night sweats, I got even less sleep. I learned paced respiration but that was not something I could do while helping passengers. A German stewardess I knew gave me some black cohosh to decrease the hot flashes, but the relief was minimal. Eventually, I consulted my gynecologist. Because I'm a nonsmoker, he suggested I try a low-dose oral contraceptive. The pill he prescribed drastically reduced the number and severity of hot flashes and also gave me shorter, lighter, and more regular menstrual periods."

Contraceptive Skin Patch

Ortho Evra is a contraceptive skin patch marketed in the United States. It releases hormones slowly through the skin directly into the bloodstream 24 hours a day, 7 days a week. A new patch is placed on the skin once a week for three consecutive weeks, followed by a patch-free week, to allow for a menstrual period. It is best to place the patch below the waist, on the abdomen or buttocks. The patch stays on during baths, showers, and swimming. In the past few years a question was raised about whether the Ortho Evra skin patch was associated with a higher risk of deep blood clots. Consider this when you discuss the contraceptive patch with your doctor.

Vaginal Ring

Nuva Ring is a contraceptive vaginal ring that releases hormones into the bloodstream through the vaginal walls. This small, soft, flexible ring is inserted in the vagina. It comes in one small size and does not require a "fitting." It is left in place for three consecutive weeks, including during intercourse. It is then removed for one week, which allows a menstrual period to occur, and then a new ring is placed in the vagina for three weeks.

Female Sterilization

Essure™ and Adiana™ are permanent birth control methods achieved by a minor surgical procedure in which a sterile coil or rod is placed in the entrance of each fallopian tube. The body's own tissue grows around the device, creating a natural tissue barrier or plug blocking the entrance from the uterine cavity to the tubes. This procedure is also called an "incision-less tubal occlusion." To place the device, a hysteroscope (a microscope for the uterine cavity) is inserted through the cervix into the uterine cavity. No incisions are needed. Three months after the device is placed, a simple dye study is done to confirm that the tubes are blocked. After that the procedure provides reliable, permanent birth control

A tubal ligation, often referred to as "getting your tubes tied," is another form of permanent birth control. Tubal ligation is a surgical procedure, usually performed with a laparoscope, a special microscope that is introduced through the umbilicus (navel). The abdomen and pelvis are filled with carbon dioxide to lift the abdominal wall off the pelvic organs and intestines. The pelvis is examined through the microscope. A tiny incision is made in the pubic area, low in the abdomen, and the tubes are sealed using cautery, or clipped, to prevent sperm from entering them and making contact with an egg.

Another option is to perform a tubal ligation at the time of a cesarean section birth if the woman has decided in advance that she doesn't want more children or within the first three days after a vaginal birth (referred to as a postpartum tubal ligation). In the past, there was a concern that tubal ligations cause abnormal menstrual bleeding. This has been disproved; having a tubal ligation will not alter your menstrual cycles.

Tubal ligation lowers the risk of ovarian cancer by 30 to 50 percent. If a woman has no family history of ovarian cancer, her lifetime risk of getting ovarian cancer will go from approximately one in 100, to one in 200, after a tubal ligation. The underlying theory here is that, after ligation, environmental toxins (though which toxins are still unknown) can no longer reach the ovaries and therefore cannot influence the ovaries to develop cancer.

Male Sterilization (Vasectomy)

Vasectomies (male sterilizations) are performed by a urologist, a surgical specialist knowledgeable about the male urinary system, kidneys, and reproductive system. It is done in the doctor's office using sterile technique. In this minor surgical procedure, the male sperm "tubes" (vas deferens) are tied off, resulting in permanent sterilization, analogous to a tubal ligation in a woman. After the procedure, at one or two different intervals, the sperm count is rechecked to confirm the procedure was effective. Although some refer to vasectomies as a nonpermanent form of birth control, it is important to note that procedures to reverse vasectomy are not always successful. Research is under way to find new birth control methods for men, including a birth control pill.

RESOURCE

The American College of Obstetricians and Gynecologists (ACOG) (www .acog.org) has 10 different pamphlets that discuss types of contraception, from hormonal contraception to emergency contraception to natural family planning and barrier methods to sterilization procedures. Many are also available in Spanish. You may be able to obtain a free copy of up to five different printed pamphlets, or request those that interest you from your gynecologist. Site last accessed December 15, 2008.

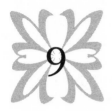

Moods, Memory, and
Mental Health

Men and women of any age are susceptible to changes in their moods, memory, and mental health. So why include this chapter? As a woman experiences perimenopause and postmenopause she undergoes complex changes in these areas. Researchers are beginning to shed light on the types of changes involved. One difficulty in understanding these changes is that each of us has our own individual biology and temperament, as well as our own physical health and psychological factors in our lives that affect our mood, memory, and mental health.

Until now, shifts in the emotional outlook or mental function of women over the age of 40 were attributed to hot flashes, night sweats, lack of sleep, or life changes such as the "empty nest syndrome." While these are all legitimate sources of stress, we now know that the whole picture is even more complex: biologic, hormonal, genetic, and social changes are at play, and they influence each of us differently.

As you no doubt know from your own life, there are wide variations in how individual women experience aging. In addition, important differences exist between the phases of menopause, making it hard to sort out which changes are linked to what. As a matter of fact, there is still no uniform definition of perimenopause itself. Studies at different research centers are performed using diverse criteria, which makes it even harder to draw universal conclusions.

It is important to note early in this chapter that, for some women, perimenopause and postmenopause pose no psychological difficulties. Many perimenopausal and postmenopausal women are pleased with the new opportunities open to them at this stage of life. They can further their education, develop new interests, plan a new career, or pursue an established career more vigorously.

Just as graduation from high school has a very different feel than graduation from college, postmenopause is biologically distinct from perimenopause in the realm of mental health. Each phase of menopause has its own distinct landmarks, including changing biology, hormone environment, and social context. This chapter describes what a woman leaves behind when she shrugs off the biology of perimenopause and dons the biologic cloak of postmenopause.

Some women are more vulnerable to stress and depression during perimenopause, regardless of whether they experience hot flashes or irregular bleeding. Anxiety, irritability, and difficulty sleeping are common. A panic attack may be difficult to distinguish from a hot flash. And minor health problems may surface, even in women who up until this stage have enjoyed exceptionally good health. All of these factors can affect mood, memory, and mental health.

A postmenopausal woman is usually relieved that she is no longer at risk for an unplanned pregnancy. Postmenopausal women also no longer experience erratic hormone fluctuations, and this stability contributes to greater resilience against stress and depression. After the heightened differences between the sexes seen during perimenopause, in postmenopause gender differences in brain function between men and women ease and the sexes become more similar. When you reach postmenopause, you are less susceptible to depression related to erratic estrogen levels because your estrogen levels are low but constant. However, during postmenopause you are more likely to have a major health issue or become more socially isolated, have financial difficulties, or experience a lack of resources. These challenges can contribute to depression in their own right.

Scientists had to begin somewhere, so they started with hormones. Focusing exclusively on hormones, though, is like cropping a digital photo of an entire extended family to include only one person's face. The big picture of menopause includes genetic components, social context, and much more. For each woman, there is a complex relationship between the physical, mental, and emotional shifts that occur with each stage of menopause, as well her lifestyle choices and social context. When women compare notes, they can be fooled into thinking they have the same problem because their cluster of concerns is so similar. In reality, the cause and the treatment may be very different for each of them.

Hormones and Moods

Today the genetic underpinnings for mood changes, depression, and even susceptibility to hot flashes have been partially unearthed. A woman who has had postpartum depression is at higher risk for depression during perimenopause. Other perimenopausal women at high risk for depression include those who experience more volatile hormone peaks and troughs, particularly if they occur over longer periods of time.

Estrogen affects mood by influencing neurotransmitters in the brain. Estrogen increases serotonin levels. Serotonin is associated with positive feelings and has a calming effect. Low levels of estrogen will result in diminished serotonin levels and worse moods. There are also other ways that low serotonin can occur, such as problems with the receptor for serotonin or inadequate serotonin production.

Receptors are the body's way of capturing specific hormones and locking onto them so they have a designated place to act. It is like having your own personal prescription for eyeglasses or contacts; it will not help someone else. With hormone receptors, the fit is even more precise. Picture a jigsaw puzzle piece fitting exactly into the opening of the master puzzle. That is how a hormone fits into its specific receptor. The color, contour, size, and orientation must match exactly for the right fit.

Estrogen receptors occur in many cells of the body but are particularly prominent in the brain, the breasts, and the genital system.

Estrogen receptors prevalent in the hippocampus and other areas of the brain important for emotions suggest that we'll be learning more about emotional changes associated with menopause. We do know that some women are particularly sensitive to the changes of estrogen during perimenopause because of these influences.

Researchers have now linked sensitivity to stress and "blue" moods with intermittent low estrogen levels. During the reproductive years, the pattern of low estrogen occurs monthly at specific predictable times during the menstrual cycle. In perimenopause, in contrast, the low estrogen levels are irregular and unpredictable.

The hypothalamus also has progesterone receptors. Progesterone can decrease anxiety and produce a hypnotic effect. At times, however, it can also worsen mood or cause irritability. Some forms of progesterone are helpful in controlling moods, especially when there is too little progesterone during perimenopause.

Genetics play a role; some women are more sensitive than others to hormones. Genetics research points to differences in how an individual's receptors function. A woman who inherits weak or ineffective receptors for a specific hormone is unable to use that hormone effectively. For example, if you have weak or ineffective receptors for serotonin, a "feel good" hormone, you will be more prone to depression. Even if you have enough serotonin, it will not produce the desired calming effect because it is not able to bind to a defective receptor.

Biologic differences between women in perimenopause and postmenopause also determine how susceptible they are to stress or depression. If you do not manufacture enough serotonin due to a biological processing problem, you will be prone to anxiety and depression even if your serotonin receptors are normal. Whether you have a problem with serotonin that is genetic (receptors) or biologic (processing), you will be prone to depression.

The debate over whether you should take hormones during perimenopause or postmenopause cannot overshadow other aspects of your health and well-being. While hormones are certainly an important issue, other aspects of your health merit attention in their own right.

Should Low Hormone Levels Be Corrected?

Perimenopause and postmenopause are normal phases of life that present unique opportunities for preventing disease and enhancing health. There are at least two polarized views about mental health and menopause that crop up perennially. Neither view serves women well.

One view rationalizes that because perimenopause and postmenopause are healthy phases, not diseases, they do not warrant diagnosis or treatment. Women should simply weather the changes. This shortchanges women who develop a treatable mental condition that is written off as a side effect of menopause.

The other view is that in order to preserve sanity and mental acuity (in addition to youth, long-term health, and sexual function) hormones are warranted. This view shortchanges a woman by advising hormones without discerning whether the benefit to her is greater than the risk at any particular time.

The balanced view is this: menopause is a healthy state in which women are at risk for certain physical and psychological problems. First, you and your doctor must identify your specific vulnerabilities based upon your personal and family history. Then, prevention and treatment efforts can be custom tailored to you—first in perimenopause, with its changing landscape of hormones, and then in postmenopause.

Hormones are trees in the forest of menopause research. In the realm of mental health, we have been losing the forest for the trees.

Changes in Perimenopause and Postmenopause

Perimenopause and postmenopause are normal phases of life, not illnesses. But even today, a woman may still feel that she needs to be "fixed" because she lacks estrogen or notices she is more forgetful or sadder. Rather than feeling broken or needing to be fixed, she deserves to know that this may be a vulnerable time for her mental and physical health. She is at higher risk for problems with her memory, depression, susceptibility to stress, trouble with sleep, and worsening of premenstrual syndrome (PMS). Specifically, she will experience changes in:

- *Hormone secretion.* The hormonal peaks and valleys of perimenopause cause more than hot flashes and mood swings; they may be associated with depression that hormones will not alleviate. In postmenopause hormones are stable, but at lower levels. Dealing with physical illness or social isolation may increase the risk of depression.
- *Reproductive status.* In perimenopause, fertility is drawing to a close. In postmenopause, having any more children is impossible. This is not just a physical change. If a woman's life has been defined by childrearing, she may feel a terrible sense of loss and confusion. On the other hand, she may feel emancipated.
- *Appearance.* Our culture does not value the aged. Women feel they must go to great lengths to continue looking as young as possible. We have almost completely lost the concept of growing old gracefully, which makes it difficult for older women to feel confident.
- *Sexuality.* Women in perimenopause and postmenopause can and do have sex (for more information, see Chapter 7), but many women have difficulty with the fact that they may become less desirable to men as they age. When 60-year-old men commonly date much younger women, where does that leave the 60-year-old women?
- *Social context.* A woman is often defined by her roles—partner or spouse, daughter, mother, sister, and/or member of a professional group. Her roles are likely to change later in life. Sometimes the changes originate within her and radiate outward; other times, shifts may be forced upon her by circumstances. Having an "empty nest" after decades of childrearing may come as a shock. A woman's relationship with her partner or work situation may change. This is the time of life when people retire and move to new communities. Some women are surrounded by loving family and grandchildren; others are isolated and alone.

Tend and Befriend: The Unique Biology of Female Stress

Gender differences exist in mental health and in how men and women respond to stress. These differences are not fixed, though, and vary with a woman's individual biology and the phase of menopause she is in. Gender differences also change with age. For example, a perimenopausal woman reacts to stress differently than a man her age (she is more vulnerable). In postmenopause, her reaction morphs and her stress response becomes more robust and more similar to that of her male counterpart.

Our understanding of women's response to stress has changed dramatically in the past few years. "Fight or flight" is the traditional understanding of human response to stress, but it is not an accurate description. For men and women there are actually three stages of response to stress:

1. the alert, or alarm phase, in which one feels disrupted
2. resistance while making biologic and behavioral attempts to adapt to, or eliminate, the stressor
3. exhaustion or decompensation (deterioration in coping abilities), if the individual cannot successfully deal with the stressor

Notice that the second step is neither "fight" nor "flight." The female stress response is more accurately described as "tend and be-friend." *Tend* involves nurturing activities that protect a woman and her offspring. These activities promote safety and reduce distress. *Befriend* involves creating and maintaining social networks that aid in the process of tending.

Gender studies provide a new lens through which to view how differently women and men deal with stressors. In one study, researchers looked at the ways in which men and women responded to the stress of being diagnosed with cancer. Men who were diagnosed with prostate cancer avoided disclosing the diagnosis to others. In contrast, the majority of women, when told they were diagnosed with breast cancer, sought opportunities to discuss it with others and to share their emotional reaction to the diagnosis. Women used more "tend and befriend" mechanisms to deal with the cancer diagnosis than their male counterparts. When researchers looked at men and women's reaction to losing a partner—which is, of course, associated with very high stress levels—the women sought more social contact. The men avoided social contact and distracted themselves with activities such as drinking more.

There are sex differences in the psychiatric realm as well. More women get depressed than men, and they report more stressors. Women are also more likely to experience post-traumatic stress disorder (PTSD). Both men and women report less stress as they age, but elderly women still report more than their male counterparts. In general, women recall more details of negative life events than men do. Women also have a greater subjective response and more behavioral changes to stress than men do. Women's increased susceptibility begins in childhood when the changes of puberty amplify their sensitivity to stress. Although women have a more pronounced *psychological* reaction to stress than men do, they have less of a *physical* reaction to it than men do.

✠ ZELDA'S STORY ✠

Witness to a Car Accident

"My husband and I are both 73 years old. We're in good mental and physical health. We witnessed a fatal car accident involving an acquaintance. Afterward, I developed what my doctor called post-traumatic stress disorder. My husband did not. I continually recalled details of the accident, and since then I have refused to drive. My husband is still comfortable driving."

THE STRESS RESPONSE IN MEN AND WOMEN

Other gender differences have emerged while examining how men and women respond to stress. Researchers are scratching the surface of a very interesting phenomenon. Basically, men and women find different things stressful because they tend to value different things.

Men and women differ in their response to stress on four levels:

1. *Subjective or psychological reaction.* In general, women tend to recall and share information about negative experiences and emotions. Women tend to express both positive and negative more often and more intensely than men.

2. *Biologic responses* including measuring the blood level of cortisol, a stress hormone. In tests, men had greater cortisol responses to the cognitive challenges. Women had greater cortisol responses to social rejection. Other studies have shown that epinephrine (another indicator of stress that mediates the nervous system) increases in response to an intellectual challenge more in men than in women.

3. *Behavioral responses,* some of which are influenced by culture and family.

4. *Mental and physical health consequences* of stress. Examples of these include changes in blood pressure, pulse, heart attacks, depression, anxiety, and post-traumatic stress disorder. These consequences are not distributed evenly. As you read earlier in this book, heart attacks are more difficult to diagnose in women. Depression and anxiety are more readily diagnosed in women, as they are more likely to talk about it. More data is needed.

On some levels women are more vulnerable to stress than men are; on other levels, they are more resilient. It's important to note that gender differences are not consistent, and they also vary over time. In postmenopause, women's behavior tends to "cross over" and become more like that of their male counterparts.

Women and Oxytocin

Oxytocin is a hormone secreted by the pituitary gland in the brain. It is secreted by men and women in response to many types of events, including stress. It also regulates and dampens other neurologic systems activated by stress. When oxytocin is released, there is a sedative effect. It produces relaxation and more maternal and caretaking behavior.

Androgens—male hormones—block oxytocin from being released. In contrast, estrogen enhances oxytocin release. Women have a greater release of oxytocin in response to stress. When estrogen wanes, women release less oxytocin and experience less of its sedative effect, less relaxation, and less friend-seeking and maternal behavior. As a result, postmenopausal women move more in the direction of the "fight or flight" stress response that males have throughout their lifetime.

Women have long reported that spending time with friends offers unique stress reduction benefits. Now there is a scientific basis for this. Oxytocin is released when women are stressed. Oxytocin release encourages a woman to gather with other women and tend to her children. Once she "tends and befriends," more oxytocin hormone is released, which dilutes the stress and calms her. Oxytocin is also high during labor and when a woman nurses her infant.

Women working in a laboratory noticed that when they were stressed, they came in to clean the lab, have coffee, and bond. In contrast, when their male colleagues were stressed, they went off on their own.

Numerous studies have found that social ties lower the risk of disease by lowering blood pressure, heart rate, and cholesterol. Those with no friends increase their risk of death over a six-month period. Those with the most friends over a nine-year period cut their risk of death by more than 60 percent.

The Harvard Medical School's Nurses' Health Study showed that women were less likely to develop physical impairments while aging if they had more friends. They were also more likely to be happy. The magnitude of the effect was so significant that the study determined not having close friends or confidantes was as damaging to one's health as smoking or being overweight.

In the book *Best Friends: The Pleasures and Perils of Girls' and Women's Friendships*, coauthor Ruthellen Josselson, Ph.D., noted that women frequently let go of their friendships with other women as soon as they get overly busy with work and family. By setting friend-ships aside, they deprive themselves of sources of strength and nur-turing.

Women outlive men in North America, on average, by 10 years or more, but whether or not they are married or have a partner, women's friendships are key to their enjoyment and their health. Jean Baker Miller, a researcher who studied positive relationships between women, found that five good things could be generated from these relationships:

1. a sense of zest
2. increasing clarity of thinking
3. productivity/creativity
4. a sense of worth
5. a desire for more connection

Women grow through connection. Relationships also influence psychological resilience. When we receive and provide support for each other, we become more resilient. The bottom line is that there is biologic proof that friendships are an important part of weather-ing perimenopause and postmenopause.

Cyclic Mood Changes, Premenstrual Syndrome, or Worse

PREMENSTRUAL SYNDROME

Premenstrual syndrome (PMS) differs from illnesses such as chronic fatigue syndrome or depression. With PMS, a woman feels well and functions normally for the first half of her cycle; then for one or two weeks before her menstrual period, she has mood changes along with physical changes that make her uncomfortable. Women with chronic illnesses do not get a reprieve every month, although they may find that their symptoms worsen before a men-strual period. These subtleties can make PMS difficult to identify. A correct diagnosis is important, as treatments differ.

PMS may worsen in perimenopause. By definition, PMS cannot take place in postmenopause when the menstrual cycles are no longer present.

Several medical problems imitate PMS. Thyroid disease is one of them. Checking the thyroid with a blood test in a woman with PMS symptoms is important. If thyroid disease is the sole cause, her symptoms will resolve with thyroid medication. In addition to thyroid disease, depression, anxiety disorders, and perimenopause may also mimic PMS. Other medical conditions with similar features include migraine headaches and irritable bowel syndrome.

The exact causes of PMS are unknown. There is probably a chemical basis for it, in addition to the hormonal effect of transient low estrogen. Ovarian hormones interact with serotonin, the neurotransmitter that promotes feeling good and calm feelings. A woman with PMS may have lower blood serotonin levels the second half of her menstrual cycle. This chemical imbalance would prevent her from feeling good and staying calm. She will improve with medications that increase serotonin. Other women who are prone to PMS may lack tryptophan, an amino acid needed to synthesize serotonin.

PMS is common, affecting up to 30 percent of women with regular menstrual cycles. The presence and severity of PMS may be influenced by:

- culture
- genetics
- family example (your mother's premenstrual behavior)
- individual biology (you may metabolize or process estrogen too quickly)
- diet
- exercise

The symptoms of PMS include:

- mood changes
- forgetfulness
- difficulty concentrating

- increased appetite
- anger
- crying easily
- gastrointestinal upset
- hot flashes
- heart palpitations
- dizziness
- abdominal bloating
- extreme fatigue
- breast tenderness
- headaches

Premenstrual syndrome is limited to the second half of the menstrual cycle. Your menstrual cycle officially begins with the first day of bleeding. Therefore, the second half of your cycle occurs immediately *before* the bleeding starts. By definition, PMS symptoms resolve when the menstrual bleeding itself begins. Keeping a diary of PMS symptoms and their timing through the month for at least two menstrual cycles is helpful to clinch the diagnosis. Include daily ratings of your physical symptoms, moods, and feelings, with their intensity. These ratings include the timing and severity of bloating, headaches, mood changes, anxiety, and other features in relation to the timing of your menstrual bleeding.

A diary of symptoms is the only way your doctor can accurately diagnose PMS. A retrospective recall of symptoms is not accurate enough. The timing of the symptoms must be precisely recorded in relation to the menstrual bleeding. Symptoms that spill over into the first half of the menstrual cycle or that persist throughout the cycle are not characteristic of PMS.

During the second half of the cycle, estrogen and progesterone are produced. When estrogen and progesterone levels fall, the menstrual period starts. The low estrogen and progesterone levels can set off PMS in some women.

As you have read earlier in this chapter, women are more sensitive to stress when estrogen is intermittently low. Estrogen levels drop during the second half of each menstrual cycle and intermittently during perimenopause as well. Both are times when women are more vulnerable to stress. A woman with PMS may shrug off a stressful situation that occurs during the first half of her menstrual cycle. When the same woman experiences the same stressful situation during the second half of her cycle, it causes considerable distress. One way to view PMS is as a heightened sensitivity to stress.

A woman is more likely to express her anger, unhappiness, or anxiety during the week before her period. At this time, low estrogen renders her more emotionally fragile. Our society does not tolerate women's feelings of anger or unhappiness. Nor does it validate these feelings when they are more likely to be expressed premenstrually, even if they are justified.

Tolerance for the moods of PMS is needed. Society's tendency to dismiss women's negative feelings does not serve women, or society, well. This denigrates a woman's negative thoughts and feelings. Remember that adage, if you do not have something nice to say, say nothing at all? While women feel more intense anger premenstrually, and are more likely to express it, they are seldom validated and heard.

ɴ DAVIDA'S STORY ℣

Not Just PMS

"I'm 45, have two teenagers at home, and am in a happy, stable marriage. My husband has been saying lately, though, that during the latter half of my menstrual cycle I'm extremely anxious. He notices that the two weeks before my period I'm intolerant of the kids and impatient with him. He always liked the fact that I've been a 'cool customer' and says that now he only sees that side of me for two weeks a month. The change in my moods has compromised the relationship I have with my children, my husband, my co-workers, and my boss. I feel depressed for the two weeks each month before my period. I also have had little energy to do normal things like make dinner. In the daytime, during this part of my cycle, I avoid business meetings that I'm expected to attend. My office has an open-door policy, but I keep my door shut for those two weeks. Recently, my husband and co-workers encouraged me to see my

doctor about it. She took a detailed history and ordered a thyroid blood test. The thyroid test was normal. She also asked me questions relating to my moods. Because I function so well for two weeks out of the month, and the impact of the mood changes on my life is devastating, she suspected I had premenstrual dysphoric disorder (PMDD). She asked me to keep a chart for the next two months, recording my moods and the timing of my menstrual cycle. She also advised increasing my calcium intake to 600 milligrams twice a day over this time period, and since my PMDD is more severe, I may need prescription medication to manage it."

PREMENSTRUAL DYSPHORIC DISORDER

Premenstrual dysphoric disorder (PMDD) is a more severe form of PMS that compromises the way a woman functions socially and at work. The timing of PMDD symptoms is the same, so like those of PMS, PMDD symptoms disappear when the menstrual period begins. The severity of the symptoms and the degree that they impact a woman's functioning are what differentiates PMDD from PMS.

Criteria for PMDD include:

- worse or more mercurial moods
- marked anxiety
- marked anger
- irritability
- more frequent and severe interpersonal conflicts

A woman with PMDD must have at least one of the above criteria as well as four or more additional features, such as:

- poor concentration
- fatigue
- appetite changes
- feeling out of control
- physical symptoms

- substantially depressed mood (for two weeks or less)
- decreased interest in usual activities

PMDD, unlike its mild sister, PMS, dramatically compromises a woman's ability to function well at work, home, school, and in social interactions during the second half of her cycle.

Problems with concentration and memory occur in women with PMDD as well as those with major depression. The difference is that the concentration and memory problems in women with PMDD are restricted to the second half of the menstrual cycle. A woman has more pronounced mental changes with PMDD, even if she has no physical symptoms.

PMS is 10 times more common than PMDD. The biology underlying PMDD was recently discovered: it is believed that women with PMDD do not bind serotonin normally, so serotonin cannot act as effectively to improve their mood. This makes them susceptible to problems during the second half of the cycle. Anxiety is the most specific emotion a woman with PMDD experiences during the second half of her cycle. This makes sense biologically, since she cannot bind and use serotonin, the calming neurotransmitter, effectively.

TREATING PREMENSTRUAL SYNDROME AND PREMENSTRUAL DYSPHORIC DISORDER

Lifestyle changes that provide relief from PMS symptoms include:

- limiting daily salt intake
- limiting daily caffeine intake
- increasing daily exercise

Additional remedies comprise:

- *Calcium*, 600 milligrams, taken twice a day
- *Vitamin D*, 800 international units daily for PMS
- *Vitamin B₆*, less than 100 milligrams per day
- *Magnesium*, 200 milligrams three times a day

- *A low-fat vegan diet,* which decreases symptoms of PMS and PMDD by reducing the amount of estrogen in the blood. A high-fiber diet and roughage helps carry estrogens out of the body through the bile duct and the liver, soaking up estrogen and stabilizing estrogen levels.

  Note: To reduce PMS symptoms by following a strict low-fat vegan diet, it must be followed for the entire month, not just before the menstrual period. It includes avoiding oily salad dressings, French fries, potato chips, butter, margarine, cooking oils, and shortening in most cookies and pastries. It may take one to two months to notice the benefits. Other benefits may include loss of excess weight and a reduction in the number and severity of migraines.

- *Avoidance of caffeine,* which aggravates PMS. Staying away from coffee, tea, colas, and chocolate helps decrease PMS severity.

- *Use of PMS Escape.* Some studies have shown that PMS Escape, a specially formulated, complex carbohydrate-rich beverage, reduces psychological and appetite symptoms in those with PMS. It is available over the counter without a prescription in pharmacies and supermarkets. The drink increases the amount of the tryptophan, an amino acid, thus increasing the production of serotonin in the body; it also contains vitamin B_6.

- *Use of the fruit of* Vitex agnus castus. This fruit from the chaste berry tree is an herbal remedy that may treat PMS. It is available as Vitex or Chasteberry or Agnus Castus fruit extract. It may help treat the symptoms of PMS by antagonizing prolactin. In one study of 170 women with PMS, it decreased irritability, anger, and breast fullness. Vitex or Chasteberry may be effective but it may have unwanted effects as well. Chasteberry is reported to lower sex drive (I don't know if that is why "chaste" is in the name). Extensive studies of Vitex or Chasteberry have not been done, and the Food and Drug Administration (FDA) does not regulate this substance.

- *Evening of primrose oil,* which was used for years to enhance mood for those with PMS. More recent studies have not confirmed it is effective.

- *Cognitive behavioral therapy* (CBT), which is a helpful counseling approach. It provides tools to blunt the sharp increases in mood changes and anxiety.

Prescription Treatments for Premenstrual Syndrome and Premenstrual Dysphoric Disorder

In the past few years, a low-dose oral contraceptive (brand name Yaz) has been approved to treat PMDD and PMS. It also includes a diuretic ingredient that decreases bloating by promoting water excretion.

Prescription treatment of PMDD may include cyclic administration of certain antidepressant medications that control serotonin (selective serotonin reuptake inhibitors, or SSRIs). SSRI antidepressant medications may also be given daily for the entire cycle to assist with regulating mood, anger, and other signs of PMDD. SSRIs are very effective because they allow more serotonin to stay in the body. Treating PMS symptoms may not be effective if underlying medical or psychological disorders are not identified and addressed.

It may be helpful to try exercise, relaxation techniques, and vitamin and mineral supplements to treat PMS, prior to taking prescription medication. These approaches can also be effective for PMDD, although PMDD will often require a prescription for an SSRI.

Depression

As we have already seen, society influences a woman's feelings about postmenopause. Women ask themselves (consciously or not): What lies ahead after perimenopause? What can I look forward to?

A woman who lives in Japan will answer this question very differently from a woman in North America. Different cultures provide different environments for mature women; some are more welcoming than others. The Japanese greet a woman entering postmenopause with increasing respect and authority. In contrast, the youth-centered culture in North America is discouraging. There are negative connotations for women as they age, gain weight, or acquire wrinkles. Is it surprising that a North American woman is more likely to be depressed as she leaves behind her status, youth, and beauty?

Culture counts. Societies that respect women recognize that a woman's intellectual and social expertise increases with her age and experience. We have more to offer as we age; the value of our experience increases over time. This respect is associated with smoother perimenopause transitions. A woman who lives in a society where she garners more respect for her experience as she ages is less likely to have hot flashes, night sweats, and depression. More than one study has shown that those who are depressed during perimenopause will be more disrupted by hot flashes than those who are not depressed. Hot flashes can cause insomnia, and the resulting sleep deprivation can cause mood swings and memory issues—all are associated with high levels of depression.

Before puberty, the prevalence of depression is the same in girls and boys. As we become adults, anxiety disorders occur twice as often in women than men. And major depression is three times more common in women than men.

During the reproductive years, women have twice the frequency of depression of men. They are also more likely to have seasonal affective disorder (SAD). Throughout the world depression is more common in women than men. It is unclear how much this is due to women's willingness to talk about their feelings or their readiness to seek help. Anxiety disorders are also more common in women, including phobias, such as agoraphobia, and panic disorders, which are twice as common in women.

Women are more likely to be sexually abused as children. Abused children are more likely to suffer depression as adults. Women's higher rate of victimization also makes them prime candidates for depression.

Role overload is another contributor; with more than 50 percent of women working full time and still doing 70 percent of the housework and childcare, it's safe to say that the overload contributes to their sense of exhaustion, a factor for depression. Those with young children who work outside the home may experience role conflict.

Married men are less likely to be depressed than single men. In contrast, married women are more likely to be depressed than married men or single women. Married men, in general, have *fewer* demands on them than when they were single. For married women, the demands increase. Women's socialization involves looking after others and minimizing their own needs or dismissing them. And women who are financially disadvantaged are more likely to be depressed.

Frequency of Depression in Perimenopause

For women in perimenopause, risk factors for depression include gender, a history of depression in a first-degree relative (a parent, sibling, or child), and a prior episode of major depression. Other risk factors for depression include lack of social supports, significant stressful life events, and current alcohol or substance abuse.

Depression is more likely to occur in perimenopausal women with a history of PMS, PMDD, or postpartum depression. Early perimenopause (before age 40), surgical menopause at an early age, and short perimenopausal transition may also lead to depression. Women with these conditions have hormone shifts that are more dramatic and sudden, and there is less time to adjust to the low estrogen levels.

There also may be a link between depression, early perimenopause and postmenopause, and cigarette smoking. Cigarette smoking hastens postmenopause by one to two years.

While early perimenopause is a risk factor for depression, the reverse may also be true. A few studies even suggest the possibility that depressed women may have an earlier perimenopause. Their follicle-stimulating hormone (FSH) levels rise sooner than in other women.

Frequency of Depression in Postmenopause

Based on her biology, a postmenopausal woman is less susceptible to depression than when she was perimenopausal because her low estrogen levels are stable and steady. She has adapted to them.

Although postmenopausal women are biologically more resistant to depression than when they were perimenopausal, they are more likely to have major health issues, financial difficulties, or a lack of resources, or to become socially isolated. The pressures of society may be more potent. Postmenopausal women are more likely to lose a partner to death, become impoverished, or lack adequate physical activity and intellectual challenges as they age. Risk factors for late-life depression include social isolation; being widowed, divorced, or separated; having limited finances; having one or more serious medical conditions; chronic or uncontrolled pain; insomnia; or a compromise in mental functioning.

Depression should be addressed because it lowers the quality of life and impacts other medical conditions. Although the prevalence of depression is higher in women than men across all age groups, the difference is not as marked in elderly women, which is good news about the passage into postmenopause.

ARE YOU DEPRESSED?

Major depression means suffering from at least five of the following nine symptoms:

1. being in a depressed mood or losing interest or pleasure in normal activities for most of the day nearly every day for a minimum of two consecutive weeks
2. change in sleep (too much or too little)
3. excess appetite or loss of appetite
4. weight gain or weight loss
5. change in psychomotor activity (increased nervous energy or lethargy)
6. loss of energy
7. trouble concentrating
8. thoughts of worthlessness or guilt
9. thoughts about death or suicide

The following two-question screen for depression has been proposed by the U.S. Preventive Services Task Force (USPSTF):

1. Over the past two weeks have you felt down, depressed, or hopeless?

2. Over the past two weeks have you felt little interest or
   pleasure in doing things?

Any individual with a positive response to either question deserves a formal evaluation for depression. Depression must be diagnosed by a trained physician, social worker, or therapist. Over
90 percent of all depressed patients also have anxiety. An anxiety
disorder itself can also put a woman at higher risk for major depression. Anxiety can be diagnosed by a doctor and will respond to
antidepressant medications that have anti-anxiety features. Cognitive behavioral therapy is helpful, as well as general stress reduction techniques such as slow, deep breathing, meditation, and other
relaxation techniques.

You may not meet the criteria for major depression, but have
symptoms of depression that are significant because they persist
or because they impact your ability to function in your usual manner. Mild or moderate depression is even more prevalent than major
depression. When moderate depression is viewed as a disability or
a decrease in functioning, you realize that it is just as important to
treat it even if it does not qualify as a major depression by formal
psychiatric diagnosis.

Factors That Can Affect Depression

Depression is *not* a normal consequence of aging.

Thyroid disease can cause depression. Stress-induced subclinical
hypothyroidism can cause depression and should be evaluated with
a thyroid blood test.

Medical problems such as severe anemia, multiple sclerosis, Parkinson's disease, and Alzheimer's disease have also been found to
cause depression. Genetic factors play a role. A family history of depression can bestow on you a 70 percent lifetime inherited risk of
depression. The underlying basis of this may be an inherited sensitivity to stressful life events.

Medications that can cause depression include beta blockers, a
type of blood pressure medication, such as Propranolol or Atenolol.
Steroids can cause depression, as can chemotherapy.

Stroke victims and those who have suffered brain injury can have depression, as can individuals who have had breast cancer or other cancers.

Sadness and grief are a normal response to life events such as the death of a loved one or the changes in social status that may come with retirement. Depression can also result after transitioning from independent living to assisted or residential care or after losing physical function after an illness. Despite the increasing frequency of these types of losses with age, healthy elderly individuals who live independently in the community have a lower prevalence of clinical depression than the general adult community. Those older individuals who have medical illnesses may have higher rates of depression. Elderly patients who are hospitalized have a prevalence of depression over 30 percent. Those with stroke or heart attack or cancer have a rate of depression greater than 40 percent.

TREATMENT OPTIONS FOR DEPRESSION

Only 33 percent of women with depression receive treatment. The good news is that doctors are beginning to increase their awareness and efforts to identify and treat depression. As the stigma recedes, women who are depressed may be more receptive to acknowledging their depression and participating in treatment.

⚔ DAHLIA'S STORY ⚔

"Empty Nest" or Depressed?

"About a year ago, I had to admit that I had stopped participating in a number of activities I used to enjoy. For two years, since around the time my doctor said I had entered postmenopause, I just haven't felt the same enthusiasm for life in general. At my age, 53, I thought this was just part of life and the 'empty nest syndrome.' I used to volunteer five days a week teaching English as a second language and also worked for my congressman, but I gave that up. I've stopped writing letters to my daughter in college, an activity I used to enjoy every week. My husband and friends are concerned that I'm no longer 'myself,' and have encouraged me to see my doctor about it. When I saw my doctor, our conversation brought up the fact that I remembered my mother feeling blue when I left home to go away to college. I had to admit I hadn't felt this hopeless since the birth of my daughter, when I was diagnosed with postpartum depression.

"My doctor used a screening tool to assess me for depression, saying that my lack of motivation and withdrawal from activities also pointed to depression. He recommended cognitive behavioral therapy and counseling. I felt better after starting these, but also needed a prescription for an antidepressant to feel like myself again. It's been over a year now and I do feel like myself again. Eventually, after I felt like myself for six months, I was able to taper off the antidepressant medication under my doctor's supervision."

Treatment may include an over-the-counter remedy, prescribed medication for depression, and counseling/psychotherapy. Exercise has a therapeutic benefit as well; it can prevent or decrease depression.

Over-the-counter Remedy: St. John's Wort

St. John's wort is a natural remedy that affects levels of neurochemicals in the brain and is somewhat effective against depression, although its long-term effectiveness is not known. Because it is not

FDA-approved, when a box of St. John's wort was tested, these findings were reported:

- some pills contained too little of the active ingredient; there was not enough of it to help the user
- some of the pills contained no active ingredient at all
- some pills contained an excessive amount of the active ingredient that could be toxic or harmful to some individuals

This does not mean that St. John's wort is not effective. Nor does it mean that no one should try it. Just be forewarned that you may be taking a substance that has not been manufactured and marketed to a high quality standard. It should never be taken with prescription antidepressant medication, including SSRIs.

Side effects of St. John's wort can include gastrointestinal symptoms, dizziness, confusion, sedation, fatigue, and dry mouth. The skin can become overly sensitive to sunlight. It reduces the effectiveness of birth control pills as well as other medications, including those used to treat HIV and cancer.

Prescription Medications

Currently, there is a trend to prescribe medication for depression. Medications such as Wellbutrin, Prozac, Paxil, Effexor, Lexapro, or Cymbalta are usually effective. Smaller doses are often needed for those over 70 years old, as they may be more sensitive to medication. Normally, medications for depression can take six weeks to be effective. In those over 70 years old, the complete response may not occur until 12 or 16 weeks.

Antidepressant medications influence the brain and modulate neurotransmitters. In women, SSRIs are especially effective since they act on the neurotransmitter serotonin. As you read earlier in this chapter, serotonin is key to a woman's sense of well-being. For those who also suffer with anxiety, some combination of counseling, cognitive behavioral therapy (CBT), or medication to reduce anxiety may also be helpful.

Counseling/Psychotherapy

Counseling has taken a back seat to prescribing medicine for depression during the past decade. Today, it is common for a doctor to prescribe antidepressants and rely on their benefit alone. This is unfortunate. Counseling offers critical tools and approaches to difficult situations women face on multiple fronts. Providing a woman with different ways to frame her situation and address her challenges is invaluable, and providing her with different tools to do so is empowering. Treatment of general depression can include psychotherapy (talking therapy) or counseling. I find it fascinating that psychotherapy itself changes brain chemistry, in a different way than antidepressant medications do. So, the benefit of therapy is distinctly different from the benefit of taking an antidepressant. Many individuals benefit from both approaches.

One counseling approach that can be helpful is CBT. This technique uses specific interventions to make individuals more aware of their feelings, their circumstances, and their responses to them. They can also employ relaxation techniques to decrease anxiety in stressful situations. In my opinion, it's extremely important to get some counseling for depression to give the individual tools to deal with her stress or difficult situations she encounters. At times, though, counseling alone is not enough to treat the depression.

Older postmenopausal patients who are depressed may benefit greatly from psychotherapy. In addition to individual therapy, couples or family therapy may be helpful. CBT or problem-solving therapy can be offered over two to four months and produce significant results in older postmenopausal patients.

In perimenopause, volatile hormones increase the vulnerability to stress at a time when the number, type, and severity of stressful events multiply. In postmenopause, the hormone storm quiets, but social stressors increase. Ideally, each woman would have access to a trained social worker or psychologist to provide fresh perspective, tools, and support for dealing with the multiple challenges she faces at this time. Researchers have demonstrated that counseling is particularly effective in postmenopausal women.

Exercise

Exercise can alleviate depression but may take longer than antidepressant drugs. One study showed that 16 weeks of exercise provided the same relief from depression as an SSRI prescription. Exercise can be difficult to start or maintain when one is depressed. Nevertheless, it can be a very important intervention for those who are depressed and, more important, can help ward off future episodes of depression.

Using Estrogen to Treat Depression

Some women with depression in perimenopause may improve with estrogen treatment, but this is controversial. Treating depression with counseling and/or antidepressant medication is the well established approach. Taking estrogen does not help postmenopausal women with depression. In postmenopause estrogen levels have already stabilized.

Mental Decline in Postmenopause

Cognition embodies many aspects of our thinking. It includes mental processes such as reasoning, thinking, evaluating, remembering, perception, and problem-solving. It is separate from emotional reactions to events or automatic responses. It is the core of our most sophisticated and creative thinking, as well as our ability to analyze and plan.

Perimenopause and postmenopause are often associated with poor memory or more sluggish thinking. In one study more than 62 percent of women reported that their memory had worsened during perimenopause and early postmenopause. It is difficult to sort out the reasons for this shift in memory and mental processing because many factors could be responsible.

A common fear I hear expressed by colleagues as well as patients is that of "losing one's mind." This fear can be set off by losing keys or glasses (representing forgetfulness or short-term memory problems). Other triggers may include difficulty retrieving a person's name or finding the right words, an inability to focus or sustain attention, or becoming more distractible.

☪ NADIA'S STORY ☪

"I'm Losing My Mind"

"I'm 58, and had my last menstrual period six months ago. Although I no longer have hot flashes, I am concerned about my memory. It has definitely worsened over the past three years. I've always been organized. My memory lapses used to be associated with episodes of hot flashes, or my menstrual cycle—I was especially forgetful the week before my period. Now I'm even more frustrated. I forget my keys, lose my glasses, and cannot remember appointments I've made. I have difficulty retrieving names of people I know. These episodes of forgetfulness are more noticeable some months than others. I've begun to fear that I'm developing early Alzheimer's disease.

"I've spoken with my doctor about these concerns. Now that I no longer menstruate, the memory lapses are more random; they don't follow a cycle. My doctor said they are most likely related to the periodic low estrogen levels I still experience. He also wanted to review the number of things I try to keep track of. I keep a mental list of my priorities. Recently, I have taken on additional responsibilities at home and at work. This has increased the number of people to whom I'm accountable and the number of projects I need to monitor and complete. According to my doctor, the number of tasks is too great. I have information overload, and multitasking is making my memory problems worse. My doctor advised me to dedicate myself to one project or task at a time and to keep written lists of my priorities to decrease my mental load and improve my memory."

Nadia is an example of a healthy perimenopausal woman who is overextended, stressed, and multitasking. The multitasking is further taxing her memory and compromising her ability to think clearly. Once she narrows her focus and stops stretching herself too thin, she can function well again. For Nadia, as for many of us, focusing on one thing at a time, and keeping written records of commitments, may free up our brains to function more as we wish they would.

Memory Loss in Perimenopause

MEMORY LAPSES VERSUS COGNITIVE DECLINE

People who nurture their mental health and stay physically active can establish a mental reserve to draw on, so that losing some speed and capacity still leaves them with plenty of mental horsepower.

Permanent memory difficulties do not wax and wane. A woman whose memory worsens with her hot flashes, PMS, or PMDD, and then resolves or improves at other times, is not likely to have a cognitive disorder. If there is any doubt, a formal assessment for memory impairment may be performed by a neurologist, neuropsychologist, or other specialist. For example, a neuropsychologist may administer particular tests to determine if a memory problem is due to normal aging, dementia, brain injury, stress, anxiety or depression, attention disorder, or excess alcohol. If the diagnosis confirms a thought process problem, memory deficit, or other compromise in cognitive function, there are tools a specialist can provide to manage these difficulties.

While traveling years ago, I met an intelligent woman with a Ph.D. who had fallen and suffered a serious brain injury. She was able to function in her profession using the tools provided by a neuropsychologist that included organizational and memory aids as well as regular note-taking. She confided that she felt she was an even a better professional than before her accident because her notes were more specific and detailed.

Today, women interact with more individuals than ever on a daily basis. These interactions take place in person and remotely, by email, phone, or BlackBerry, with people who could be down the hall or in another time zone. Women maintain a growing number of pivotal social connections inside and outside their homes. I know that when I was single and working in obstetrics and gynecology, I was able to keep my schedule in my head for more than a week. I could also remember what I needed to bring to each different office or clinic as well as the hospital each day that week. I was also able to remember my social and on-call commitments without difficulty. Once I married and had children, the ability to keep the schedules of colleagues, spouse, children, and employees diminished. It was also easier when I only had to check my phone messages and my beeper, whereas now I have to check my email at home and at the office, the faxes at work, and the cell phone in addition to the beeper and the regular phone messages.

Today, there are too many "tools" for connecting. These tools generate overwhelming demands. Being available and accessible by cell phone and email 24/7 has not contributed to peace of mind, happiness, or satisfaction. Today, it is more difficult to end the day feeling satisfied that you have fulfilled your responsibilities and met your commitments. These additional burdens flood our minds and cloud our thinking. It's no wonder we can't remember things as well.

In addition to the hectic distractions we have, there are also other environmental and lifestyle choices that can decrease memory and compromise cognition. Alcohol kills brain cells, dulls thinking (when consumed in excess), and disrupts deep sleep. Lack of physical activity will also decrease cognition, as will lack of mental stimulation.

WHO GETS DEMENTIA AND ALZHEIMER'S AND WHY

Dementia is characterized by impairment of memory and one other cognitive domain such as aphasia (inability to speak), apraxia (inability to move), and agnosia (inability to think, reason, or remember). Dementia represents a decline from previous function severe enough to interfere with daily function and independence.

The strongest risk factor for dementia is age. This is particularly true for Alzheimer's disease. The estimated annual incidence of Alzheimer's disease goes from less than one percent for those age 65 to 69 years to one percent for 70- to 74-year-olds; 2 percent for 75- to 79-year-olds; slightly over 3 percent for 80- to 84-year-olds; and slightly over 8 percent for those 85 years and older.

In addition to age, family history can also be a risk factor for developing Alzheimer's disease. Those with a first-degree relative with dementia have a 10 to 30 percent increased risk of developing it.

Vascular dementia—disease of the blood vessels in the brain—is another risk factor for dementia and Alzheimer's. Still other risks that can increase the chance of getting Alzheimer's disease include diabetes, high blood pressure, heart disease, and smoking. High blood cholesterol also increases the risk of dementia in some studies. Diabetes has been associated with a 50 to 100 percent increase in the risk of Alzheimer's disease and dementia, and a 100 to 150 percent increase of vascular dementia. It's possible that diabetes impairs cognitive status mainly in those older than 70. The relationship between diabetes and the increased risk of dementia is not well understood and is being explored.

STAYING SHARP

Three lifestyle components help ward off dementia and Alzheimer's disease:

1. *An active social life.* Social interactions boost one's "resistance" to dementia or Alzheimer's. Interacting with others emotionally and intellectually stimulates brain function in a different way than solitary intellectual pursuits. Relating to different people challenges our social skills and forces our brain to read cues from people's expressions. One theory suggests that mental activity, learning, and social interaction prevent or reduce cognitive deficits by activating brain plasticity (flexibility) and enhancing synaptogenesis and neurogenesis (good communication in the nervous system).

2. *Mental challenges.* Intellectual stimulation can include activities such as learning a new language or reading in an area of interest such as history or literature. Doing puzzles (crossword puzzles, number puzzles, or jigsaw puzzles) challenges the brain, as does learning or practicing a musical instrument. Higher levels of education are associated with a reduced risk of Alzheimer's disease. There is more developed brain capacity so the reserve brain function is more generous. Even in the face of some loss of brain function with age, there is plenty of mental capacity left to function well.

3. *Regular physical activity.* Physical activity, including both exercise and daily activities, correlates with good cognition. Physical activity increases blood flow to the brain as well as the rest of the body. It enhances vascular and non-neuronal brain components that support neurons. The blood flow to the brain is better, and the nerve centers are healthier.

There are other theories as well. The vascular hypothesis suggests that social, mental, and physical activity prevents or reduces dementia and Alzheimer's disease through reduction of heart disease and stroke.

The stress hypothesis suggests that active individuals maintain a more positive emotional state. Reduced stress leads to a lower susceptibility to Alzheimer's disease. In contrast, increased stress changes the feedback to the adrenal glands, a stress hormone center. The adrenal glands interact with cortisol stress receptors in the brain. As the imbalance worsens, the stress receptors in the hippocampus portion of the brain are affected, and this part of the brain actually atrophies and shrinks, impairing mental function, including reasoning, memory, and judgment.

Difficulties in studying the impact of lifestyle and activity on dementia include the fact that those with higher cognitive activity and functioning have higher baseline intellectual function. Even with Alzheimer's, they are still left with adequate cognitive skills to avoid the diagnosis of dementia. This implies that keeping active intellectually and staying intellectually challenged lessens the effect of dementia if it does occur.

Just as these positive interactions and activities stimulate the brain, there are activities that compromise brain function. They include poor quality sleep or inadequate amount of sleep; alcohol consumption, which destroys brain cells; and stress.

⚥ ESTHER'S STORY ⚥

Making the Move to Assisted Living

"I'm 68 years old and lived alone for years with no problems, even though my closest family member is 45 minutes away. I have a bad

hip that's been limiting my activity so I no longer go to my stretching class at the YMCA three times a week. Since the hip has become painful, I have trouble getting in and out of the car and have not gone to lunch with my friends. I've had trouble paying my bills and I make more mistakes doing the arithmetic. Plus I've been misplacing the bills and actually forgetting to pay them. Occasionally I forget to call to have my groceries delivered. My daughter visited and noticed there was no food in the refrigerator, and she found unpaid bills in unusual places in the apartment. She was alarmed and scheduled a medical evaluation for me. A neurologist diagnosed 'early dementia' after performing a history and physical exam. Testing showed that I had had a transient ischemic attack, or 'mini stroke.' I agreed to move to an assisted living community and to build regular activity back into my schedule. Since walking was difficult for me, I agreed to do aqua jogging. This did not put pressure on my hip joint. Even though I don't swim, I've been able to participate in this activity, which involves wearing a float around my waist and moving my legs in the water to music. The doctor says the physical activity has improved my mental and physical health, and the increased social interaction in the assisted living community has also been beneficial."

Estrogen and Cognition

The Women's Health Initiative Memory Study (WHIMS) was part of the Women's Health Initiative (WHI). (For more background information about WHI in general, see Chapter 3.) In this portion of the WHI study, 4,000 postmenopausal women, with no dementia at the start of the study, were followed on a combination of estrogen and progesterone. Postmenopausal women, age 65 and older, were at higher risk for dementia after taking estrogen and progesterone for four years. Hormone treatment did not prevent mild cognitive impairment in these women.

Another large study in the United Kingdom, the Women's International Study of Long Duration Estrogen after Menopause (WISDOM), was also stopped due to concerns about estrogen promoting dementia in older women.

It has become clear that estrogen is not beneficial to women over

65 years old and more than 10 years from their final menstrual period: it will not help their memory at this age and stage of menopause.

Neither of these studies refutes the benefit of prescribing estrogen for younger women (under age 60) in perimenopause or early postmenopause who have had their final menstrual period within 10 years or less. In this group of women, estrogen has not increased the risk of dementia, and may well decrease it. No one is recommending prescribing estrogen for this purpose but only for relief of debilitating hot flashes. If a younger woman with severe hot flashes meets criteria to take low-dose estrogen and wishes to take it, she will not increase her risk of dementia.

Estrogen may help ward off cognitive decline in some individuals who start taking it before they turn 60, but it is not prescribed for this purpose. In contrast, starting or restarting systemic estrogen in a woman over 60 is not advisable; it may worsen her mental health.

RESOURCES

AARP (www.aarp.org). You may be too young to join, but you are eligible for membership in this nonprofit when you turn 50. *AARP the Magazine* and the corresponding website cover wellness tips for mental and physical health in addition to a wide range of other topics that impact your quality of life.

Beating the Menopause Blues: Distinguishing Mood Swings and Depression. This tool is available to download and print on the North American Menopause Society website, www.menopause.org/. Look under Consumer Education Materials. Last accessed December 14, 2008.

Brehony, Kathleen. *Awakening at Midlife: Realizing Your Potential for Growth and Change.* New York: Riverhead Books, 1996. This book captures the imagination and provokes you to think of new possibilities that will break you out of your current mold.

Gordon, Barry, M.D., Ph.D., and Lisa Berger. *Intelligent Memory: Improve the Memory That Makes You Smarter.* New York: Viking, 2003.

LaRoche, Loretta. *Kick Up Your Heels . . . Before You're Too Short to Wear Them: How to Live a Long, Healthy, Juicy Life.* Carlsbad, CA: Hay House, 2007. If you ever have a chance to hear Loretta LaRoche give a talk, do not miss out. You may laugh for a week. The book will keep you laughing even longer. And there is research to show that those who laugh live longer.

Legato, Marianne. *Eve's Rib: The New Science of Gender-Specific Medicine and How It Can Save Your Life.* New York: Harmony Books, 2002. This Columbia University medical professor is an international expert on gender medicine and helped start the field. Her book provides insights into how the structure and function of men's and women's brains differ. And yes, the men's brains are bigger, but the different regions do not communicate with each other as well.

More magazine (www.more.com). As its headline reads, this magazine "celebrates women over 40." I was a fan long before the North American Menopause Society gave the magazine's editor an award for excellent health coverage in 2007. It has articles about health, fitness, relationships, fashion, finance, and careers, as well as books and movies. © Meredith Corporation.

Sheehy, Gail. *New Passages: Mapping Your Life across Time.* New York: Random House, 1995. Written by a world-class expert, this book covers life's transitions.

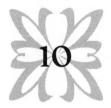

10

Successful Sleep

In the past, sleep problems in a midlife woman were attributed to hot flashes or night sweats. The medical community has only now become aware that some sleep disorders are specific to perimenopause, while others are more common with increasing age. Perimenopausal women find it harder to fall asleep. When they do get to sleep, the quality of their sleep is less satisfying.

The two most common types of sleep disorders associated with menopause and aging are insomnia (inadequate sleep) and sleep apnea (disturbed breathing during sleep). A woman who has premature menopause at age 30 might be at higher risk for apnea or insomnia because of her menopause status, even though she has not yet reached midlife. Independent of age, perimenopause influences the risk of insomnia even if a woman does not have hot flashes, although hot flashes and night sweats can increase insomnia.

While the relationship between changing hormone levels and insomnia is unclear, researchers have found a clear association between changing hormone levels and sleep apnea. There are other sleep disorders, such as restless leg syndrome, but their relationship to perimenopause and postmenopause is not well established, so they are beyond the scope of this chapter.

The Biology of Sleep

There are two phases of sleep that represent two distinct activity states. The first is non-rapid eye movement (NREM) sleep. During the NREM sleep, the body repairs tissues and builds bones and muscle. It's also a time when the immune system is strengthened. The second is rapid eye movement (REM) sleep. REM sleep is the deep sleep when dreams occur. REM usually begins 90 minutes after falling asleep, but the first period of REM lasts only 10 minutes. Each time a person enters REM after that, it will last longer, up to one hour. Normally, the body will cycle between the two stages.

As a woman ages, deep sleep is less intense and the periods of deep sleep become shorter. An infant spends 50 percent of its sleep time in REM, while an adult will spend only 20 percent of her sleep time there. So aging will produce both a shorter time in REM and less deep sleep even while in REM.

There is a popular misconception that older people don't need as much sleep. Although a mature adult needs the same amount of sleep as she gets older (seven to eight hours), her body spends less time in each period of sleep. For men and women, the quality of sleep also changes with age; becoming lighter.

Many people are sleep deprived during the work-week, then try to make up for it by "sleeping in" on weekends. Unfortunately, this doesn't work. The body adapts poorly to missed sleep and cannot "make up" the loss.

If you are sleep deprived, there is nothing else that can meet your body's needs. You can *function* on less sleep, for example, by drinking coffee or tea, or eating chocolate, but your body doesn't need caffeine, it needs sleep. Your body cannot adapt to less sleep than it really needs. Those who try to get by on less than seven hours of sleep on a regular basis are taxing their bodies.

Sleep patterns change with age, but quality sleep is critical to maintaining optimum health. When evaluating your sleep, it's helpful to look at the quality as well as the quantity. Quality sleep includes a certain amount of deep sleep. Both perimenopausal and postmenopausal women have problems with the quality of their sleep after they have fallen asleep.

The relationship between estrogen, serotonin, and sleep is being explored. So far researchers have found that estrogen influences serotonin production. Serotonin is needed to produce melatonin, the "sleep hormone." Deficiencies in serotonin and/or melatonin disrupt the length, timing, and quality of sleep. They also disrupt the body's internal clock.

Sleep and Weight

Sleep loss leads to hunger. It affects metabolism in a way that makes it more difficult to lose or even maintain weight. Sleep loss affects the stress hormone cortisol. Cortisol plays a role in regulating appetite, so sleep-deprived women will feel hungry even when they are full. In addition, a sleep-deprived woman will store more fat because her body's ability to metabolize carbohydrates is compromised. Her body will overproduce insulin, leading to the storage of more body fat. The insulin will not be as effective, and her body will not respond to it as it should. This is when she may develop insulin resistance.

The hormones ghrelin and leptin work together to control appetite as well. Ghrelin, produced in the gastrointestinal tract, stimulates hunger. Leptin, produced in fat cells, decreases hunger. When you don't get enough sleep, your levels of leptin are lower, allowing your hunger to grow out of control. Your levels of ghrelin rise, stimulating your hunger when you might otherwise feel satisfied. With sleep deprivation, high ghrelin and low leptin create the perfect scenario for overeating—and it occurs after as little as two nights of sleep deprivation. People who sleep less than seven hours per night are more likely to be overweight. In fact, in one study, those who slept the fewest hours per night weighed the most.

During deep sleep, growth hormone is released. Growth hormone helps the body regulate its proportion of fat and muscle. This is another way that sleep affects weight.

Thinner people sleep better than heavier people. Researchers looking at patients who had lost weight or undergone weight loss surgery noticed a dramatic improvement in the quality of their sleep after a significant weight loss. For example, 82 percent of obese patients snore, but only 14 percent snore after losing weight. While 33 percent of obese women suffer from sleep apnea, only 2 percent of these women have sleep apnea after weight loss. Abnormal daytime sleepiness and poor sleep quality also resolve dramatically with weight loss.

Burning the Candle at Both Ends

"I work full time and also care for my elderly parents. I've always heard that you need less sleep as you get older, and at 54 I'm finding I'm getting by on a lot less sleep. In order to fulfill all my obligations, I usually do chores until 11:00 at night and get up at 5:00 in the morning. I get a Grande coffee at 3:00 p.m., and this mid-afternoon caffeine surge keeps me going. Dinner is my big meal of the day, which I usually eat around 8:30 at night or later. I often have trouble unwinding after my long, busy day, so I usually have two glasses of wine with dinner to help me relax. When I have a chance to exercise, it's usually 9:00 at night, while I watch TV. I never feel rested, even if I sleep later on the weekends.

"At my annual physical, I mentioned to my doctor how exhausted I was. My blood pressure was normal, but I was still 15 pounds overweight. I lost 10 pounds since my previous visit, by adding exercise to my routine. My doctor ordered a thyroid blood test and a hematocrit to check for anemia. They were normal. My physical exam was also normal. The doctor asked more details about my sleep habits. He advised me to develop better sleep routines and said if that did not help, I should schedule another appointment and we could talk about other alternatives, like a formal sleep study to see if there was a medical cause for the poor quality of sleep I was experiencing. I learned that many of my routines put me at risk for insomnia."

Insomnia

Insomnia is the most common sleep disorder. As many as one out of every three women have insomnia. Especially in women, the association with depression, anxiety, and other psychological mood changes is very strong.

The risk of insomnia increases with age. Before age 40, men and women have similar experiences with insomnia. Once a woman is over 40, she has a much higher risk of insomnia than a man her age.

Beginning with perimenopause, women also have a higher risk of insomnia, even without hot flashes or night sweats. As you read in the previous chapter, women have a higher risk of depression than their male counterparts. In women, depression itself contributes to the high risk of insomnia. Finally, a woman over 40 is much more likely to have a psychological cause for her insomnia, such as depression, than a man over 40 with insomnia.

Insomnia involves difficulty falling asleep and/or staying asleep. It is characterized by:

- difficulty falling asleep
- awakening frequently during the night and having trouble going back to sleep
- early awakening, or waking up before you planned to end your sleep period
- feeling tired when you wake up
- sleepiness during the day
- problems with concentration and memory as well as irritability

Sleep problems typically begin or worsen during perimenopause and postmenopause independent of age. Add to that the fact that aging itself also affects men's and women's ability to sleep. This places even more importance on improving sleep habits to avoid insomnia. For optimum mental and physical functioning, plan on seven or eight hours of good quality sleep each night.

A National Sleep Foundation poll of American women showed 70 percent of them reported sleep problems some nights. They looked at insomnia reported by different women who woke up not feeling refreshed, woke up too early, or were unable to go back to sleep. While 33 percent of women ages 18 to 24 reported sleep problems, 48 percent of women ages 55 to 64 reported sleep problems—an increase of nearly 50 percent.

Primary insomnia is not related to a discernable cause. *Secondary insomnia* has an identified cause related to medications or illness. Insomnia can be a chronic/long-term issue or an acute/recent one. Chronic insomnia, lasting more than a month, is extremely common in women who are depressed or anxious. It can also occur in those experiencing chronic stress or those with pain at night. Before you or your doctor blame menopause for your insomnia, it is important to have a thorough evaluation of the quality and quantity of your sleep, and to have an assessment for depression.

Some possible causes of insomnia include:

- medication for allergies or a cold
- blood pressure medication
- asthma medications
- antidepressants
- thyroid disease
- depression
- job-related stress
- relationship stress
- moving
- death of a family member or close friend
- jet lag
- changing work shifts
- a new physical discomfort (such as pain from an injury or arthritis)

Decreasing emotional stress or modifying the medication regimen may help. One approach to consider is cognitive behavioral therapy (CBT). In this instance, CBT is used as a form of short-term therapy to correct thoughts and beliefs that are not helpful to an individual and reroutes one's thinking to a more positive, adaptive path. It is available through trained therapists.

Sleep Apnea

Sleep apnea is a term for disturbed breathing patterns that occur when there is an interruption in breathing during nighttime sleep. People stop breathing on multiple occasions during the night, sometimes as often as 300 times. In some cases, an obstruction in the upper airway prevents air from flowing freely into the lungs. When someone has sleep apnea, carbon monoxide can build up in the blood because it is not being properly oxygenated.

There are three types of sleep apnea:

1. *Central sleep apnea (CSA).* Normally, the brain automatically instructs the muscles involved in breathing to take a breath. Central sleep apnea occurs when the brain does not send the signal to the muscles to take a breath, and there is no muscular effort to do so. As a result, breathing stops.
2. *Obstructive sleep apnea (OSA).* This occurs when the brain sends the signal to the muscles, and the muscles try to take a breath, but the airway is blocked (obstructed), usually due to the collapse of soft tissue at the back of the throat.
3. *Mixed sleep apnea* (both central sleep apnea and obstructive sleep apnea).

Sleep apnea is common in those who snore and who are sleepy during the day. It is also more common in people with central obesity. Type 2 diabetes, insulin resistance, and polycystic ovarian disease are conditions also associated with a higher risk of sleep apnea. Early perimenopause and postmenopause are risk factors for sleep apnea. Advancing age is a risk factor for sleep apnea, up to age 60.

Sleep apnea is associated with heart attacks, heart failure, stroke, obesity, depression and mood disorders, excess daytime sleepiness, injury from accidents, poor quality of life, and alterations in sex hormones. Blood pressure and sleep apnea are very closely related. Their relationship is as perplexing as that of the old "chicken and egg" conundrum. High blood pressure is a major risk factor for sleep apnea. Sleep apnea exacerbates high blood pressure.

Sleep-disordered breathing becomes more common in midlife. As a woman ages, the muscle tone in her neck weakens. She is more likely to snore or get disrupted breathing during sleep. Researchers have been trying to determine whether hormone changes during perimenopause cause sleep disturbances.

Sleep apnea is confirmed using specialized testing and evaluation by a sleep expert. The testing may include a formal sleep study done at a sleep center, where breathing, body movements, heart rate, and oxygen levels are monitored.

There is relief for those with sleep apnea. Controlled positive airway pressure (CPAP) is a therapeutic technique where air pressure is used to keep the airway open at the back of the throat. A CPAP machine pumps slightly pressurized air into a face mask or nasal pillows that sit in your nostrils while you sleep, keeping air flowing into your lungs.

Apnea also diminishes with weight loss and exercise. Apnea does not respond to hormone treatment.

⚜ MARLA'S STORY ⚜

Sleep Apnea

"Six months ago, I was diagnosed with obstructive sleep apnea, and it's nice to have an explanation for why I was having trouble concentrating, and why it was always so hard for me to lose weight. I was at least 50 pounds over my ideal body weight, even though I walked regularly and went to the gym twice a week. I was having trouble sleeping, but it wasn't from night sweats, like those that bother many friends my age. My husband tells me that I snore at night, but I am unaware of it. During a recent physical examination, I was told I have high blood pressure, and laboratory tests showed I had a high cholesterol. Fortunately, my doctor asked if any members of my family have sleep apnea. My father does, and my brother is undergoing a sleep test next month. So, she recommended I have a sleep evaluation. The sleep study showed I stopped breathing 30 times an hour. My doctor explained how this compromises and interrupts my deep sleep. She sent me to a sleep specialist, who reviewed my sleep study results, examined my nose, throat, and lungs, and prescribed a controlled positive airway pressure (CPAP) mask, which I wear to keep my airway open at night. After six months of using it, I've been able to lose weight! I have also successfully modified my portion sizes—something I always had trouble doing—and am continuing with regular physical activity. My mood and concentration *are also vastly improved since the sleep apnea has been treated with CPAP."*

Both men and women have less ability to get quality sleep with advanced age. As you read earlier, they have less deep REM sleep. One reason for the reduced amount of deep REM sleep is the increase in stress hormones such as cortisol, and in middle age, the body becomes more sensitive to cortisol.

The Effects of Hormone Treatment on Sleep

Estrogen may improve the quality of sleep in perimenopausal women, but not in women who have been in postmenopause for more than a few years. Treating debilitating hot flashes or night sweats with estrogen during perimenopause may help prevent sleep apnea. However, estrogen will not treat sleep apnea once it is present.

How to Have a Good Night's Sleep

If you cannot fall asleep in 20 to 30 minutes, sleep experts recommend that you get out of bed and do something else. Avoid lying in bed worrying. It's best to go to a different room for a relaxing activity and return to bed when you feel you can go to sleep. This way, your body associates your bedroom with sleeping (or sex) instead of tossing and turning.

Sleep quality is influenced by sleep habits and routines (in medical lingo, "sleep hygiene"). Beneficial sleep routines are healthy measures that can be tried to improve the quality of sleep, especially if you turn them into habits. Healthy sleep habits help your body ritualize the pre-sleep preparation in anticipation of quality rest and adequate sleep. If you are experiencing sleep problems, try these measures first for a restful sleep. If you still wake up tired, your physician can determine what aspects of the sleep process are disturbed. Problems like difficulty falling asleep, difficulty staying asleep through the night, and waking up before you plan to are all likely to respond to improved sleep habits.

Following are some steps you may take to improve your sleep.

Food Intake

Avoid spicy foods for dinner, and avoid eating within three hours of bedtime. If you have gastritis (inflamed stomach lining) or gastroesophageal reflux disease, or GERD (stomach acid rising up into the esophagus and irritating the lining of the food tube), you are prone to acid reflux when you lie down. Avoid going to bed extremely hungry. If you do not have GERD, have a small snack that includes tryptophan, an amino acid that is sleep-inducing. Milk has tryptophan, as do bananas. An Australian study showed that eating starchy carbohydrates four hours before bedtime helped individuals fall asleep faster. The carbohydrates increased tryptophan and serotonin. Carbohydrate-rich snacks would include a bowl of oatmeal, yogurt with a graham cracker, or an apple with some pretzels. Some people benefit from a cup of soothing herb tea. Avoid protein or a heavy meal at bedtime. Eating too much sugar at bedtime will cause your blood sugar levels to spike, then fall.

Exercise

Exercising regularly helps the quality of sleep. The timing of the exercise may negatively affect your sleep, though, so it's best not to exercise vigorously within three hours of bedtime. Exercise decreases stress, increases energy and overall well-being, and may help you to sleep well as long as you have not exercised too close to your bedtime.

Caffeine

Caffeine can make it hard to fall asleep, even 12 hours later. Half the amount of caffeine that you consume is cleared in 6 hours. Drinking large quantities of caffeine and/or consuming caffeine later in the day ensures that the caffeine will be in your system after you go to sleep. Caffeine will increase the number of times that you wake up at night, as well as decreasing the total amount of time that you sleep. If you are sensitive to caffeine, avoid coffee, tea, chocolate, and soda. Green tea does not have as much caffeine as black tea, but it is not caffeine-free. Try slowly cutting back on caffeine over time and see if your sleep improves. (See Chapter 2 for tips about tapering your coffee consumption.)

FLUIDS

Dehydration is associated with insomnia, so make sure you stay hydrated during the day. Some people can wake up to go to the bathroom and go right back to sleep again, while others never recover from the interruption. If nighttime urination is a problem for you, stop drinking fluids two hours before bedtime, or finish drinking most of your fluids at dinner.

SMOKING/NICOTINE

Nicotine disrupts the quality of sleep. Although low doses of nicotine from smoking are relaxing and produce a mild sedative effect, high doses of nicotine have a stimulant effect in the bloodstream at night.

ALCOHOL

Initially, alcohol (beer, wine, or liquor) is calming, relaxing, and slightly sedating. As alcohol is metabolized or processed, however, withdrawal causes poor sleep quality and sleep disruption. Deep REM sleep is disrupted and compromised by alcohol. Even two to three hours after the alcohol is completely eliminated, there is an after-effect of sleep disruption and awakening.

NAPS

A daytime nap can interfere with your overnight quality of sleep. If you have trouble sleeping at night, avoid daytime naps. If a nap is unavoidable, it's helpful to limit it to 30 minutes or less. That way you won't fall into a deep sleep, but you'll wake up refreshed.

Pre-sleep Rituals

De-stressing for 10 to 60 minutes before bed is helpful. Relaxing pre-sleep rituals cue the body that it's time to wind down. These could include a warm bath, light reading, relaxing, or meditating. Some people can fall asleep watching late-night TV, but most experts advise taking the television out of the bedroom. They also advise using the bed for sleep and sex alone, and not other activities. For those with sleep problems, training your body to associate the bed with sleep and sex alone helps ingrain good sleep habits. Avoid stimulating or disturbing practices such as reading or viewing upsetting news, having stressful discussions with family members, or doing demanding work. Some experts advise not using any type of electronics, such as working on your computer, and avoiding TV for an hour before bedtime because computer use and TV watching stimulate the brain and keep it from unwinding. Falling asleep is associated with a drop in body temperature. If you take a warm—not hot—shower or bath, you can hasten this process.

Making a Schedule and Sticking to It

Select a regular time to go to bed and a regular time to wake up seven days a week. Yes, even on weekends. This helps your body habituate to a healthy sleep routine and gets it accustomed to having enough sleep beginning at a particular time.

Sleep Environment

Make sure your bed and pillow are comfortable. Open the window for some fresh air. Turn down the thermostat; it's easier to sleep in a cool room. Use layers to adjust to the room temperature so that you're comfortable. For some, this will mean no night clothes and only a light blanket. For others, this may mean breathable night clothes and a sheet or an electric blanket that regulates your part of the bed. A pleasant sleep environment is dark and quiet. Darkness not only hides distractions but is also essential for your body to make melatonin. Liquid crystal displays (LCDs) on alarm clocks or other electronics should be covered or turned away from you. Room darkening shades may be helpful. Eye masks may help. Ear plugs may help in more active households on different timetables. Use a small night light if necessary.

Some women have their sleep disrupted by restless leg syndrome (their legs move uncontrollably during sleep). This can be associated with iron deficiency and can be diagnosed with a sleep study.

Certain medications, such as steroid medications or over-the-counter cold remedies or allergy remedies, can disrupt sleep. Thyroid disease can also decrease sleep quality.

Pets probably should not join you in bed, unless you find them soothing. They move about, and allergies to pets may influence the quality of your sleep.

RESOURCES

American Sleep Apnea Association (www.sleepapnea.org).

Medline Plus; Sleep Disorders (www.nlm.nih.gov/medlineplus/sleepdis orders). This site is sponsored by the U.S. National Library of Medicine and the National Institutes of Health. It is a comprehensive site that has a great deal of information about various sleep disorders as well as links to additional resources. It is available in 12 languages.

National Sleep Foundation (www.sleepfoundation.org).

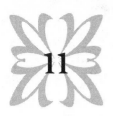

Better Bones

I f you're a physically active woman with no bone pain, you're likely to assume that your bones are healthy and strong. You may be right. If you are in postmenopause, however, you may be seriously mistaken. Postmenopause sets into motion silent, invisible changes that weaken bones over time, even if you continue to look strong and healthy. These silent changes take place, to one degree or another, in each and every postmenopausal woman. This chapter exposes the silent, invisible process of bone thinning.

For many, the thin bones of osteoporosis may be prevented. Lifestyle choices as well as adequate amounts of mineral and vitamin supplements can help the majority of women prevent this weakening and thinning of the bones. For those who already have osteoporosis or have suffered a fragility fracture, thin bones can be strengthened using prescription medication. Whenever possible, weak bones should be strengthened before they break.

A national survey in 2008 revealed that American men and women age 45 and over are not discussing bone health with their health providers. And primary care providers are also not as concerned about osteoporosis as needed to prevent this condition. Given this new statistic, 55 percent of people over age 50 are living with osteoporosis, or are at risk for osteoporosis. This survey also demonstrated that 40 percent of women age 45 and older had little or no concern about osteoporosis and its impact on their daily lives and their independence. After all the media coverage of osteoporosis, this is quite surprising and disturbing. Since one in two women over 50 years old will break a bone due to osteoporosis in her remaining lifetime, awareness of bone health and concern about prevention and treatment need to increase.

Why Should I Worry about My Bones?

For your grandmother or great-grandmother, bone strength was not a big concern since they spent less time in postmenopause, when dramatic bone loss starts. Now that women are expected to spend a third of their lives in postmenopause, bone health has become a major issue.

In the past decade, there have been substantial advances in bone research. We now know a great deal more than we used to about bone health and bone thinning. The new information has enhanced your doctor's ability to help you have healthy bones.

Achieving or maintaining bone health is critically important to you as a postmenopausal woman. Healthy bones are essential to your physical health and well-being, as well as your independence and ability to be self-sufficient. Bone health influences the quality of life you will enjoy from the time of your last menstrual period until the end of your life.

Osteoporosis: The Scary Statistics

Osteoporosis, a condition of weak bones or having bones so thin that they are at high risk of breaking, is increasingly common. According to the National Osteoporosis Foundation, one out of every two women over age 50 will have an osteoporosis-related fracture in her remaining lifetime. In fact, a woman's risk of hip fracture is equal to her *combined* risk of breast, uterine, and ovarian cancer. In 2005, osteoporosis was responsible for more than two million fractures, including hip fractures, vertebral spine fractures, wrist fractures, and pelvic fractures as well as those at other sites.

Women with mildly thin bones, the condition called osteopenia, should still pay attention to prevention measures because the majority of fractures occur in women with osteopenia (low bone mass), not osteoporosis. This means that *all* perimenopausal and post-menopausal women should attend to their bone health from a prevention stance as well as treatment. You should consider your bone health seriously; it's key to your longevity.

How serious is it? Once you break a bone in your hip or spine, you are likely to lose your mobility and independence, severely compromising your quality of life. One in five of those who were ambulatory before their hip fracture requires long-term care afterward. Six months after a hip fracture, only 15 percent of hip fracture patients can walk across a room unaided. Half of the women over age 70 who have an osteoporotic hip fracture never regain the degree of function they enjoyed before the fracture. Women who do not regain their pre-fracture level of functioning need outside assistance in their home or require nursing home care.

Osteoporosis can be life threatening. If you get an osteoporotic fracture, you may die prematurely from complications that follow. Some of the complications are related to being bedridden. Once bedridden, a postmenopausal woman often develops other medical problems, such as pneumonia, particularly with advancing age. About 24 percent of hip fracture patients age 50 and over die in the year following their fracture. For women over 70, this figure goes up to 40 percent.

It is tempting to rationalize that these numbers do not apply to you personally. Neither my female colleagues, my patients—who usually walk into my office under their own steam to see me, even if they are in their eighties or nineties—nor I envision becoming victims of osteoporosis. But statistics show that 50 percent of us are wrong. You may not experience a fracture yourself, but half of your female friends and relatives over age 50 will have osteoporotic fractures.

Osteopenia

Osteopenia is the term for low bone mass that may progress to osteoporosis but is not yet that severe. Osteopenia is a diagnosis made from measuring bone thickness on a DXA, or Dual Energy X-ray Absorptiometry, test. Usually, a woman with a mild degree of bone thinning as seen in osteopenia may choose lifestyle modifications alone to improve her bone strength. In contrast, a woman with severe bone thinning usually requires prescription medication to strengthen the bones, in addition to lifestyle modifications.

A SILENT PROBLEM

Unlike a broken bone resulting from a traumatic fall or accident, an osteoporotic fracture occurs due to weak bones, often without warning. The fragile state of the thinner, weaker bones is usually invisible to a woman and her doctor. It is not necessary to fall down or to experience a physical trauma such as a car accident to get an osteoporotic fracture. Weak bones in the spine or hip may break even in the absence of a fall or injury.

Most women never realize they have critically thin bones until they actually get an osteoporotic fracture because osteoporosis is painless until a fracture occurs. A fracture that occurs without trauma or a fall is called a "fragility fracture" or a "non-traumatic fracture." Osteoporotic spine fractures can also cause height loss and, in severe cases, may compromise lung capacity.

Natural Bone Formation

There are two major types of bone in the body: trabecular bone and cortical bone. These two types of bone respond to postmenopause differently.

Trabecular bone is more porous bone, like a spider web, which is found in the central core of a bone. It is the central inner marrow you see when you break a chicken bone in half. Trabecular bone weakens with the loss of connections, much as a spider web weakens when it is torn or broken.

Cortical bone is the hard, smooth compact layer of bone that covers the outer surface. Cortical bone is affected by muscle strain as well as changes in blood supply, nerve connections, and vitamin D levels.

Just as skin replenishes itself throughout a lifetime, bone is restored by a process called remodeling. Older bone is removed, and newer bone is laid down. The two types of bones remodel differently.

Trabecular bone remodels quickly, showing a 25 percent turnover within a year, while cortical bone changes slowly, at 2 percent. In trabecular bone the rapid changes may produce loss of struts and connections, weakening the structure and compromising the bone strength.

It's tempting to think that once adulthood is reached, the bones are formed for life and remain unchanged. In fact, although we no longer gain any height, our bones continue to form, dissolve, and re-form throughout our lifetime.

Bones are built by osteoblast cells that lay down the bone, forming new bone. Osteoclast cells dissolve or clear away bone. Both osteoblasts and osteoclasts are involved in remodeling because both bone formation and bone removal are part of this process.

Early in life, bone formation is rapid and exceeds the amount of bone that dissolves. During the teenage years, bone is built quickly and then stabilizes. In the stable phase of bone building, when a woman is in her twenties, bone formation and bone dissolving are in balance. Then, as a woman progresses into her late thirties, the balance begins to shift. Closer to postmenopause, the osteoclast cells dissolve bone faster than it is formed. More bone is lost than built.

Bone Thinning

A slow process of bone thinning is associated with aging. Both men and women experience slow bone thinning as a gradual process that generally starts around age 35. Unlike men, though, postmenopausal women experience two types of bone loss.

In addition to the slow bone loss associated with aging, a woman has a second type of bone loss when she enters postmenopause. Because of low estrogen, a rapid decline in bone strength and thickness occurs during the first five years after her final menstrual period. A woman can lose up to 20 percent of her bone mass during the first five to seven years in postmenopause. In addition to these two bone-thinning processes encountered by all postmenopausal women, an individual woman may have additional risk factors that will make her bones weaker or thinner before those of her peers.

The rapid bone loss seen in early postmenopause mainly affects trabecular bone first. This is why women commonly fracture the vertebrae of their spine long before men do. Vertebrae consist mostly of trabecular bone and are most sensitive to the estrogen loss of early postmenopause. Stress fractures of the vertebrae in the spine and radius bone of the forearm are the first to occur.

After the initial rapid weakening of the bone, there is a slower decrease in bone density and strength that continues for the remainder of a woman's lifetime. This slow, age-related bone thinning, which occurs in both men and women, is called Type 2, or senile, osteoporosis. This affects both trabecular bones and cortical bones equally. A woman's anatomy, particularly as these changes take place, puts her at greater risk of fracture than a man. Her lighter, more delicate female skeleton is more vulnerable to damage and breakage than the heavier, more robust male skeleton.

Bone loss in the early postmenopausal period results from the rate of remodeling or bone turnover, which increases by 300 to 400 percent at this time, wrecking havoc with bone quality. Increased bone turnover compromises bone quality on a microscopic level. It decreases bone mass, so the bone becomes lighter, even if it remains the same size. It disrupts the trabecular cross struts that provide strength throughout the bone. It also decreases the amount of calcium and other minerals in the bone, and makes the bone more porous.

After a woman turns 50, her cortical bone becomes weaker and more porous. Researchers theorize that the cortical bone recedes from the inside during postmenopause and beyond, meaning it thins "from the inside out." If you put a heated stick into an ice pop, the inner core becomes a larger cavity, while the outer portion of the ice pop stays frozen. The overall thickness of the ice pop decreases as it melts from the inside out. This is analogous to cortical bone becoming hollowed and weakened from the inside. It decreases in diameter, thickness, and strength. In addition, it becomes more porous, further decreasing its strength. When the normally solid cortical bone suffers from thinning and gets more porous, it starts to look more like trabecular bone. For cortical bone, even a small increase in porosity substantially decreases the bone strength.

If healthy bones look like cheddar cheese, then osteoporotic bones look like Swiss cheese. They are no longer solid, strong, or thick. Another way to think of the difference in bone quality is by imagining two hand-knit sweaters of the same size. The first is knit with fine yarn, small needles, and tight stitches. This sweater represents strong bones that are less likely to tear or unravel. Their architecture is robust. The second sweater is knit loosely with large, loopy stitches and lots of spaces. The loopy sweater with more holes will tear or unravel sooner. It is more fragile, just as weaker bones have a weaker architecture and greater susceptibility to fracture.

In addition to the poorer, less robust quality of the bone itself that comes with age, there are other circumstances that increase the risk of falls. With age, eyesight worsens and it becomes more difficult to negotiate stairs and uneven terrain. Coordination becomes compromised. Muscle strength weakens. Balance is worse. The brain processes signals more slowly. Over time, the risk of falls rises as the bone becomes more fragile, increasing the likelihood of a fracture—which is why prevention is vital.

Who Is at Risk for Osteoporosis?

All women over the age of 50, and all postmenopausal women, need to be concerned about the health of their bones. Additional risk factors for women include:

- *A family history of osteoporosis* (or broken bones, even if there is no diagnosis of osteoporosis). This increases a woman's individual risk of osteoporosis, but the *absence* of a family history of osteoporosis should not be interpreted as immunity. It is common for a woman to have osteoporosis even if there is no family history.
- *Being small-boned and thin.* Slender individuals weighing less than 127 pounds are at higher risk of osteoporosis. Similarly, a woman whose weight falls in the lowest 25th percentile for her height is at higher risk for fragility fractures. A woman who is underweight should be followed closely and assessed for her

risk of osteoporosis. On the other hand, being "big-boned" is not protective against osteoporosis.

- *Low estrogen levels*
- *Missing periods* (amenorrhea), as it is associated with lower estrogen
- *Low calcium intake*
- *Low vitamin D intake*
- *Anorexia or bulimia,* either now or in the past (a poor diet is also a risk factor for weak bones)
- *High-protein diet or high-protein weight-loss diet* (such as the Atkins diet). Excess protein alters kidney function and increases calcium loss from bone.
- *Lots of salty foods.* Foods with high sodium or salt content thin bones, probably by leaching out calcium and decreasing bone strength.
- *Lots of caffeine.* Caffeine is an insult to healthy bones.
- *Lots of soda.* Soda weakens bones in different ways. The high phosphorous content increases calcium loss from bones, weakening them. This is true if the soda is diet or regular, with or without caffeine. All types of soda also have high sodium content. High salt leaches calcium from bones, decreasing bone strength.
- *Sedentary lifestyle.* Those with a sedentary lifestyle or who experience long periods of inactivity develop weaker bones. Less physical activity weakens muscles and bones because bones that are not exercised and muscles that don't work against gravity become thinner and weaker. Weight-bearing exercise is needed to maintain bone health. The type of exercise, how often she does it, and the number of years she has exercised all have an impact on a woman's bone strength.
- *Smoking.* Cigarette smokers have weaker as well as thinner bones.
- *Alcohol.* The exact threshold of alcohol consumption is unclear, but it may be as little as one drink a day.
- *Certain medical conditions.* Any disorder or procedure that affects your ability to absorb calcium adds to the risk of osteo-

porosis—for example, inflammatory bowel disease/syndrome (IBS), celiac sprue disease, and gastric bypass surgery. Diabetes and hyperthyroidism are associated with a higher risk of osteoporosis. Certain types of anemia, including sickle cell anemia, cause osteoporosis as well. Rheumatoid arthritis is associated with thin bones. Kidney disease may also be responsible for osteoporosis.

- *Certain medications.* Seizure medications (such as Depakote or Dilantin) increase the risk of thin bones. Glucocorticoids (steroids) cause osteoporosis over time, when given by mouth, injected, or inhaled (for asthma). Chemotherapy, including aromatase inhibitors used to treat breast cancer, can also thin bones. Long-term use of heparin, a blood thinner, causes osteoporosis. Lithium, a medication used to treat those with bipolar disease, causes osteoporosis. Other antidepressants such as the SSRIs (see Chapter 9) may also be associated with osteoporosis, but it may be difficult to determine because depression itself is associated with osteoporosis. Finally, proton pump inhibitors, used to treat those with ulcers or gastroesophageal reflux disease (GERD), are associated with osteoporosis.
- *Certain hormones.* Depo Provera (a long-acting progesterone injection for contraception) thins bones.
- *Anti-estrogen medications.* The long-term use (beyond six months) of Lupron or other anti-estrogen medications will produce osteoporosis. These anti-estrogen medications are often used to treat fibroids and endometriosis.
- *Vitamin A.* Even an over-the counter supplement, such as vitamin A, can cause osteoporosis when used in excess.

Your personal medical history may harbor clues that predict an increased risk of osteoporosis, independent of laboratory testing or bone measurements. The first feature is age. The second feature is a history of a prior fragility fracture, such as a vertebral spine fracture or a hip fracture. A personal history of a prior fracture, particularly after age 50, increases the risk of osteoporosis and future fractures. Height loss of more than one inch may signal the presence of osteoporosis in the spine or a spinal fracture. Breaking a bone may be a sign of osteoporosis.

If a woman's nutrition is poor, or has been poor in the past (including a history of anorexia or bulimia), her bones may be compromised. A woman is at higher risk if her bones never achieved their peak mass while she was in her twenties or early thirties (for example, because she was pursuing a career as a professional athlete, gymnast, or dancer and the extremely rigorous exercise caused her menstrual periods to vanish). Untreated depression is associated with osteoporosis, particularly if it persists long term.

Ethnicity is also a factor. Asians have weaker bones than Caucasians, but both Asians and Caucasians are at higher risk for osteoporosis than African Americans. Even with stronger bones, one in four African American women still gets osteoporosis.

⚔ SHOSHANNA'S STORY ⚔

History of Steroid Medications

"I've been taking steroid medication for severe asthma for many years. That, plus my slender build, sedentary lifestyle, and family history of osteoporosis, put me at risk for compression fractures. My doctor suggested improving my calcium intake with calcium-rich foods and calcium supplements, to reach a total of 1,200 milligrams of calcium a day. She advised me to get most of the calcium from food, if possible, and to avoid consuming more than 600 milligrams of a calcium supplement at once. She told me about common 'bone robbers' that could speed up bone loss and sabotage my efforts to strengthen my bones, including soda, cigarettes, alcohol, coffee, and high-sodium foods. Although I've never smoked, I do drink a lot of soda. She also recommended that I begin bone-building exercises, particularly for my spine. Without these interventions, she told me that my bone thinning would progress to a severe level, leading to fractures of my spine."

Measuring Bone Health

In the past, medical experts could only identify who was at risk for thin bones, but this did not tell an individual woman if she already had thin bones. Fortunately, today there are tests to identify those who have thin bones and are at risk for having a fragility fracture.

DUAL ENERGY X-RAY ABSORPTIOMETRY (DXA)

The gold standard for testing and assessing whether you have osteoporosis or significant bone thinning is a Dual Energy X-ray Absorptiometry (DXA) scan. Other tests, such as a chest X-ray or bone scan, cannot yet match the accuracy of this test. Currently, DXA is the test of choice to diagnose osteoporosis, and its precursor, osteopenia, by measuring bone mineral density (BMD), an indicator of bone strength.

The DXA scan is a painless test using low-dose X-rays. DXA assesses bone mass by measuring the amount of low-dose radiation that passes through the tissue. It is a precise measure of bone thickness at the hip and the spine. Ideally, a woman will have her bone densities measured using the same machine in the same facility over time to compare to the baseline evaluation. This minimizes differences between machines and technicians. The machine does not touch the body. If you wear clothes and undergarments with no metal hooks, snaps, or zippers, you can keep all of your clothing on during the test.

While many experienced physicians recommend a DXA for a woman over age 50 who is postmenopausal, this is earlier than the recommendations of some health care organizations, including the National Osteoporosis Foundation (NOF). The NOF advises a DXA be done at age 65, but sooner if there is a family history of osteoporosis or other risk factors such as hyperthyroidism, a malabsorption disorder, corticosteroid use, seizure medications, prior anorexia, or bulimia. But menopause clinicians—and menopausal women themselves—don't see the wisdom in delaying a test that is vitally important to a woman's overall health and longevity. Reliable DXA data for premenopausal women is not yet available; a healthy woman under age 50 is extremely unlikely to suffer a hip or spine fracture unless she has an unusual medical history.

To plan treatment and prevention strategies for thin bones, a postmenopausal woman and her doctor need to know the degree of bone thinning present and the location of the weakest bone. The treatment may include lifestyle modifications and/or medication. Questions you and your doctor may discuss include: Is the thinning at such a critical stage that the weakened bones may fracture without warning at any time? Or are the bones in the process of early mild thinning, allowing time for preventive measures?

Although DXA measures bone mineral density for individual vertebrae in the spine and various locations in the hip, reports are issued using comparisons expressed as T scores, not BMD values. The T score compares the measurement of bone density that represents bone strength to a healthy woman in her early thirties with strong bones. In general, a woman who has strong bones will have a score of zero or a positive number. A woman with thinning bones will have a negative T score.

Part of the DXA test involves entering a woman's precise height and weight to adjust the calculations and standardize them for her particular build. Those with T scores from zero to –1.4 have minimal thinning or normal bones. Those with positive T scores above zero most likely have dense bones. A woman with a T score between –1.5 and –2.5 has osteopenia or mildly thin bones. A woman with a T score of –2.5 or below (that is, –3.5) has osteoporosis. A T score showing osteoporosis means that a woman's BMD is more than 2.5 standard deviations below that of a healthy 35-year-old, and the woman is at high risk of a fragility fracture.

Even if your average T score is okay, you may still have early osteoporosis in an individual vertebra or specific location on your hip. Averaging a weak bone density in one area with stronger densities elsewhere may mask the presence of the weaker area. To prevent fractures, treatment is based on "the weakest link," the worst or thinnest of the individual measurements.

The average T score may be falsely reassuring. If you have had a bone density test and your doctor is deciding whether you need treatment for thin bones, it is helpful to ask the doctor to specify the thinnest area on the study. Do you have any measurement on your DXA that shows severe bone thinning or osteoporosis in one area of your spine or hip? If you do, you will want to discuss the pros and cons of treatment based upon the weakest bone measurement in your DXA study, even if the average bone density on your study is within the normal range. For example, if one of the vertebrae in your spine shows osteoporosis with a T score of −2.7, but the other measurements in your spine are reassuring, you may still benefit greatly from treatment. It is possible that arthritis with bone spurs is causing the other vertebrae in your spine to appear denser or stronger than they really are.

Ask your doctor to clarify whether you have osteopenia or osteoporosis on your most recent DXA scan. While osteopenia can require treatment with medication to prevent osteoporosis, it is usually amenable to lifestyle changes. This will be determined by the most negative T score on your DXA report and your age. A T score of −1.5 in a 55-year-old woman indicates osteopenia or mild thinning. A 70-year-old woman with a T score of −1.5 has a high risk of developing an osteoporotic fracture in the next 10 years based upon her age.

Find out the thinnest area of bone on your DXA. You will want to base your discussion with your doctor on the weakest area so that the treatment or prevention plan is rigorous enough to reverse the most severe area of bone thinning. The area with the thinnest bone is the area most likely to fracture. Strengthening the bone at that point will decrease your risk of fracture there, even if your DXA measurement stays the same after treatment. If you focus your interventions on the most negative T score, you will have the best outcome. Often, a woman hears that her average T score is close to normal or in the osteopenia range. She breathes a sigh of relief. In reality, there may be an area of osteoporosis in her hip or spine that needs more aggressive management. She may not be receptive to her doctor's advice to take medication because she is not convinced of the severity of the bone thinning. She is falsely reassured by the average value. Is your weakest T score measurement in your hip or your spine, or are they both equally affected by thin bones? Certain medications are more effective in targeting the spine; others are more effective in strengthening hip bones. Some are appropriate for both.

⚑ KASEY'S STORY ⚑

Focal Osteoporosis of the Spine

"I'm 54 and have been postmenopausal for five years. I'm lactose intolerant and do not consume milk or other dairy products. I only recently started to drink calcium-fortified soy milk and calcium-fortified orange juice. I was not enthusiastic about taking calcium pills and rarely took them. My DXA showed a T score of −2.9 for the L4 vertebra (the fourth lumbar bone in my lower back) in my spine. The average T score for my spine, compared to that of other women my age, is only −1.2. I concluded that my −1.2 score was only osteopenia, but my doctor had a different perspective. He was concerned about the −2.9 measurement at L4. He explained that treatment is based upon the weakest bones that are measured, not just the average. Part of my spine had already progressed to osteoporosis, not merely mild thinning prompting preventive measures, but more severe thinning pointing toward treatment. Treatment would prevent me from suffering a fracture or break of the vertebral bone in my spine. I asked my doctor if I could correct the thin area in the spine by being more consistent in taking calcium and vitamin D supplements and exercising. He told me that taking calcium and vitamin D would certainly help in preventing further thinning, but would not address the severe thinning that had already taken place."

Limitations of Dual Energy X-ray Absorptiometry

Limitations of DXA include not taking a woman's age into account. Age is an independent risk factor for fracturing a hip, distinct from bone mineral density. A woman who is 70 years old with a T score of −1.5 has a higher risk of fracture in the next 10 years than a woman who is 52 with a T score of −2.5.

In addition to not accounting for age, DXA does not account for other risk factors that thin the bones or increase a woman's chance of a fracture. Weakened bones from illness or medications may not be reflected by the BMD result or T scores because illness or medications may change the quality or architecture of the bone before they alter the actual bone density. The gold standard for predicting your risk of fracturing a bone in your spine or hip in the next 10 years is FRAX, the fracture risk assessment tool, discussed shortly.

T scores on DXA scans are misleading if a woman has had a prior fracture, if she is older, if she has arthritis in her hip or spine, or if she has been treated with steroids. For these reasons it is important for a woman and her doctor to review her medical and family history and not just plan treatment based upon the DXA results alone.

The Z score is also reported on DXA studies. The Z score tells a woman how she compares to others her age. This is not helpful clinically, since 50 percent of women over age 50 suffer an osteoporotic fracture in their lifetime. Treatment, therefore, should not be based upon a Z score.

Bone density measurements can also be misleading and actually falsely reassuring at other times. They can underestimate the risk of fracture. The test can be "fooled" by arthritic changes or scarring from a previous fracture. For instance, a woman who has arthritis may have thickening or spurs in her bones that create a falsely elevated bone density and do not actually show the quality and strength of the bone. She may be at risk for osteoporosis but have a reassuring bone density on DXA.

DXA does not factor in a prior fracture. Both increasing age and a history of a prior fracture significantly increase the risk of a future fracture. The DXA T score will not reflect the degree of this increased risk accurately.

In the past few years, researchers have learned more about bone's properties. Bone thickness is still an important feature and can be measured to assess bone health. Mineral content is another characteristic of bone that plays an important part in bone health. For example, even if the bone is thick enough on a measurement, it will fracture if there is not enough calcium or vitamin D in it. But even bone thickness and mineral content do not completely explain how bone behaves. Bone architecture, or microscopic internal structure, is an important factor, but it is difficult to measure.

The strengths of the DXA test are that it provides information about the amount of bone and some information about bone strength. DXA testing cannot, however, provide information about the number and type of trabecular connections or properties of the cortical bones. Picture a broken ladder that is missing rungs; it becomes unstable and unsuitable for weight bearing. Trabecular bone that is missing connections or struts will not provide adequate support. In women, loss of trabecular connections is a more frequent cause of fractures than decreases in bone mineral density as identified by DXA studies. As researchers and clinicians are able to monitor the loss of trabecular connections more closely, they can assess whether individual medications are stopping the loss of trabecular connections to treat osteoporosis.

At present it is not possible to monitor the loss of trabecular connections closely, or to evaluate the effects of various medical treatments. Fortunately, this technology is being developed by researchers, even though it is not yet ready for clinical use. In addition to using technologies that identify these kinds of changes and developing medications targeted at correcting them, norms must be established to understand the range of values healthy bones express compared to compromised osteoporotic ones in different individuals.

Bone Density Result with a Prior Fracture

"I'm 60 years old and have a history of a compression fracture in my spine, even though my spine T score is normal. I was pleased by the normal test results and was not receptive to taking bone-building medication to prevent future fractures. But I've since learned that DXA does not represent my true risk of fracture. While DXA is a helpful tool to evaluate a woman who has not experienced an osteoporotic fracture, it underestimated my risk of another fracture. My doctor has told me that I am at high risk of another osteoporotic fracture by virtue of my first one. DXA does not take my high-risk history into account, and, in this case, is falsely reassuring. I have a higher risk of fracture than a 60-year-old woman with no prior fracture, even though my bone density shows no osteoporosis. My doctor and I have been discussing medications to strengthen my bones. He says I will also benefit from having my blood vitamin D level checked to be certain that my body can use all of the calcium I take to strengthen my bones."

DXA of the Arm

Portable DXA scans image the forearm and wrist. In women over 70 years old, a DXA measurement of the arm or wrist may be a reasonable predictor of fracture risk and may be similar to analyzing the spine and hip. But in younger postmenopausal women, a DXA measurement of the arm or wrist is not predictive of hip or spine fracture. There is a lot of metabolic activity in the spine and the large amount of trabecular bone will show osteoporosis earlier than in the hip. In women younger than 70, the peripheral DXAs that measure a wrist will not be an accurate predictor of the spine or hip fracture risk.

❧ Katrina's Story ❧

Portable DXA Arm Test

"I am 55 and postmenopausal. A health fair where I work featured a portable DXA. They offered to assess the bone density of my radius [a forearm bone]. I was pleased that it showed no osteoporosis and brought the report to my annual gynecology exam two months later. My gynecologist was not reassured by this finding. He ordered a central DXA to check the thickness and mineralization of my spine and hip bones. It showed that I had osteopenia, mild thinning, in the spine. He explained that as a younger postmenopausal woman, I can't rely on the findings about my forearm because they doesn't correlate well with the health of my spine and hip. At this time in my life, he advised me to have DXA evaluations to accurately assess my bone strength. He also reviewed preventive lifestyle choices with me."

BONE ULTRASOUNDS

Ultrasounds of the calcaneous (heel bone) have been used to predict bone mineral content and fracture risk. Quantitative ultrasounds are less expensive and more portable, so you may see these used at health fairs. This test poses the same concerns as the DXA of the arm. For younger postmenopausal women, a calcaneous ultrasound result does *not* correlate well with the risk of fracture in the spine or hip.

Quantitative ultrasound measures the speed of sound waves moving through the bone. It is a less expensive test than DXA, involves no radiation, and is portable. At this time, the normal values and standardization for quantitative ultrasound are not well established. It can be useful in postmenopausal women over age 70, when the thickness of the calcaneous bone (heel bone) correlates better with spine and hip strength than it does in younger postmenopausal women.

❧ Bertha's Story ❧

Ultrasound Test

"I'm 75 and live in an assisted living facility. I have painful osteoarthritis in my knees that impairs my mobility and makes it difficult for me to get to appointments. The assisted living facility offers ultrasound of the heel to check for osteoporosis; a van with the ultrasound comes by every six months. I've mentioned this to my doctor and she has told me that although she would not recommend it for a younger woman, it might be an adequate screen for me."

FRACTURE RISK ASSESSMENT TOOL

In February 2008, the World Health Organization (WHO) published an interactive tool, the Fracture Risk Assessment (FRAX) tool, to help predict a woman's personal fracture risk for the next 10 years. This is a more comprehensive approach to managing fracture risk than using the DXA alone. The DXA result is still helpful and is included in the WHO fracture risk tool as one of the variables that predict fracture risk.

FRAX is the most comprehensive assessment tool to date. It includes variables such as bone mineral density, age, family history, history of hip fracture, and history of fractures over age 50, as well as smoking, corticosteroid use, and a history of rheumatoid arthritis. The tool also takes into account ethnic differences in bone fragility and fracture risk based on specific epidemiology that includes statistics about illness and mortality for different groups, increasing the accuracy of the fracture risk predictions. The predictions will be more accurate for African American, Latino, Asian, and Caucasian men and women. Using these additional factors, not accounted for in a DXA study alone, allows more accurate predictions of your fracture risk over the next 10 years. This tool may be accessed online at www.shef.ac.uk/FRAX/ (click on Calculation Tool).

In the future, DXA machines will include the "FRAX patch"—a way to incorporate the FRAX predictions by entering the appropriate data at the time of the DXA study and including the FRAX estimate of fracture risk for the next 10 years along with the DXA report.

FRAX is a big step in the right direction. There are some limitations in its use. First, it is designed to predict fracture risk for the next 10 years only for patients who have not been treated before. Second, it is most accurate in predicting fracture risk for those with thinning mostly at the hip, since it does not have an entry for a vertebral T score. If bone thinning occurs mainly in your spine, your doctor will most likely use the guidelines of T scores from your DXA scan as well as the rest of your clinical assessment as the basis for recommendations for treatment.

Promoting Bone Health

Today, maintaining bone health includes these strategies:

- *Get adequate calcium* intake daily in food and, if necessary, divided doses of supplements.
- *Take adequate vitamin D* daily.
- *Participate regularly in weight-bearing and muscle-strengthening exercises.*
- *Avoid "bone robbers,"* such as excess alcohol, cigarette smoking (active or passive), high salt consumption, soda, caffeine, excess vitamin A, and aluminum (found, for example, in antacids).
- *Minimize your risk of falls.* Minimizing the risk of falls, particularly as age increases and eyesight and coordination decrease, includes using good lighting, keeping walking paths free of obstacles inside the home and out, avoiding loose throw rugs, and avoiding slippery outdoor conditions whenever possible. Improving your balance through specific exercises also helps.
- *Talk to your doctor about bone health,* when to have a bone density test, and whether you would benefit from prescription medication to prevent or reverse osteoporosis.

CALCIUM

Your skeleton contains 99 percent of your body's calcium reserves. If you do not consume enough calcium daily, especially after age 50, your bones will leach out calcium to keep the calcium level in your blood at a healthy level.

For more than 20 years, I have been recommending calcium to my patients, encouraging them to get more in their food and then to use supplements as needed. This advice is based on long-standing conclusions supported by years of research and clinical experience.

For the past two years, patients have been telling me, "I guess I don't need to take that calcium anymore, since it doesn't help prevent bone thinning after all. Didn't you see the news?"

They were referring to news headlines that read: "Calcium supplements do not prevent bone thinning!" As it turns out, this news flash was based on an Australian study in which the participants were asked to take calcium supplements, but they did not take them regularly or reliably. Therefore, the authors concluded, calcium supplements are not an effective intervention to prevent osteoporosis in the group of postmenopausal women studied. The fact that the calcium did not work because the women did not take it did not deter the author of the catchy but misleading headline. A more representative headline might have read, "Women who remember to take calcium supplements daily, strengthen their bones; those who forget or do not take them reliably, do not." That, obviously, is not an appealing sound bite.

The point of the study was to alert doctors to the fact that a significant number of women do not take calcium supplements as they are advised. The reality is that calcium and vitamin D do strengthen bone if they are taken several times a day in divided doses. Women who take them regularly and reliably will strengthen their bones.

In a different study, women were advised to take calcium supplements in addition to calcium they were already taking on their own. The additional calcium supplements did not show an added benefit, because the women were already taking enough before the study. The conclusion of the study was that calcium supplements do not improve bone health if you are already getting enough calcium in your food to meet your needs.

⚡ AMANDA'S STORY ⚡

Low Calcium Intake

"I am 55 and lactose-intolerant. I recently started drinking calcium-fortified soy milk after a lifetime of avoiding dairy products. I swim once every week. My first bone density test was done two years ago and the result showed a T score of -1.5 in the hip and spine. I was placed on calcium supplements and vitamin D, but often forgot to take them. Two years later, my T score on a repeat DXA test was -2.5. My risk of fracture had doubled in two years! At this time my doctor prescribed Fosamax and emphasized the need for calcium and vitamin D on a daily basis. He planned to recheck my bone density and evaluate my progress in two years. He has encouraged me to continue swimming, since I enjoy it and it is an excellent aerobic activity for heart health. He also advised starting a strength-training program either at a gym or on my own at home using Miriam Nelson's book Strong Women, Strong Bones. *He told me this would also improve my balance over time and decrease my risk of a fall, as well as improving my muscle and bone strength."*

The Benefits of Calcium

Calcium is critical to maintaining bone health. It is an essential ingredient for strengthening bones in preventive strategies and treatment regimens.

Imagine that your bones are like a brick wall. To build a brick wall, you need bricks and mortar. Calcium and vitamin D represent the bricks. Although calcium and vitamin D are essential to the brick-work, they will not cement the wall and provide enough strength to withstand regular use unless there is mortar to hold them in place. Medication represents the mortar that holds the bricks in place and literally cements the strength of the wall over time. Before post-menopause, estrogen acts as the mortar for women. After postmeno-pause, if osteoporosis and severe bone thinning have already set in, more mortar in another form must be supplied to do the job, as the amount of natural estrogen a woman has will not hold the calcium in the bones—and the bricks will not be held securely in place.

In addition to building bone strength, there are other benefits to be gained from taking calcium. Calcium improves blood pressure. It also decreases the risk of getting colon and rectal cancer. Preliminary research shows that calcium may even decrease the risk of obesity.

Some women are afraid that they will develop kidney stones if they take calcium supplements. In fact, there is a *lower* risk of kidney stones in those who take the recommended amount of calcium. Calcium supplements will not increase the risk of kidney stones as long as the recommended daily amount is not exceeded. Keeping the total daily intake of calcium under 2,000 milligrams per day does not increase the risk of kidney stones. And a postmenopausal woman only needs 1,200 milligrams of calcium a day from food sources and supplements combined for bone health.

How Much Calcium Do I Need? How Do I Tell If I'm Getting Enough?

The amount of calcium women require is 1,000 to 1,200 milligrams a day during perimenopause. Postmenopausal calcium requirements are 1,200 milligrams of calcium per day in divided doses. These totals include calcium in food as well as supplements.

To estimate how much calcium you are getting from food, begin with the label on the container. For example, a container of yogurt that provides 30 percent of the daily calcium requirement contributes 300 milligrams of calcium. Add a zero to the percent of the daily requirement and you have an estimate of the milligrams of calcium you are getting per serving. This only applies, of course, if you consume the entire serving.

Postmenopausal women do not absorb calcium well, particularly if they are not on estrogen replacement or bone builders such as Evista, Fosamax, or Actonel, so it is important to understand how to take it.

The Art of Taking Calcium

There is an art to taking calcium. If you take too much at once your body cannot metabolize or use it. If you greatly exceed the recommended supplement requirements, you may get kidney stones. If you don't take enough calcium, you are at risk of osteoporosis.

It's best to take calcium in divided doses, no more than 500 or 700 milligrams at a time. If you take 1,000 milligrams at once, your body cannot utilize the entire amount well. For a postmenopausal woman who gets no calcium from her food, one option is to take a 500 milligram or 600 milligram calcium supplement twice a day. Depending upon how much vitamin D was in her calcium supplement, she may need to add vitamin D to this regimen.

To enhance calcium absorption, become familiar with the best ways to absorb your calcium.

Do not take calcium supplements with iron supplements. Iron and calcium are not absorbed well when taken together, and you will not get the full benefit of either. Women over 50 or those who are no longer bleeding should choose a multivitamin that does not contain iron, such as Centrum Silver or a generic version. This way you will get the benefit of the calcium in the multivitamin, and the iron will not counteract your absorption of the calcium.

For those who are anemic or need to take iron because they bleed heavily or often, take the iron at a separate time from when you take calcium.

Calcium and fiber are also not absorbed well together. Fortunately, new types of fiber are now available that are compatible with calcium and do not decrease its absorption. There are several versions to try. If calcium makes you constipated, you may find these calcium preparations more appealing. Metamucil makes a fiber supplement that also contains calcium. Fiber Choice makes chewable tablets that contain calcium with inulin, a type of fiber that is compatible with calcium absorption. You can look for inulin fiber in other supplements and foods to maintain the calcium absorption and get the benefit of added fiber at the same time. Some foods now contain calcium and probiotics that help prevent or minimize constipation, such as Kefir yogurt with probiotics.

Two kinds of calcium that are commonly available are calcium carbonate and calcium citrate. Either one may be taken with food. Calcium carbonate is absorbed best when taken with food. Calcium citrate is absorbed better in those over 70 years old. It is also well absorbed when taken on an empty stomach. Often, with increasing age, individuals have less hydrochloric acid in their stomachs, so they may have more success with calcium citrate.

If a woman gets an upset stomach when she takes calcium, she may take calcium in the form of Tums (calcium carbonate). Calcium in foods may be tolerated best.

Are Calcium Supplements Better Than Food Sources?

In general, it's best to get as much calcium from foods as possible, and then use supplements as needed to reach the target amount of up to 1,200 milligrams daily in divided doses. There are no reports of calcium from food causing kidney stones.

Which Food Sources of Calcium Are Best?

Calcium from vegetables and nondairy sources is extremely well absorbed and preferable for many women. Vegetarians may get calcium from their foods or add nondairy supplements to achieve their calcium targets. Beans also have calcium, as do spinach and kale. The milligrams per serving tend to be lower than those in dairy products. Calcium-fortified orange juice as well as other juices, and calcium-fortified soy milk, are other ways to reach your goal of 1,000 to 1,200 milligrams per day, particularly for those who prefer to avoid dairy products.

Low-fat and non-fat dairy sources of calcium are also excellent. An 8-ounce glass of skim milk has approximately 300 milligrams of calcium. Those women who like drinking milk may drink two 8-ounce glasses of milk a day at different times to satisfy part of their calcium requirements. Avoid the third glass of milk, as three or more glasses of milk may increase the risk of ovarian cancer. For those who are lactose-intolerant, Lactaid milk is available that has lactose enzyme added and is calcium-fortified. There are other calcium-fortified milks in the supermarket that provide 500 milligrams of calcium per 8-ounce serving instead of 300 milligrams. Yogurt and cheese are other good sources of calcium. Canned salmon (with the bones) and sardines are also excellent sources of calcium.

Vitamin D: What We Now Know

Recently, researchers have shown that achieving and maintaining normal blood levels of vitamin D is essential to having strong bones and muscles and decreasing the risk of falls. Vitamin D is a substance that is produced in human skin, then transformed into its active form by the liver and kidneys.

Vitamin D enhances calcium absorption and is also critical to bone health and muscle health in its own right. Vitamin D helps keep one's sense of balance intact and thus contributes to lowering the risk of falling.

The desirable level of vitamin D in the blood is now 30 nanograms per milliliter or higher. The new adult guidelines for daily vitamin D consumption are 800 to 1,000 international units of vitamin D_3 (cholecalciferol). However, if your blood level of vitamin D is low, this amount of vitamin D may not be enough to put you into the normal range.

You may be vitamin D deficient even if you take a multivitamin and separate calcium supplements with vitamin D. A typical calcium supplement may have 100 or 200 international units of vitamin D added to it. Even if the multivitamin has another 400 international units of vitamin D, a postmenopausal woman may still fall short of her daily vitamin D requirement.

Based on the new research findings, a postmenopausal woman needs 1,000 international units of vitamin D daily if her blood level of vitamin D is to remain in the normal range.

A woman with a low blood level of vitamin D may not be able to catch up to normal levels for her muscles and bones by taking this amount. She may need a booster dose of vitamin D, available by prescription from her doctor to replenish her low reserves. After the low reserves are replenished, she can then continue to take 1,000 international units of vitamin D a day to maintain healthy muscles and bones during her postmenopausal years.

Researchers report vitamin D levels in different units than clinicians or clinical laboratories. A woman's bones are healthiest when her blood level of vitamin D_3 is more than 30 nanograms per milliliter. In some cases, a blood level below that will not improve without booster doses of vitamin D_3 as high as 50,000 international units once a week for 8 to 12 weeks.

Vitamin D_3 is synthesized in the skin. While wearing sunscreen is advised to minimize the risk of skin cancer, sunscreen blocks vitamin D absorption. Living in a northern latitude also predisposes a woman to vitamin D deficiency because the farther away you live from the equator, the less sun you get. Ten minutes a day of natural sunlight exposure with no sunscreen, including to the arms and face, helps keep healthy vitamin D levels in the blood, but that may not be all you need to maintain healthy blood levels.

In addition to stronger bones, women with normal vitamin D levels enjoy stronger muscles. Researchers have recently found vitamin D receptors in muscle tissue. Insufficient or deficient vitamin D levels are now thought to contribute to low BMD as well as osteoporosis, decreased mineralization of normal bone, and problems with muscle pain and weakness. In one study of women with muscle pain and weakness, 88 percent had vitamin D deficiency.

Vitamin D deficiency may also play a role in other problems postmenopausal women face, including high blood pressure, Type 1 diabetes, and rheumatoid arthritis. In the Women's Health Initiative (WHI) study, it was found that the risk of colon cancer went down as the level of vitamin D went up, suggesting there may be a potential role for vitamin D in colon cancer prevention.

WEIGHT-BEARING EXERCISE

In addition to adequate calcium and vitamin D intake, it is also important to expose healthy bones to regular weight-bearing exercise. Weight-bearing exercises, which include walking, cycling, and weight lifting, defy gravity.

Weight-bearing exercise not only maintains bone strength, but also restores it. Researchers found that even inactive senior women living in nursing homes were able to improve bone strength this way. The women (in their eighties and nineties) were given adequate calcium and vitamin D and started on an exercise program with weights. The program was designed to target major muscle groups in the upper and lower body that support the spine and hip to improve bone strength. Even the octogenarians improved their bone strength with this program. (Modifications are included for wheelchair-bound participants.) This shows it is never too late to begin an exercise program. Women also lose their balance with increasing age. Loss of balance increases the likelihood of falling, which is associated with bone fracture. Exercises to improve balance are discussed in Chapter 12.

MEDICATIONS FOR BONE HEALTH

Most women will be able to prevent fractures by eliminating "bone robbers," engaging in regular weight-bearing activity, and meeting the age-specific requirements for calcium (with food and/or supplements) and vitamin D. The majority of postmenopausal women will not need any medication to prevent osteoporosis. For those who do, there are several categories of medication.

For women who have severe thinning, calcium and vitamin D supplementation are essential but not sufficient to correct the problem. Prescription medications to keep the calcium in the bone are needed.

Ask your doctor if the medication(s) you are discussing are the best for the type and location of the most severe bone thinning you have at that location, spine or hip. A woman who focuses only on the summary of her DXA results and declines medication when the average T score is in the reassuring range may be falsely reassured about her bone strength. False reassurance or complacency will cause a woman to miss a window of opportunity she may have to prevent osteoporosis or its progression. Honesty is the best policy, as is full disclosure of the most severe thinning demonstrated by any of the measurements taken for the test.

Any of the osteoporosis medications available will strengthen bones if the DXA shows severe bone thinning is present. Not all prescription medications to strengthen bones and reduce the risk of fracture are created equal. Each has different pros and cons, risks and benefits. One key point is that the medication you see advertised on television, in a magazine, or on the Internet may not suit your individual needs because it does not target thin bone in the area that yours is the weakest. This is why it's important for the doctor to individualize his or her recommendation for each woman, and for the woman to speak up and participate in the discussion so that the doctor knows what is agreeable to her and what is practical as well as acceptable. A woman who does not "buy into" the prevention or treatment plan is unlikely to carry it out and benefit from it.

These days, pharmaceutical companies are permitted to openly promote their brand of medications and advertise them directly to you, the consumer. The companies manufacturing medications for osteoporosis are appealing to you with well-conceived, targeted ads. Of course, detailed information about your personal and family medical history and your specific DXA results are not factored into the ad campaign. Nor are the specific advantages and disadvantages of that brand of medication compared to those of other comparable medications revealed. Some medications may be overrepresented in the media, while others may be unsung "heroes" in rescuing your bones from the perils of a fracture. It is tempting to be swayed by the ads promoted by a favorite actress or by a less-frequent dosing regimen, but it is in your best interest to learn what the other risks and benefits are in view of *your* specific DXA results by discussing them with your doctor.

❧ WENDY'S STORY ❧

An Active 66-year-old with Height Loss

"At 66, I was an active woman who had always taken charge of my health. I've always walked daily. I am a vegetarian. I maintain my weight within a 15-pound range of my ideal body weight. Because I was active, I did not suspect that I had early signs of bone thinning. When *measured at my doctor's office, I learned I was one inch shorter than my previously measured adult height. He ordered a DXA bone density test. My T scores were -2.1 for the hip and -2.3 for the spine, both showing severe osteopenia. The doctor encouraged me to take a prescription bone builder to treat the changes, but I wasn't receptive. Instead, I agreed to try exercises specifically designed to strengthen my bones. I committed to doing them two times a week for 20 minutes each session. I also agreed to take calcium supplements with vitamin D to boost my daily calcium intake. After two years of this new regimen, the DXA showed my bones were no worse, but neither did they improve. I have agreed to continue the exercises and calcium supplements but also added a prescription bone builder to increase my bone strength. Now, two years later, at age 70, my DXA test shows that my bone density is closer to the normal range, and my bones are stronger."*

Bisphosphonates

These medications slow the process of bone dissolving as it remodels itself. Examples of bisphosphonates are Fosamax (alendronate), Actonel (risedronate), Boniva (ibandronate sodium), and Reclast (zoledronate). Bisphosphonate medications equilibrate these processes so that bone formation and bone dissolving are more closely matched, and bone dissolving is slowed down so less bone is lost. In this way, bone formation can "catch up," leaving more strong bone in place. Most of the bisphosphonates can be prescribed for preventing osteoporosis or treating it.

Bisphosphonates are not hormones. They do not affect estrogen levels or breast cancer risk or the amount and frequency of hot flashes. They decrease bone loss so that bone building is more lasting. In effect, bisphosphonates allow bone building that keeps calcium and vitamin D in the bone, much like mortar helps bind bricks in a brick wall.

Fosamax (alendronate) comes in two forms, Fosamax or Fosamax plus D. It is approved for prevention of osteoporosis in a lower dose (35 milligrams once a week) and for treatment (70 milligrams a week), and comes in tablet or liquid form. Fosamax decreases the number of spine, hip, and wrist fractures by 50 percent over three years in those who have already had a previous spine fracture. It lowers the risk of spine fractures by 48 percent in three years for those who have not had a previous spine fracture.

When taking a bisphosphonate, such as Fosamax, Actonel, or Boniva, be certain to take it on an empty stomach with plain water; don't consume other liquids or food for at least 30 minutes after taking it. Precautions include staying upright (sitting, standing, or walking) for half an hour after taking the medication. Bending over or lying down may cause the medication to get stuck in the esophagus (food tube), and also may cause some stomach discomfort or irritation. Side effects of bisphosphonates include trouble swallowing, inflammation of the esophagus, and gastric ulcers. Some women with a history of ulcers cannot tolerate this medication; others tolerate it well if they observe the precautions. Bisphosphonates are not intended for women who plan to have more children or who are pregnant because they can affect the fetal skeleton. They are prescribed for postmenopausal women only.

Boniva (ibandronate) is a newer, long-acting bisphosphonate. It can be taken by mouth once a month or administered every three months by intravenous injection. The oral form can be given for prevention or treatment. Boniva targets spine fractures well, and can reduce the risk of spine fractures by 50 percent over three years. If you take it by mouth, you must follow the same precautions as for Fosamax (above); also, do not drink anything but plain water (no other food or drink) for 60 minutes after the Boniva and remain upright. Your doctor will check your kidney function before giving each dose of the injectable form. Although research data on Boniva shows it helps improve bone thinning in the spine, the data is not definitive in showing substantial improvement in hip bones.

Actonel (risedronate) is a bisphosphonate that is taken by mouth. It comes in two versions, with or without calcium. You can take 150 milligrams once a month or 35 milligrams once a week. It lowers the chance of spine fractures by 41 to 49 percent and other fractures by 36 percent over three years in those who have had a previous spine fracture.

Reclast (zoledronate) is the newest of the bisphosphonates. It is given once a year by intravenous infusion over a 15-minute period and is FDA-approved to treat osteoporosis in postmenopausal women. Some women get joint aches, headaches, muscle aches, or fever, so they are pretreated with Tylenol (acetaminophen) to lower the risk of these symptoms. One out of 3 women will get these symptoms after the first dose, but only 7 of 100 get them after the second dose, and only 3 out of 100 experience them after the third dose. Reclast lowers the incidence of spine fractures by 70 percent and lowers hip fractures by 41 percent over three years. The side effects are similar to those of other bisphosphonates.

It is possible to achieve normal bone strength by taking these medications over years and monitoring progress with a DXA scan every two years or so. When the bones have returned to normal density, the medication can be stopped. The benefit of the medication lasts at least an additional five years after it is stopped. It is possible that a permanent benefit may be achieved; more studies are under way.

Concerns have been raised about the risk of osteonecrosis as a result of taking Fosamax. Osteonecrosis describes bone that will no longer heal itself. Osteonecrosis of the jaw is a rare condition that has been seen in cancer patients who received chemotherapy at the same time that they were taking abnormally high doses of Fosamax. Even in this unusual circumstance, the risk is estimated at less than one in 200,000 cases and remains rare, especially in those taking a bisphosphonate for less than five years.

⚔ FIONA'S STORY ⚔

Poor Healing after a Broken Hip

"By the time I was 58, I had already had a hip fracture. I attributed that to being clumsy, but I learned later that my hip 'gave out' prior to my fall. I was hospitalized for a week after the hip surgery. My rehabilitation was difficult; physical therapy was a struggle. The hip did not heal rapidly. My doctors were concerned that I was not active enough after the surgery. Due to the pain in my hip with walking and difficulty

using a walker, though, I spent more time in bed. This immobility caused a pulmonary embolus, a clot that formed in the blood vessels near my hip and migrated to my lungs, where it caused a blockage. I had to go on blood thinners for six months after I underwent additional surgery to prevent future formation of clots.

"It's two years later and I still walk with a cane. When I saw my gynecologist, I still had not had an evaluation for osteoporosis even though I had had bone scans and plain X-rays. When a DXA scan revealed osteoporosis, I learned that this was the most likely cause of my hip fracture, not clumsiness, as I had previously thought. I actually had fallen after my hip broke. Osteoporosis had so weakened my hip, my doctor explained, that I suffered a 'fragility fracture.'

"I had a habit of drinking three glasses of milk a day and assumed I was taking adequate measures to keep healthy. Reviewing my medical history and lifestyle in more detail made me realize that I normally drank 12 cups of coffee a day. Each mug I used was 16 ounces, really two cups. I also enjoyed diet soda—up to four cans a day. I was a former smoker of two packs of cigarettes a day for 20 years. My evening routine to unwind from a day's work included two glasses of wine while preparing dinner. I was unaware that adequate calcium intake alone would not protect me from getting osteoporosis. And I didn't know that the high amounts of phosphorous in my soda prevented my bones from absorbing the calcium I took in with food. Furthermore, I had milk with coffee or at the same time that I drank coffee. I've learned that calcium is not well absorbed by the body if it is taken at the same time you drink coffee. I had always enjoyed wine while preparing dinner and reassured myself that the wine was good for my heart. Unfortunately, the wine also thinned my bones and I learned that alcohol is associated with osteoporosis."

Estrogen and Combined Hormone Therapy

Systemic estrogen and estrogen-progesterone combinations are approved by the FDA for preventing osteoporosis. The WHI found five years of Prempro (synthetic estrogen and progesterone) lowered the risk of clinical spine fractures and hip fractures by 34 percent. As you read earlier in Chapter 3, they may be given to healthy younger women (who have been in postmenopause less than 10 years) to control debilitating hot flashes or night sweats.

Selective Estrogen Receptor Modulators

Selective estrogen receptor modulators (SERMs) are modified hormones that are cousins of Tamoxifen. Tamoxifen is chemically made by modifying estrogen so that it prevents breast cancer. SERMs, like Tamoxifen, lower the risk of breast cancer. SERMs are interesting because in some ways they act like estrogen, and in other ways they act the opposite way that estrogen normally acts in the body.

Evista (raloxifene) is an example of a SERM that increases bone strength in the spine and, like its cousin Tamoxifen, decreases the risk of breast cancer. One drawback is that it may worsen hot flashes to a small degree in some women. Evista does not influence vaginal dryness; it will not get better or worse on this prescription. Evista does not cause uterine cancer or change the uterine lining.

Evista lowers the risk of spine fracture by 30 percent in those with a prior spine fracture. Evista lowers the risk of spine fracture by 55 percent in those without a prior spine fracture.

One drawback is that Evista is associated with a higher risk of deep vein clot formation, also called deep vein thrombosis (DVT). This risk of vein clots decreases over time. The risk is small but significant (three extra people out of every 10,000 who take the medication). An active woman is less likely to get a clot. Once a woman has been on Evista for a year, her risk of developing a clot in her blood is even lower. Evista is taken once a day, by mouth, with or without food. For a woman who cannot tolerate bisphosphonates, it may be an excellent choice.

Tibolone is a newer SERM that is available only in Europe. It has not been approved by the FDA for use in the United States. Tibolone may be a desirable option for postmenopausal American women in the future because it helps reduce hot flashes while it strengthens bones. It may also improve sex drive. It is uncertain whether it will lower the risk of breast cancer.

Other Approaches, Including Parathyroid Hormone

Parathyroid hormone (PTH), brand name Forteo, is a bone builder in the newest category of osteoporosis prescription medications. Rather than slowing bone loss, it promotes bone growth by stimulating osteoblast activity. Forteo is reserved for high-risk individuals with severe osteoporosis who do not respond to the other medications or cannot tolerate them. It is given as a daily subcutaneous (under the skin) injection. In those with osteoporosis, it decreases the risk of spine fractures by 65 percent and non-spine fractures by 53 percent after approximately 18 months of treatment.

⚕ WILMA'S STORY ⚕

Healthy, Active 78-year-old with Newly Diagnosed Osteoporosis

"Even when I was 78, everyone who knew me was impressed by my vigor. I walked three miles a day at a brisk pace and had always maintained a normal healthy weight. And I felt healthy. When my doctor advised me to have a test to check my bone density, I bristled. I told him, 'But I walk three miles a day, my bones must be very strong.' Unfortunately, the DXA revealed that I had severe osteoporosis and was at high risk for hip fracture even if I didn't fall. At first, I took the news very poorly. I was crestfallen that my lifelong rigorous fitness routine had not produced strong bones. When the disbelief and disappointment abated, I was ready to consider my options. In the past, my treatment options would have been limited, but I found that I had several alternatives, all of which were acceptable to me.

"Since my osteoporosis was severe, my bone loss was already substantial. I wanted to try taking more calcium, without additional medication, to improve my bone strength. My doctor was concerned about my high risk of bone breakage since my bones were already very weak. I would have been risking further bone loss if I used calcium alone. I needed medication to help put the calcium into my bones and keep it from leaking out. After reviewing the side effects and effectiveness of Fosamax (alendronate), a bone builder that works through the calcium *system, and Evista (raloxifene), a modified synthetic hormone that does not cause any vaginal bleeding or breast tissue changes, I settled on trying Fosamax. I initially thought I did not have to change my diet if I took the medication. My doctor advised me to increase the daily calcium intake in my food as well as use calcium supplements. This would provide enough calcium for the medicine to help improve my osteoporosis. I was encouraged and surprised that my severe bone loss could actually be improved, and that I could attain strong bones again even at my age. I hadn't realized that the new medications available could reverse bone loss and allow a return to normal bone strength over time. Today, after two years of medication and conscientious daily intake of calcium, I have made substantial progress. A subsequent DXA scan shows that my bone mass is closer to normal."*

Ongoing Reassessment

DXA can be used to assess the impact of treatment on bone strength. If interventions are made, it can be helpful to redo the DXA in two years. Because bone builds slowly and there is a four- to seven-month turnover cycle, obtaining a bone density only one year after making an intervention or lifestyle modification is not always informative or accurate.

To tell if a medication, lifestyle intervention, or nutritional approach is having an effect, doctors look for a 3 percentage-point change in the spine measurement of the DXA, or a 4 percent or more change in the hip, to signify a statistically significant change.

If your DXA has not improved, that does not mean your medicine isn't working. Women who take medication to decrease their risk of fracture will have a lower risk of fracture as long as they take adequate calcium and have normal vitamin D levels. Sometimes the lower risk of fracture is not reflected in the DXA results. This may be because the medication is improving other features of the bone that the DXA cannot measure.

Once a woman has received treatment for her thin bones, the average T score for her spine or hip is more helpful in gauging her progress on the medication or lifestyle strategy than an individual measurement. Bone remodels slowly. If a woman modifies her supplement regimen or has begun a new medication, it can be helpful to redo the DXA measurement in two years.

The study and understanding of osteoporosis and menopause is changing rapidly. Soon we hope to have new criteria for predicting whose bones will fracture and who will benefit most from medication. New studies are being done to learn what supplements, lifestyle modifications, exercises, and medications are most effective to strengthen bones in a given individual. Every year, after updating your medical history and current medications and supplements with your doctor, plan to discuss your bone health. At this time you and your doctor can ascertain whether your current regimen is still the best, particularly in view of new strategies to prevent or treat osteoporosis that become available.

Marylou's Story

Which Medication Is Best?

"I'm 57 years old and travel extensively for my job. I've been postmenopausal for five years, since age 52. Because of my schedule, I had not gone in for a routine exam with my gynecologist for a few years. When I finally made the time, one of the tests my doctor ordered was a DXA scan. It showed thinning in my hip that was severe enough to meet the criteria for osteoporosis on one measurement. The average measurement of the hip was not as alarming, and the spine bone strength was more robust, but my doctor was concerned. Since I had seen one of my favorite actresses in an advertisement for Boniva, the bisphosphonate that can be taken once a month, I told my doctor I thought that would work well for me. But he explained that the most severe bone thinning was in my hip, and that Boniva, the medication that appealed to me, had research data supporting its efficacy in decreasing spine fractures. He advised I take Fosamax, a bisphosphonate with a strong track record for returning strength to the hip as well as the spine, once a week."

Future Trends

Recently, researchers have identified changes in the porosity of cortical bone associated with postmenopause as well. Cortical bone becomes weaker as its architecture is compromised. Newer research tools such as hip structural analysis (HSA) can add information not normally possible with a routine DXA. HSA software allows analysis of the topography of the bone, including hills and valleys, representing more detail about the microscopic structure of the bone. This will allow researchers to analyze the effect of various medications on the microscopic structure of the hip. So far it has shown that the cortical bone of the hip thins *and* becomes more porous with the loss of estrogen in early postmenopause. Preventing cortical bone compromise in postmenopause will involve stopping the cortical bone from becoming more porous and increasing the cortical thickness. This will lower the number of hip fractures.

A sister technology, high-resolution peripheral quantitative computed tomography (HR-pQCT), is a research technology that uses specialized software to enhance the ability of a CT (computerized tomography) scan to show the microscopic architecture of the bone. It can be used for limb bones such as the tibia bone in the lower leg or the radius bone in the forearm. It allows the researcher to determine the density of the trabecular bone, separate from the cortical bone density, and then evaluate each, determining the ratio of the two. It can even show the number and thickness of the trabecular struts, as well as their spacing. This detailed information about the microscopic structure of the bone and its microscopic architecture is enhancing clinicians' understanding of how trabecular and cortical bone change in postmenopause as well as how different treatments and medications will affect this process. Advantages of HR-pQCT include providing a three-dimensional evaluation of the architecture and density of the limb bones in a short imaging time with a low radiation dose. Another advantage is that HR-pQCT shows age-related changes. Only the radius and tibia can be evaluated, however, not the hip or the spine. No fracture data is available to correlate with the findings, and there is limited reference and therapy-related data. Therefore HR-pQCT is not ready for prime time use yet, but is in the wings as an interesting research tool.

Researchers are discovering that preserving bone quality, not just maintaining bone density, is a goal for treatment. Measuring these changes will be another challenge. As researchers and clinicians embrace these goals they will learn how new technologies can help them to achieve these goals. One is called micro magnetic resonance imaging, or micro MRI.

This research technology obtains a high-resolution image of a bone made possible with special adaptations to an MRI machine. It mathematically extracts information to reconstruct a three-dimensional model that shows the bone volume at each tiny image location. It does a topographic analysis of the trabecular architecture much like an architect's model of a future shopping complex or a topographic map of a mountain range. With a micro MRI one could distinguish between two women with the same bone volume or amount of bone per area. In one case a woman might have compromised bone architecture; in another woman, the architectural structure of the bone may be intact. The advice a doctor gives each woman would differ substantially. Micro MRI can tell the types of microscopic surfaces in the bone, such as curved versus plate-like or rod-like surfaces and the relative amount of each just as one might tell how many plates, bowls, cups, and saucers were in the microscopic cupboard of a miniature dollhouse. It can also tell the amount of erosion of the structure, or how worn the dishes are in the dollhouse.

A woman whose bones have compromised architectural structure has osteoporosis despite her reassuring bone volume. Her DXA result might be the same as her counterpart with the same bone volume but no osteoporosis, because the osteoporosis victim has compromised bone function due to structure, not volume, of bone. In her case, the DXA shows a normal bone volume and cannot detect osteoporosis that is due to compromised architecture. One advantage of micro MRI is that it is noninvasive. Second, there is no ionizing radiation. A third advantage is that it can be used to modify clinical scanners currently in use. Drawbacks are that micro MRI is only used to assess the limbs, not the hip or the spine. Further, there is very limited reference data and no data on fracture risk. Therefore it is not yet suitable for clinical use.

Prior to these new research findings, the focus has been on the rate that bone was deposited and removed. In view of the drastic increase in bone turnover at the onset of postmenopause, instability in bone structure was not recognized. Only the decrease in bone volume was understood. Now this unstable situation is known to alter the architecture and quality of bones as well as their strength. The architecture of both trabecular and cortical bones is affected.

⚥ Barbara's Story ⚥

Osteoporosis and a Family History of Breast Cancer in a 52-year-old

"I have avoided milk and other dairy products most of my life because I am lactose-intolerant. My mother developed breast cancer when she was 45 years old and died within two years of her diagnosis. I am now 52, an age I never expected to reach. In perimenopause, I had severe hot flashes but was reluctant to take any estrogen because of my family history of breast cancer. My gynecologist ordered a DXA bone density test that showed osteoporosis with enough thinning of the vertebral bones in my spine to predict that I might fracture my spine even if I did not trip or fall. The doctor was also concerned about my height loss, which can be associated with osteoporosis. So even though I had taken good care of myself, felt well, and looked healthy, I was at high risk for a vertebral spine fracture. At my doctor's suggestion, I am taking a medication, Evista, to strengthen my bones and hoping to avoid a fracture. My gynecologist says I am greatly reducing my chances of a spine fracture and height loss with the medication, as well as lowering my risk of breast cancer."

American College of Obstetrics and Gynecology (www.acog.org). This professional organization is dedicated to women's health across the lifespan. Its members are board-certified obstetricians and gynecologists who have been recommended for membership and attain a high standard of education, training, and practice by virtue of passing examinations and updating their credentials on a regular basis. They have excellent materials on most major topics in women's health that are updated frequently. Several booklets on bone health are available online or at your doctor's office.

International Osteoporosis Foundation (www.iofbonehealth.org). There is an interactive IOF One-Minute Osteoporosis Risk Test you can take online.

National Osteoporosis Foundation (www.nof.org). In addition to their other resources, you can click on FRAX™ WHO Fracture Risk Assessment Tool and estimate your risk of breaking a bone in the next 10 years. After you pull up the FRAX WHO Fracture Risk Assessment Tool, click on Calculation Tool, then your country of origin, followed by your race or ethnicity to get the most accurate estimate of your fracture risk. You will also need your DXA T scores to enter. Since this is a new tool, guidelines about its use, benefits, and drawbacks are still being developed, so check with your doctor for updates.

Nelson, Miriam, and Sarah Wernick. *Strong Women, Strong Bones: Everything You Need to Know to Prevent, Treat, and Beat Osteoporosis.* New York: Perigee Books, 2006. Miriam Nelson is a Ph.D. who did groundbreaking research on women in their seventies and eighties who strengthened their bones by doing the exercises in this book on a regular basis.

North American Menopause Society (www.nams.org). This association includes nurses, nurse practitioners, and physician assistants as well as medical researchers and pharmacists and those from other disciplines dedicated to menopausal health. They certify menopausal clinicians who have attained a certain level of expertise and require them to maintain the credential with regular educational updates. They have current information on osteoporosis.

World Health Organization (www.who.org). The FRAX™ tool was developed by this organization. They post other helpful information about bone health.

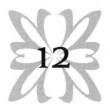

12

Lifestyle Choices for Living Longer

Age and postmenopause are kinder to some women than others. You may age well if your parents or grandparents have bestowed favorable genes on you. Yet genes alone are not enough. Perimenopause heralds the initial changes: metabolism slows, muscle mass diminishes, and hormones run riot. Thoughtful nutrition and activity choices become critical to your health. Even if you are naturally slender and never dieted prior to perimenopause, you will find you can no longer eat the same and exercise the same without gaining weight.

By the time we have reached postmenopause, many of us have lost count of all the diets we have tried and exercise programs we have abandoned. Whether you want to lose weight or maintain it, you owe it to yourself to become more informed about the type of nutrition and activity levels your body prefers at this time. Nutrition and activity influence how much independence you will preserve and how much energy you will have to do what you wish to do for the rest of your life. Even if you are well into postmenopause, the nutrition and activity door is still open. Women in their eighties and beyond can acquire additional strength and agility.

While no one can guarantee you will avoid obesity, diabetes, metabolic syndrome, heart disease, or bone thinning if you eat wisely and exercise regularly, you will be *much* less likely to be visiting your doctor for these medical problems if you prioritize strategies to lower your risk of these silent threats. With regular physical activity and wise nutritional choices you will also lower your risk of many types of cancer (see Chapter 13).

While it is good to be young at heart and to have a youthful outlook, it can be hazardous to your health to assume that your body has the same resilience against illness it once did. Your post-menopausal body (and to a lesser degree your perimenopausal one) is less forgiving of unhealthy lifestyle choices than your body was when you were in your teens or twenties. To enjoy healthy post-menopausal years, you need more information about nutrition and exercise than you did during previous decades because your risks of many different chronic illnesses are higher.

While increasing age does bring an increased risk of illness, in North America many diseases and ailments that have been attributed to aging in fact are directly related to lack of activity and poor nutrition. Although it is difficult to determine which diseases result from aging and which are specific to perimenopause and postmenopause, the medical profession has learned that illnesses formerly considered age-related can actually be prevented. Women who become overweight or obese (up to 65 percent of women in North America are in that category) are placing themselves at risk of metabolic syndrome, diabetes, cancer, heart disease, and even osteoarthritis due to the increased strain that excess weight places on joints.

Menacing Medical Conditions: Diabetes and Metabolic Syndrome (Syndrome X)

There are two major medical conditions that drastically increase the risk of heart disease and stroke, as well as death from other complications: diabetes and metabolic syndrome (or syndrome X). Being overweight increases the risk of both. As you read in Chapter 4, one out of two women over age 50 dies of heart disease. Those women who develop metabolic syndrome or diabetes are going to be in the wrong 50 percent. Their risk is even greater. Once you have either of these conditions your health is permanently compromised—unless the excess weight is lost.

DIABETES MELLITUS

This term is used to describe a group of diseases where carbohydrate metabolism is abnormal. Someone who has diabetes cannot process sugar normally and has hyperglycemia (excess sugar in the blood). Insulin, a hormone secreted by the pancreas, controls carbohydrate metabolism or sugar processing and does not function normally in individuals with diabetes. In some cases there is not enough insulin produced. In other cases the insulin is not working efficiently. Some types of diabetes are hereditary, others are not. Getting older and gaining weight both increase the risk of acquiring diabetes.

Those with advanced diabetes are more likely to suffer heart attacks. Diabetics who have heart attacks are less likely to survive them. Those with severe or advanced diabetes may also have trouble with their vision, trouble with their circulation, or loss of feeling in their feet.

People with diabetes can decrease their risk of heart attack, stroke, and blindness by working closely with their doctors to keep their blood sugar in the normal range.

METABOLIC SYNDROME (SYNDROME X)

Metabolic syndrome, or syndrome X, is a cluster of abnormalities related to obesity and high blood sugar that has grave consequences. While there is still not a uniform definition of metabolic syndrome that applies around the globe, I will give you the criteria for a few so that you become familiar with the syndrome and the concerns it raises.

When individuals have risk factors for both Type 2 diabetes and cardiovascular disease, such as abdominal obesity, high blood sugar, high blood lipids, and high blood pressure, they may be labeled as having syndrome X, or metabolic syndrome. In 1998, the World Health Organization (WHO) diabetes group proposed criteria for metabolic syndrome. The criteria include hyperinsulinemia (high insulin levels in the blood), or a high fasting glucose, or diabetes, as well as two of the following:

- abdominal obesity with a waist-to-hip ratio of over 0.9; a body mass index (BMI) of 30 or more kilograms per meter-squared; or a waist girth over 37 inches (94 centimeters)
- dyslipidemia (abnormal lipids, including cholesterol), with a serum triglyceride of 150 milligrams per deciliter or more or a high-density lipoprotein (HDL) cholesterol ("good cholesterol") of less than 35 milligrams per deciliter
- blood pressure of 140/90 millimeters of mercury or more, or taking medication for high blood pressure

Metabolic syndrome doubles the risk for heart disease and increases the risk of stroke by 75 percent. It increases the risk for Type 2 diabetes by more than five times. These adverse outcomes exceed those predicted by obesity alone. In addition to the high risk of heart disease promoted by high blood pressure and abnormal lipids, metabolic syndrome is associated with increased inflammation and a higher risk of clots, both of which are associated with heart attacks and strokes.

Risk factors for metabolic syndrome (syndrome X) include:

- being postmenopausal
- eating a high-carbohydrate diet
- leading a sedentary lifestyle

Metabolic syndrome is common in obese individuals, especially when fat is concentrated in their abdominal area. Obesity in general leads to diabetes, and abdominal obesity puts an individual at even higher risk for diabetes. Obese individuals can become resistant to insulin—they no longer respond when insulin gives the signal to remove glucose (sugar) from the blood. Insulin resistance in turn leads to excess insulin, as well as excess glucose in the blood.

You do not have to be overweight to be at risk for metabolic syndrome. Individuals can develop insulin resistance even if they are not overweight but carry their fat in an unhealthy location in their body (abdominal obesity). If core fat accumulates around the internal organs such as the liver and intestines, the risk of diabetes increases dramatically. Consequences of abdominal obesity include vascular endothelial dysfunction (poor blood vessel lining performance), vascular inflammation (inflamed blood vessels), abnormal fatty tissue function, abnormal lipids (blood fat levels such as cholesterol, high-density lipoprotein [HDL], low-density lipoprotein [LDL], and triglycerides, with low HDL [insufficient high density lipoprotein or good cholesterol])—all independent predictors of heart disease and stroke.

Heredity, body weight, abdominal obesity, and a low activity level can increase the risk of heart attack and stroke. Some experts believe that the cluster of risk factors for metabolic syndrome increase an individual's risk of heart attack and stroke more than each of the risk factors alone would predict, even when the risk is totaled for each. In other words, the total risk is greater than the sum of the individual risk factors when one accumulates them.

While different medical organizations have different definitions of metabolic syndrome, the risk factors and the adverse outcomes, including heart disease, stroke, diabetes, and death, are indisputable. Preventing metabolic syndrome, or treating it aggressively if it has already been identified, is critical to a postmenopausal woman's short-term and long-term health.

How Fit Should I Be?

Lowering your risk of metabolic syndrome (or trying to shed it if you have it) involves the need to:

- Change your exercise and nutrition routines until your abdominal girth is less than 35 inches (this is measured around the widest part of your belly at the level above the top of your hip bones).
- Achieve a serum triglyceride level of 100 milligrams per deciliter or less.
- Raise your HDL ("good cholesterol") to more than 40.
- Normalize your blood pressure to less than 120/75.

- If you already have Type 2 diabetes, a more aggressive goal is advised: 80 milligrams per deciliter for LDL, or less. This reflects the substantially higher risk of heart disease in those with Type 2 diabetes.

While a healthy goal of a waist measurement under 35 inches for a woman is becoming a new standard, some experts still use the waist to hip ratio of 0.8 as a healthy target. Another healthy target that can be used is a body mass index (BMI) of less than 25.

There are a number of measures of fitness and heart health that are available to women and medical professionals. They range from the ability to walk 10,000 steps a day, to passing an exercise stress test while the function of the heart is being monitored, to a normal waist measurement or a cholesterol blood test. A normal glucose (blood sugar) is another sign of health and suggests that the body is handling sugar normally.

BMI has been used for some time to gauge if an individual is in a healthy weight range for her height. It has limitations to its usefulness; specifically, it does not account for those who are very muscular. To determine your BMI, divide your body weight by the square of your height. Or you can use a BMI table: look for your height on one axis and your weight on the other. The table will show what range your BMI falls into. A healthy BMI falls between 19 and 25. A BMI over 25 indicates the person is overweight, and a BMI over 30 suggests the individual is obese and has even higher medical risks than weight alone may suggest.

A waist measurement greater than 35 inches is associated with too much central fat and correlates with a high risk for heart attack, stroke, and diabetes. Still another guideline you may come across is whether you have gained more than 10 pounds since your high school graduation weight. Today, with so many teens overweight, this rule of thumb may no longer hold fast. To me, based upon a review of the literature and opinions of experts in this field, the easiest guide is to measure your waist; if it's larger than 35 inches, you almost certainly have core body fat to remove. Central body fat, sometimes described as an apple-shaped physique, is strongly correlated with heart disease and diabetes, more so than heavy thighs or arms or a large chest.

In perimenopause, women are predisposed to acquiring fat around their middle. This is a worrisome place to acquire it. If it is just five pounds or so, one can view it as a "menopot." Dr. Pamela Peeke coined this term, reassuring women that a small amount of fat acquired during perimenopause or early postmenopause comes with the transition. After the ovaries stop manufacturing estrogen, the body's principal source of estrogen is from body fat. So a small amount of extra body fat supplies a natural source of estrogen that offsets hot flashes and thin bones.

Researchers now understand that being lean is associated with longevity. That said, it is not necessary to be *thin* to be healthy. You do not need to have an unrealistic goal of losing an overwhelming amount of weight if you are overweight. Losing even 5 percent or 10 percent of your current weight (if you are overweight) produces measurable benefits for your overall health and can lower your blood pressure. This kind of weight loss is an attainable goal for many.

Liposuction to remove abdominal fat does not improve insulin sensitivity nor does it lower the risk of heart disease or improve lipids. There is no short cut. An improved nutrition plan and daily exercise are *the* way you can achieve optimal health and proper weight.

When improved nutrition and activity levels do not achieve the desired goal of weight removal or improved glucose or lipids, your doctor may prescribe medication to control glucose levels and normalize lipid levels. This may be done before or during the time that lifestyle changes are being put in place. Medications to control high glucose levels and high cholesterol levels may keep heart disease, stroke, and diabetes at bay. Sometimes, even normal-weight or thin individuals require medications to control their cholesterol levels, particularly if they inherit a risk of heart disease, high blood pressure, high cholesterol, or more than one of these.

The Mystery of Vitamin X

The most frequent request I hear as a doctor is, "Just give me a pill to fix everything." I will tell you about a magic cure-all that I call "vitamin X." It is not on the market with this name, but you deserve to know about it so you can look for it.

Women in perimenopause and postmenopause benefit from vitamin X whether they have hot flashes, irregular menstrual periods, or no symptoms at all. Vitamin X lowers the risk of diabetes, obesity, heart disease, and stroke. Vitamin X lowers a woman's risk of breast cancer as well as other cancers. It strengthens bones and helps prevent osteoporosis and Alzheimer's. It also improves your sex life. Vitamin X is inexpensive. It comes in many forms. If you select the right version for you, it rarely has adverse side effects. Every woman can benefit from some type of vitamin X, regardless of her medical history, physical condition, or phase of menopause.

What is vitamin X? If you guessed exercise, you are correct. Research has shown that perimenopausal women who exercise up to 40 minutes a day, four times a week decrease their risk of breast cancer by 60 percent. If vitamin X could be packaged and sold as a pill, cream, or powder, it might be the only supplement most people would need.

Why Exercise Is More Important Now Than Ever

Women who do not exercise during perimenopause must accept that they will have a higher risk of breast cancer, osteoporosis, obesity, diabetes, and heart disease than they would have otherwise. Why is exercise so critical at this time of life?

Women begin to lose muscle mass in their mid-thirties. From that time on, even if a woman eats the same amount and exercises the same way, she is still likely to gain weight. Muscle tissue burns more calories per hour than fat, 24 hours a day, while awake or at rest, and even during sleep. Loss of muscle mass means fewer pounds of muscle are burning fewer calories all day long. As you have just read, once additional weight accumulates around the waist, the risk of diabetes, heart attack, and stroke increases dramatically.

A woman's body composition and her metabolism both change as she progresses from perimenopause to postmenopause. The gradual loss of muscle mass is one of the changes that contribute to a slower metabolism that naturally occurs with age. Also, most of us begin to accumulate more fat around the waist and abdomen. This provides our bodies with natural reserves of the weaker estrogen, estrone, which is converted in the fatty tissue. It offsets the loss of the ovarian estrogen, estradiol, which is diminishing.

Rapidly accumulating medical evidence suggests that attaining and maintaining a lean, healthy physique and a healthy level of physical activity dramatically increases the likelihood that you will enjoy many years of good quality life. This evidence of healthy longevity through healthy eating and regular activity flies in the face of our sedentary culture. Perhaps the excesses of food consumption and our tendency for passive sedentary activities (such as email and web surfing) make these goals seem unattainable. We are trending toward becoming workaholics compared to our global counterparts. We may not have enough time off from work to think about these goals. If we did, we might be able to embrace them and enjoy our time on the planet to a greater extent.

Choosing Your Activities

"Activity" is a term that includes exercise, but encompasses much more than that. For many, the thought of exercise is off-putting, overwhelming, and exhausting. Exercise is the last thing on many a woman's "to do" list, if it makes it on the list at all. While women who are not active may remain fairly healthy in their twenties and early thirties, they will not remain healthy over 40 without some form of regular activity.

The activity you select should be enjoyable for you, and doable. Start with what you enjoy, and figure out how you can do it regularly. After that, things will fall into place more readily. Once you are moving, and you have considered what is appealing to you, you can begin to assess whether you are incorporating the types of activity that will maintain your physical and mental health.

Exercise improves blood pressure, promotes weight loss, and removes abdominal fat, especially in women. Exercise helps remove weight and keep it off. Thirty minutes of brisk walking most days is the minimum recommendation, but you can break this up into shorter intervals if you are pressed for time. If the aerobic or weight/resistance sessions are at least 10 minutes each, you will get more aerobic benefit. That doesn't mean you cannot add shorter spurts of activity whenever possible. Every bit counts. More exercise is even better—ideally, we would all do 60 minutes or more of daily activity—but it is better to start with a realistic goal. It's important to do at least 10 minutes of an activity at a time that requires effort, raises your heart rate, and makes you sweat. A casual stroll is good for your health, but it won't help you lose weight or build muscles as effectively.

FOR WOMEN WHO DON'T EXERCISE

If you do not exercise or get regular physical activity at least once a week, start slowly. Start small. See your doctor first and get the green light to exercise. Do not go from parking next to the front door to parking a mile away. Consider any small habits that you can change on a daily basis. For example, if you take a train or bus each day, can you get off one or two stops early and walk the rest of the way? Can you take a walk during lunch? Are there stairs you can take as often as possible, instead of the elevator? Can you choose to take extra flights of stairs rather than avoiding them? Can you deliver a message in person instead of sending an email?

Do you like to garden? That counts. Do you like to dance? Put on the radio or a CD and dance to your heart's content. Use a DVD or take a dance class. Inexpensive classes are often available in adult education programs or community centers. Go with a friend or partner, or meet one there. Dancing is an excellent form of exercise, *and* it is good for the brain. It increases blood flow, and remembering the routines requires mental sharpness.

Do you like to walk? Consider wearing a pedometer, a small device attached to your waist that counts your steps. Eventually, the goal is to take 10,000 steps a day. In our sedentary society, some individuals take as few as 1,000 steps a day.

If you are not walking regularly, but like to walk, consider starting with five-minute walks in the morning. Perhaps you can walk for five minutes when you go to get your newspaper. Then add another five minutes at lunchtime and before dinner.

Consider cycling or walking to work, or to do your errands.

For Women Who Exercise in Moderation

Women who are somewhat active may use the strategies I've just reviewed to add to their activity level. Motivation may be an issue. Sometimes a woman chooses activities that do not appeal to her. She may "force" herself to do them because they are "good" for her. Incorporating adequate amounts of activity into your schedule to enhance your mental and physical health is difficult enough without asking yourself to do things that are not enjoyable.

I have found it helpful both personally and professionally to think about the social aspect of exercise and look at individual preferences through that lens. Do you like to have time alone when you walk or garden? Do you like to let your thoughts roam, or listen to music or a book on tape? Would you like to watch a show you've taped or a movie while you use an exercise bike or a treadmill? Free exercise tapes are available at most public libraries. You can borrow one or two and experiment to see what types of routines appeal to you.

Or do you prefer company? Would you rather go for a walk with a friend, or join a group class that meets at a fixed time? Do you prefer the flexibility of a gym or an exercise franchise that has open hours for exercising? Some of these facilities have other exercisers there to chat with if you wish, but you are not committed to a particular time/schedule each day. Sometimes seeing others exercising can be personally motivating.

For Women with Physical Restrictions

Even those with physical restrictions can find a suitable, enjoyable activity. There are aqua jogging classes. You do not need to be able to swim, nor do you need to put your head in the water or get your hair wet. A flotation device around your waist keeps you buoyant while you move your legs in the water to music. This does not stress your joints and may appeal to you if you have problems with your feet, ankles, knees, or hips. Those who are wheelchair-bound may also enjoy aqua jogging. If you have not tried aqua jogging or aqua aerobics, you may be surprised by the range of people enjoying these activities: they encompass many ages and sizes of women—do not feel intimidated if you do not wear a small-size swimsuit.

If you have hip, knee, ankle, or foot issues, water aerobics is another alternative. Exercises are conducted in shallow water. The water provides resistance and buoys up your body so that there is minimal stress on your joints. The classes I have seen or taken at the YMCA enroll women of all shapes, sizes, and health statuses.

When checking out classes, see if there are modifications provided to the standard routine that accommodate whatever physical restrictions or discomforts you may have.

⚡ Rita's Story ⚡

Social Exerciser

"I am a genetic counselor who talks to people all day long at work. I relax by doing quiet, solitary things like reading or playing the piano. Although I am disciplined in my professional life, I was having difficulty sticking to an exercise regimen. My cousin suggested I compile a list of friends and acquaintances that became my 'walking buddies.' Different friends were available during the week and on weekends. I try to make three or four walking dates a week, some planned ahead, and some spur of the moment. I no longer struggle to make myself go for a walk because I look forward to seeing my friends and enjoy their company."

Solitary Exerciser

Sharon is a friend from high school whose approach is opposite to Rita's. "I know Rita and wouldn't like her approach. I don't want to bother calling anyone. I would rather hop onto a treadmill each morning. I borrow books on tape from the local public library, and only listen to them while I am on the treadmill. This way, I am motivated because I want to hear what happens next. Occasionally, for variety, I record a favorite show and watch that while I am on the treadmill. I seldom miss a session."

WE ALL NEED THESE FOUR TYPES OF EXERCISE

As you begin to exercise more and try out different activities, keep in mind that there are four kinds of exercise that should be a part of your routine after you warm up. A warm-up can be as simple as walking in place for two to three minutes prior to stretching. "Warming up" means getting your circulation going and your muscles limber.

Stretching

Stretching is often overlooked. With age, we lose flexibility. Stretching helps to preserve flexibility and range of motion. Not only does stretching keep you flexible, but it also helps prevent injury and preserve range of motion. If you stretch regularly, it is less likely that you will get stiffness that limits what you can do. Recently I learned that stretching also enhances muscle strength by an additional 18 percent.

It is best to stretch after you have warmed up. Bob Anderson's book, *Stretching*, has a variety of stretches, which may help you warm up or cool down and ease the muscles you use most during the activities you enjoy.

Yoga naturally incorporates stretching with relaxation, and enhances flexibility and strength. T'ai Chi and Pilates also incorporate stretching.

Strengthening

Working with dumbbells or weights increases muscle strength and tone. Weight-bearing exercise may be done on weight machines, with free weights, or with exercise bands. It is also possible to work against your own body weight to build strength, as in doing push-ups.

Weight-bearing activity forces your body to work against gravity, strengthening your bones as well as your muscles. Targeted strengthening will help to preserve and replenish healthy muscle mass that is naturally lost with increasing age. Muscle conditioning helps ward off osteoporosis. It also helps keep your body trim and may decrease your waist and hip size by inches even before you lose any weight. Most important, muscle conditioning helps to preserve a woman's independence. She can continue to lift her own grocery bags and travel independently if she preserves her physical strength. Now we know that aerobic activity alone is not as important to heart health as including muscle conditioning and strengthening. Rowing indoors or outdoors is becoming more popular and strengthens the upper body in addition to providing aerobic benefits. Indoor rowing machines are available at health clubs and gyms. Light kayaks, rowboats, or skulls are fun for those with access to the water.

Remember, there is an added bonus: muscle tissue burns more calories per minute, even when you are not exercising.

Working out with weights does not create bulky muscles and will not make you look like a bodybuilder, unless you strive to look like one. And you are never too old to begin a weight-bearing exercise regimen.

Aerobic/Cardiovascular Activity

Raising the heart rate is sometimes referred to as "cardio" for short. You do not have to be a runner or triathlete to attain cardiac fitness. Cardiac exercise can be as simple as marching in place as fast as you can or using the stairs more at home or at work. It can consist of doing your own housework or gardening. It can be using a treadmill, stationary bike, or ellipse machine, or a variety of these. It can be dancing. Using a jump rope helps to prevent spine fractures from osteoporosis, but avoid jumping rope if you have already had an osteoporotic fracture. A nontraditional sport such as fencing can be enjoyed well into your eighties. Convenience and the appeal of the activity are key to entice you to do it on a regular basis.

Balancing

Maintaining a healthy posture and preserving your balance become increasingly important as you age. With age, your posture may deteriorate, and you lose your sense of balance. Now we know that specific types of exercise can help us regain our balance. One of the simplest balance exercises I know of is this:

1. Stand on one foot while you brush the top row of teeth.
2. Stand on your other foot while you brush the bottom row of teeth.
   (Do not try this while wearing sandals or shoes with heels.)

Exercises to regain balance range from walking on rugged uneven terrain, to doing Pilates, to working on an exercise ball or on a rubber disc placed on the floor. Improving your balance decreases your risk of falling. Fewer falls mean fewer fractures of the hip or the wrists when you reach out to break a fall. Activities that contribute to standing tall and preserving straight posture as well as balance include T'ai Chi, yoga, and Pilates, all of which can be practiced well into the senior years.

T'ai Chi is an ancient form of slow movements that enhance one's posture, alignment, and range of motion. You may find a class taught by a certified instructor, or you can borrow a videotape or DVD from the library. (You will find a good website and catalogue with a large variety of dance and exercise tapes at the end of this chapter, including tapes for those with handicaps.)

Yoga combines exercises that incorporate stretching and strengthening with breathing. It originated in India thousands of years ago. Yoga develops strength, flexibility, and a steady mind. It can be as gentle or demanding as you make it.

Pilates was developed by Joseph Pilates, a German boxer. When he was interned in England during World War II, he devised a system of pulleys and resistance exercises on the bunk beds to stay in shape. These exercises were designed to work the core of the body from the ribs to the pelvic area and stabilize it. Pilates differs from muscle training in that the core of the body is stretched, strengthened, and stabilized with each movement. Alignment of the body is also stressed. Pilates can be performed in a vigorous way on special machines or on mats on the floor. A certified instructor will assist you in learning the subtleties of the technique and enhance the benefits you will derive, but there are also books, tapes, and DVDs available at various levels of difficulty.

Optimal Nutrition

To recap, if you enter perimenopause and keep eating the same way you always have, and exercise as much as you always have, you will gain weight as you age. You may already have noticed your metabolism slowing down over time. You may also have noticed that your muscles are not as strong as they were, especially if you do not do weight-bearing exercise. Losing muscle mass results in fewer calories burned per hour.

Perimenopause and postmenopause bring other variables to the weight/balance picture. In addition to the decrease in metabolism associated with aging, and the fewer calories needed as one ages, there are other effects that are related to perimenopause and postmenopause that are difficult to sort out.

Dr. Pamela Peeke, an expert on menopausal activity and nutrition, reports that women metabolize smaller meals better than larger ones beginning in perimenopause and lasting into their postmenopausal years. She also found that a perimenopausal or postmenopausal woman needs fewer carbohydrates than she did before perimenopause. Since we cannot metabolize larger meals as well during perimenopause and postmenopause, she advises smaller portions. These smaller portions should include whole grains (no white sugar or flour) and high-fiber carbohydrates that provide longer lasting satisfaction and superior nutrition. She also recommends enjoying your carbohydrate servings early in the day. Consuming smaller portions of high-fiber carbohydrates earlier in the day matches our metabolic needs best.

Consuming more calories than the amount of energy you expend will cause weight gain, even if you only overestimate your calorie needs by a modest amount. Cutting calories too drastically to lose weight will not serve you well either. Cutting calories drastically (below your body's healthy requirements) will prompt a "starvation response." When this happens, your body will conserve calories and store them as fat because it thinks you are "starving." While this was originally an adaptive response when food was scarce in caveman times or during a famine, it is not adaptive for a postmenopausal woman. The last thing you want is to store extra fat while eating too few calories.

Another factor to consider is that as you lose weight, your calorie requirements decrease. A smaller body that has decreased in size has smaller energy demands. Activity can offset this so that your minimal calorie requirement is not too restrictive.

Researchers have recently shown that those who eat 80 percent of their body's requirement live longer. Those who are leaner and consume fewer calories (1,800 or less a day) also have lower body temperature; they are literally "cool customers," and the lower body temperature is associated with longevity. Leaner individuals who consume fewer calories are less prone to poor eyesight such as the kind that results from macular degeneration. Those who are thinner—due to eating healthy foods and adequate activity levels—*do* live longer, healthier lives. On the other hand, excessive dieting and even anorexia is surfacing in perimenopausal and postmenopausal women. This kind of "thinness" is not healthy.

INSTEAD OF COUNTING CALORIES, MAKE EACH CALORIE COUNT

Keep in mind that all calories are not created equal. Some foods are "nutrient-dense," meaning there is a high ratio of nutrients to calories, and you get more bang for the buck. Processed, sugary, commercially prepared foods have few nutrients, but lots of calories.

Proteins, carbohydrates, and fats are all essential to health. Different fad diets will discount one while overemphasizing another, but the body needs a balance of all three.

- Protein is needed for your body to build and repair cells, tissues, organs, hormones, antibodies, hair, fingernails, and so on.
- Carbohydrates are used primarily for fuel but also contribute to healthy moods.
- Fats are used by every cell in the body. Healthy fats are incorporated into cell membranes.

Healthy carbohydrates include whole grains that contain fiber to help digestion and elimination. Further, whole grains help to maintain healthy levels of serotonin, essential for good moods. Whole grains also help to prevent heart disease and several types of cancer, including bowel cancer. Whole grains should be in every woman's shopping cart.

Do not feel you must use the traditional Food Pyramid to govern your food choices. The government dietary guidelines represent input from special interest groups, including the dairy industry, the meat industry, and those who grow corn, to name a few, not a consensus of the latest developments in medical research on nutrition. Dr. Walter Willett, an internationally respected M.D., Ph.D., at Harvard School of Public Health, reviews some of the issues in his book *Eat, Drink, and Be Healthy.*

Similarly, be wary of diet books; their content is not regulated or monitored. Their recommendations are not necessarily based on good science. Celebrities in the diet and exercise domain are akin to Pied Pipers mesmerizing the attention of adult women. A celebrity need only provide a charismatic book cover photo, exuding sex appeal, to draw women in. The implication is, "Do what I say, and you will achieve my looks and appeal for yourself!" There are also books that have intrinsic appeal but no evidence backing them up. For example, the book *Eat Right for Your Blood Type* has an enthusiastic following. Although it is an interesting book, not a single research study is cited by the author. Published articles are needed to validate this theory. Perhaps blood type is the key to how we should eat, but some proof is in order.

FOODS TO AVOID

"White stuff" is a term that has been coined to encompass carbohydrates that are not good nutritional value for the calorie punch they pack. White stuff includes white flour, white sugar, and starch with minimal fiber and vitamins. The downside of eating white stuff is that it is digested too quickly, leaving you with a "sugar low" after the carbohydrate sugar rush suddenly vanishes from your bloodstream. After quickly digesting white stuff, you may feel weak and especially hungry, and crave even more white stuff. The nutritional value of white flour has been stripped away in the process of preparing it. Further, white stuff has no fiber so it can lead to constipation. White stuff is calorie-dense, so you don't have to eat a very large portion to pack in many nutritionally empty calories that will only leave you begging for more.

Colas, whether they are diet, sugar-free, or regular, lead to thinner bones, and should be minimized or eliminated from your diet.

Alcohol (beer, wine, or liquor) can decrease inhibitions and compromise judgment about how much to eat and what to select. Alcohol is also calorie-dense. Lastly, it disrupts sleep, which disturbs the body's ability to tell when it is satisfied with the amount of food that's come in (see Chapter 9).

⚥ JANELLE'S STORY ⚥

Changing Eating Habits

"I'm 53 and newly postmenopausal. I've been keeping a food diary for three weeks and adjusting portion sizes of protein and carbohydrates. I used to skip breakfast, but now I have yogurt in the morning. I try to have carbohydrates more often at lunch. A month ago, I would eat a whole chicken cutlet for dinner, but I've reduced my portion size

to four ounces. Now I only buy whole wheat pasta and measure out a one-cup serving. When I eat out, I request brown rice instead of white. I know I'm on the right track: I'm moving away from the white stuff and increasing my whole grains. This increases my fiber consumption and provides extra nutrients in my diet. I am also becoming more aware of what I eat by keeping a food diary and trying healthier portion sizes, especially for my protein and carbohydrate servings."

STRESS EATING

Janelle's story illustrates the role of keeping a food diary to learn more about your eating patterns. Often we are unaware of what we put in our mouths. Even the process of keeping a food diary can help awareness and decrease stress eating.

If you are prone to stress eating, try to reduce your stress by meditating for 5 minutes a day, and then gradually increase that to 15 or 20 minutes a day. Meditating can be as simple as repeating a word to yourself over and over. When your mind wanders, bring it back to the word you are repeating in your head.

Sometimes food preferences or stronger cravings influence you to have food with a particular texture or flavor. If you are stressed, you may succumb to the urge to eat a certain type of food, but you may be able to make healthier substitutions that satisfy you as well. For example, crunching on baked potato chips, instead of fried potato chips, might be a healthy substitution. Crunching on an apple instead of baked potato chips might be a helpful next step. If you are looking for a smooth, creamy texture, a sugar-free, fat-free pudding might work instead of chocolate mousse. Substitutes for your favorite treats may also help. Ice cream lovers may find a low-fat, frozen yogurt that they like. Alternatively, you can use portion control to enjoy the original form of the foods you like, but in smaller servings.

Experiencing stress releases the stress hormone cortisol. Cortisol promotes storage of abdominal and core fat around the internal organs. This type of fat storage is the most hazardous. It increases one's risk of heart attack, stroke, and diabetes as well as metabolic syndrome. Those who are stress eaters may find that stress reduction is a critical component of their improved nutritional plan.

Identifying whether you are a stress eater is helpful. Before eating a meal or snack, try asking yourself if you are hungry, bored, nervous, or stressed. Or, are you stimulated by the appealing food? Did you just walk past a bakery and smell the special of the day? If you admit to being a stress eater, you've identified important information. This means you'll need to find and use strategies to neutralize stress and stress eating, which include meditation, cognitive behavioral therapy, hypnosis, and acupuncture, to name a few. Exercise is also an excellent stress reducer.

Support from others is a stress reducer as well as an independent factor in attaining and maintaining a healthy weight. Support may come in different forms. Some women find support from meeting with their doctor or a nutritionist. Others may find that an online forum works for them (online programs are available through Weight Watchers, E-diets, and WebMD, to name a few). These online programs provide nutritional information as well as recipe suggestions and support. The support may be individual feedback or chat rooms. Meetings are another way to get regular support. Weight Watchers has meetings run by trained leaders that include a weekly (private) weigh-in and nutrition and behavioral strategies for weight removal and maintenance. Overeaters Anonymous also provides group support at meetings.

❧ SAMANTHA'S STORY ❧

A Speed Eater

"I'm a 'speed eater.' I grew up in a large family where those who ate fast got more of what they wanted! Throughout school, I kept up this rapid eating pace. Plus, I always had somewhere else to go. When I'm hungry, I can eat a lot of food quickly without realizing how much I've eaten. This way of eating is why I've never really developed the ability to tell when I'm full. Now, at 65, I'm 40 pounds overweight and having trouble with my knees. My doctor diagnosed osteoarthritis of the knees *and told me that the arthritic changes in my knees were a result of the extra stress they bore from my added weight. He said the bony changes would continue to create further damage and increasing pain if I did not remove the excess weight. He recommended that I consider Weight Watchers. I was under a lot of stress at the time and was not ready to begin the Weight Watchers program. I wanted to try to modify my eating on my own. The doctor recommended a food diary where I record every-thing I eat—before, during, or immediately after I eat it, including the portion size. In addition, he recommended that I eat more slowly. Taking at least 20 minutes to eat a meal allows me to begin to appreciate when I'm no longer hungry. My doctor explained that's how long it takes for the stomach to sense that it's full. During the period of ongoing stress in my life, I've continued to keep my food diary and to eat more slowly. When I'm mentally ready, I will start the Weight Watchers program, which I will do by attending meetings or using the online program."*

WEIGHT-LOSS DIETS

The pure definition of diet originally encompassed the food that you ate, not the food you had to give up or restrict yourself to eating. Anything you put in your mouth constitutes your diet. Diet is now synonymous with attempts to lose weight. Unfortunately, the term "diet" has been distorted to connote depriving oneself of foods one wants.

The term "nutrition" can help shift our thinking toward how to best nourish our bodies. Long-term nutrition with healthy choices is the goal.

Women are constantly enticed in our culture to become un-reasonably slim or to attain an unrealistic shape. The unrelenting pressure and exposure to painfully thin models are enough to drive a woman to drink, smoke, or eat an entire carton of ice cream in frustration and rebellion. Eating nutritious foods and developing a routine of regular, enjoyable, healthy activities is more realistic and sustainable, not to mention effective.

Before starting a new nutrition plan, decide if this is a good time for you to start one. Pick a time in your life when you are likely to succeed. It is better to stay the same than make a lukewarm effort and "fail" or binge and regain the weight. If you are under extra stress due to a relative or friend's illness, unusual demands inside or outside your home, or not in a favorable mindset for weight loss, you may want to maintain your current weight until you are ready to make some lifestyle changes. On the other hand, don't wait *too* long for the right time to begin.

One way to start gradually is to make one change a month. For example, you could commit to keeping a food diary every day. Even though you may not change your choices deliberately, keeping a daily food log has been shown to contribute to weight loss. It makes eating more conscious. By increasing awareness of what you are actually consuming, you have more detailed and accurate information on which to base your future food choices. If you like cream in your coffee, you could switch to low-fat or non-fat half-and-half. Alternatively, you could try low-fat milk and then skim milk. If you are an ice cream lover, you could try individual prepackaged servings of a frozen treat, or try low-fat or fat-free frozen yogurt instead of regular, full-fat ice cream. If you are wed to full-fat ice cream, consider individually wrapped servings or stopping for a small or "kid-size" scoop once a week.

Maintaining a healthy weight also requires effort. Some menopause experts say that maintaining your weight in perimenopause and early postmenopause is a victory in itself. As metabolism slows during the perimenopause and future decades, weight maintenance becomes challenging.

⚡ LINDA'S STORY ⚡

The Low-fat Maven

"Ten years ago I lost 30 pounds, and I have maintained my weight over that time by eating low-fat foods and monitoring my portion sizes. I eat whole grain carbohydrates. I do eat breakfast, but often miss lunch. I get very hungry in the evening and crave carbohydrates. My weight is good but my nails have become more brittle, and my hair

Linda is a victim of the low-fat era. She lacks healthy fats. All individuals need some healthy fat. Fats help to digest essential vitamins and minerals. Fat-soluble vitamins include vitamins A, D, E, and K. Vitamin A is important for eyesight. Vitamin D is important for bone health. Vitamin K is important for blood clotting. Without sufficient fat, these vitamins are not adequately absorbed by the body. Taking excess amounts of the vitamins will not correct this problem if there is not adequate fat to promote their digestion and absorption. Linda's doctor found that she had a vitamin D deficiency that contributed to thin bones. He prescribed supplemental vitamin D by mouth, and recommended that Linda have two teaspoons of olive oil each day or a few nuts to give her adequate amounts of healthy oils in her diet. Over time, Linda noticed that her hair was not as dry, and her nails were less brittle several months after she added the healthy oils to her diet. She also found she was not as hungry after dinner; the oils helped her to feel more satisfied.

HOW TO EVALUATE A WEIGHT-LOSS DIET

Weight reduction is the cornerstone of treatment for metabolic syndrome, as well as diabetes and heart disease for those who are overweight. Nutrition strategies that address this increasingly common threat to menopausal health include the Mediterranean diet. There are many versions of the Mediterranean diet that vary by country and cuisine. In general, they emphasize lean protein, olive oil, nut oil, or canola oil, as well as fresh fruits and vegetables. One version of the Mediterranean diet is presented in the *Sonoma Diet Cookbook* by Connie Guttersen and includes a detailed description of the program as well as recipes. Although the Sonoma diet is not promoted as a low-carbohydrate diet or a low-calorie diet, it has features of both. The healthy fats in this program, including olive oil along with the fruits, vegetables, and whole grains, promote lower blood pressure, weight loss, more normal lipid profiles, and less severe insulin resistance as well as less inflammation of the blood vessels.

Another program that addresses metabolic syndrome is the DASH diet, which limits daily sodium intake to 2,400 milligrams and promotes a higher dairy intake compared with the Mediterranean diet. It also may improve triglycerides and diastolic blood pressure as well as fasting glucose. A program with low carbohydrates and a low glycemic index will improve glucose control as well as blood lipids.

When you are considering a weight-loss plan, your doctor may be able to help you answer these questions, or she or he will refer you to a nutritionist.

- What is the nutritional value of the program?
- Does it promote heart health and strong bones?
- Are there enough healthy carbohydrates to sustain serotonin levels and maintain good humor as well as maintain healthy digestion and elimination?
- Are there enough fruits and vegetables to keep the risk of cancer and heart disease at bay?
- Are there enough fats allowed to maintain skin, hair, and nail health? Are the fats healthy ones such as those from nuts, avocados, and olive and canola oils?
- If you are diabetic, does the program meet your needs, or should you consult a nutritionist or diabetic expert as well?
- What prep work is involved for the program? For example, the South Beach diet is a heart-healthy program that also has cancer prevention features and is nutritionally sound, but substantial preparation is needed to create the dishes it advises. Are you someone who will devote the time and energy to chopping and assembling the foods ahead? The Sonoma diet is another program that emphasizes a Mediterranean cuisine. The food is delicious, but it helps if you like to cook, and often.

Conversely, there may be minimal or no prep work with a program such as with Jenny Craig, where the meals are provided for you. To be successful, you need to be committed to the maintenance phase when you will no longer have the portion control built into the premade dinners.

- Do you have the option of eating out and still staying on the program?
- How do you feel about eating the way the weight-loss plan advises for the rest of your life? Is there a maintenance phase built in? Are you willing to commit to the maintenance program? Would it fit into your lifestyle? Committing to the weight-loss plan without a maintenance plan just sets you up to regain the weight. You will need to commit to long-term lifestyle modifications and new nutritional choices to allow your hard-won progress to stick to you permanently. Researchers have shown that Weight Watchers followers do not achieve larger or faster losses than followers of other nutritional programs such as Atkins or South Beach, but Weight Watchers members do keep the weight off longer if they follow the maintenance program faithfully.
- What is the appeal and flavor attraction of the program that you are considering? Do you like the foods in the program and the way they are prepared? Are you open to trying the foods they suggest? Is there enough variety for you to experiment or create healthier versions of your favorites? Flavor and appeal count. If you are not accustomed to eating vegetables, and do not like them, switching to a vegetarian diet should not be your first move. Eventually, your palate may become more accustomed to enjoying the taste of vegetables, perhaps after several transitions. When you decrease the amount of white stuff you eat, you will probably notice fewer sugar cravings, and your tastes may shift to enjoying the nuances of various sensations other than the sweet ones. Varying textures and taste may help. Many women stick to sweet or salty, and creamy or crunchy. At some point you can expand your horizons to include sweet, sour, salty, savory, or bitter. Textures can include crunchy, chewy, or creamy, as well as combinations of these.
- Is there a behavioral piece to the program? Are there strategies

for coping with various roadblocks you may encounter, such as cravings, urges, parties, or emotional eating? Consider adding other behavioral tools such as hypnosis or meditation to reduce stress, or even cognitive behavioral therapy to give you insights as to why you may be a stress eater or an emotional eater.

- Is there an adjustment for decreasing your food intake as your weight loss progresses? You will need fewer calories as you remove weight. Beware: if you eat too little at first, your metabolism will slow down to guard you against starvation. Your body thinks you are starving it and will hold on to the calories and store them as fat to prepare for the famine.

As every woman probably knows all too well, if you eat too much, you will not lose weight. The problem that sets in during perimenopause and persists throughout postmenopause is that the range between eating just a little too much (resulting in unwanted weight gain) and eating too little (with its inevitable slowing of metabolism and calorie burn) is that the range between the two narrows at this time.

ꙮ MARILYN'S STORY ꙮ

Likes Protein and Carbohydrates

"I was brought up on meat and potatoes. I grew up eating salty, soggy canned vegetables that held no appeal. I've tried low-carbohydrate diets such as Atkins in the past and found my moods plummeted without the carbs. I've tried low-protein diets and found that I couldn't think straight and felt weak. My husband is also fond of meat and potatoes, so we always returned to that tried and true pattern. Recently, my doctor found I had high blood pressure as well as high cholesterol. I'm ready to make a change and make healthier food choices. Even though I'm 70, he said it's not too late.

"He recommended a low-sodium diet as well as one that includes more fruits and vegetables. He advised me to fill half of my plate with non-starchy vegetables, one-quarter with carbohydrates (preferably whole grains), and one-quarter with lean meat, chicken, or fish. He referred *me to a nutritionist who suggested I try to have one or two vegetarian meals each week. The nutritionist recommended a few programs with ideas about serving raw vegetables, in addition to those that include lightly steamed ones as well as frozen vegetables. Also, vegetarian versions of some of my favorite recipes were suggested. For example, I've found I like low-fat moussaka, a recipe with no meat, found in the American Heart Association cookbook. I also was surprised how much I enjoy vegetarian lasagna made with tofu crumbles (found in the freezer section of the supermarket) instead of ground beef as one of the fillings. Low-fat soup, another of my new discoveries, leaves me feeling full and satisfied with fewer calories and better nutrition."*

Comparing Diet Plans

Remember to consider how you feel as a result of different choices. Ideally, the food you select will allow you to feel full for some time and provide some satisfaction. The amounts should meet your metabolic needs without causing you to gain weight. Also, whatever choices you make should allow you some flexibility so that you do not feel so restricted that you cannot enjoy special occasions with your friends, co-workers, or family.

The Atkins Diet

Atkins emphasizes unlimited protein and fat, with minimal vegetables and carbohydrates and almost no fruit at first. Nutrition experts have voiced concerns about the types of fat Atkins promotes. Full-fat dairy and saturated fat products are not heart-healthy, and may promote cancer over time. For some Atkins devotees, adding back carbohydrates and fruits results in unwanted weight gain.

The advantage of Atkins is that it is simple to understand. One does not have to measure portion sizes or track food. To me, it is ironic that nutrition experts attribute the success of all diet programs, Atkins included, to calorie restriction. In the end, they say, one can eat only so much steak and full-fat dairy.

Some of Atkins's sound principles include minimizing the white stuff (simple carbohydrates and sugars). But healthy carbs with whole grains are not incorporated in the initial phases. The down-side is that Atkins may lead to heart problems. It may also be associated with constipation (because of very low fiber consumption), ketosis (bad breath resulting from breakdown of muscle tissue), and bad moods because carbohydrates are needed to have an adequate blood level of serotonin for well-being (calming and feel-good hormone levels).

Another concern raised about the Atkins high-protein program is that it may be associated with osteoporosis. Very high-protein diets promote bone loss. That is not an acceptable outcome for perimenopausal or postmenopausal women.

The South Beach diet, introduced by Dr. Arthur Agatston, is a healthier, more nutritionally sound, balanced low-carbohydrate program. Programs like the South Beach diet, the Core Program in Weight Watchers, and the Sonoma diet (Mediterranean diet) all stress healthy high-fiber carbohydrates and heart-healthy fats in small amounts (olive oil and canola oil), with liberal amounts of lean protein and non-starchy vegetables and fruits. These are all heart-healthy strategies.

Volumetrics

Volumetrics emphasizes your ability to select larger portions of food with good nutritional value and fewer calories, rendering it "less dense." This translates into lots of steamed vegetables and fruits that have high water content, which helps you feel full and satisfied longer.

Currently, according to one survey, Volumetrics is the most popular diet plan. The book was written by Barbara Rolls, a Ph.D. nutritionist, and incorporates many sound nutritional principles. Some of these principles are found in other diet programs. Mainly, Volumetrics emphasizes eating a large quantity of healthy food that is satisfying and of low calorie density. These types of foods include mainly non-starchy vegetables and many fruits that have very high water content as well as high fiber content. As long as they are not fried or prepared with butter or excess oil, this is a very healthy strategy. For some women, it will not be easy to transition to Volumetrics. They may not be willing to devote the time required to prepare these foods. Others may find this strategy satisfying immediately after eating, but then feel hungry two hours later. Certainly, from a nutritional standpoint, all women can benefit from eating more vegetables and fruits.

The Flavor Point Diet

Theories about selecting foods by taste to regulate appetite abound. Some experts advise a variety of tastes and textures to avoid boredom. They rely on variety to keep the program appealing. The approach of the Flavor Point diet differs in that it advises saturating your senses with a particular flavor so that you are not tempted to eat too much of that flavor. In this diet program, you select a flavor theme for the day. Each meal of the day includes that flavor as the major food. For example, at the end of the day, you will not be eager to eat extra turkey with cranberries after you have had a cranberry muffin for breakfast and a cranberry and spinach salad for lunch. After your body adjusts to one flavor a day, the program expands your options. It is another way to adjust portion sizes and expectations. The variety of food is there, but the uniform taste/ingredient of the day curbs the appetite and decreases the chances you will overeat.

Vegetarian Diet

Low-fat vegetarian diets are associated with excellent health, including a lower risk of many types of cancer, in particular, bowel or colon cancer. Further, a low-fat vegetarian diet lowers the risk of heart attack and stroke. In addition, consuming fewer calories, as associated with low-fat vegetarian choices, can mean living longer. Dr. Dean Ornish is an international expert on very low-fat vegetarian nutrition. He has done pivotal research showing that regular exercise combined with a very low-fat eating program lowers the risk of heart disease and even *reverses* existing heart disease. A woman who is not ready to completely embrace very low-fat vegetarian fare on an exclusive basis will benefit from adding vegetarian recipes or restaurant choices to her repertoire. You will find a list of books with vegetarian recipes and strategies at the end of this chapter.

Keeping a Food Journal for Weight Loss

You have already read about food diaries. If you are on a budget, or do not wish to set aside the time or devote the effort to a formal program just yet, you can use this simple, low-cost option. Record everything you eat, just before or after you eat it, on a piece of paper, or in your computer or hand-held device. Merely recording your food intake makes you more conscious of what you are eating, how much, when, and where. Understanding the circumstances of when and where you eat will assist you in identifying the issues you want to address. Studies show that recording food intake causes the recorder to change her eating habits even if she does not consciously commit to changing them.

⚡ MARINA'S STORY ⚡

Reasonable Food in Unreasonable Portions

"I've always made healthy eating choices and I'm quite knowledgeable about nutrition. I bake or grill chicken breasts without the skin, I buy whole wheat bread and brown rice, and I often have fresh fruit for dessert. But I was brought up to clean my plate. Although my choices were usually healthy, my portion sizes were outsized. When I had whole wheat pasta, I'd serve myself as much as I wanted. I knew that it was healthier than white pasta and didn't force myself to gauge the servings. Even though I walk one mile with a co-worker twice a week during lunch, my waist size has gradually expanded to 36 inches, and I weigh 45 pounds more than I did in high school. I thought it might be my age, 59, and just an inevitable part of menopause. I talked about it with my doctor and she recommended several options. Because she also took the time to explain the negative health consequences of the excess weight I was carrying, I listened.

"I can begin a program such as Weight Watchers that includes guidelines for portion sizes. Or I can choose a program such as the South

Beach diet or the Sonoma diet that also have portion guidelines. She said Volumetrics would also meet my needs as it would educate me about the energy content of the different types of foods I eat and change the amount of vegetables and fruit I eat compared to the amount of protein and carbohydrates. I could learn the portion sizes on my own, measure them out, and record them in a food journal. For example, if I choose to have frozen yogurt, and a regular portion of that brand is one half of a cup, I would measure out the half cup for a serving. If I choose to have two servings, I would have to measure out the second half cup and show myself that I was eating a second serving, rather than blithely eating one cup more and, in my mind, thinking of it as one serving. Writing down the amounts and types of foods that I eat makes me more accountable to myself."

Can't Lose Weight?

At times, you can be making your best effort to develop a healthy pattern of nutrition and exercise, yet not see results. In perimenopause in particular, this may be due to hormonal shifts affecting serotonin and sleep as well as disparate estrogen levels, the full effects of which are still not understood. There are other medical conditions that undermine weight-loss efforts. Identifying and addressing these conditions may remove these barriers.

Medical Saboteurs

Thyroid disease may prevent weight loss despite one's best efforts. An underactive thyroid will slow the metabolism so calories are not burned off at a normal rate. Correcting the thyroid imbalance with treatment will enable weight-loss efforts to succeed, but it is not a rapid "fix"; it can take more than six to eight weeks to even begin to see the difference. Although an overactive thyroid often burns more calories and leaves a woman lean, it can also stimulate appetite and promote unwanted weight gain in some cases.

Sleep problems may promote obesity. Sleep apnea, insomnia, or other causes of an insufficient amount of sleep disturb the body's ability to judge satiation and control eating (see Chapter 10).

Insulin resistance promotes obesity, as the body cannot respond normally to sugar.

Age weighs in, as there is a natural loss of muscle mass over time, and muscle burns more calories per minute than fat. Age and activity must be factored in when considering the amount of food required to be healthy and to maintain normal energy levels.

Medications that sabotage weight loss efforts include corticosteroids. They cause the body to store extra fat. Some types of antidepressant medication, such as the SSRIs, are also associated with unwanted weight gain.

Assessing Your Progress

Like other aspects of menopausal health, reassess your nutrition and activity patterns at least once every year. Reevaluate them sooner if your schedule changes, you lack energy to do the things you enjoy, or you have a change in your health status such as trouble with your hip, knee, or ankle that forces a change in your routine. Nutrition and activity choices impact your health significantly at this time; wise choices will enhance the health of your heart and your bones and add to your general sense of well-being in addition to helping you to achieve or maintain a healthy body size.

In some cases, an exercise stress test will be part of the assessment of your general fitness level and cardiac health. If your doctor does not think you need one based on your medical history and exam, there are other fitness goals. Those who take 10,000 steps each day, as measured by a pedometer, are likely to be healthy and/or physically active enough to maintain their health. Other guides to signal physical health include your stamina and energy level. Do you have the stamina and physical energy to do the things you enjoy on a regular basis? Does your exercise or activity pattern match your schedule? Does it meet your social preferences or needs? Have you changed from a solitary exerciser who works out or walks on her own to someone who enjoys a class or a walking companion more?

Are your exercise expectations too rigorous? Are you demanding so much of yourself that you throw up your hands in defeat? For example, do you tell yourself that you either work out at the gym every day after work or not at all? Do you have alternatives that you enjoy if the weather foils Plan A for your activity that day? Regular tweaking and a set of Plan B alternatives can save you. Also, keep in mind the variety of activities that provide benefit. If you do not feel like walking or getting on a treadmill, stepper, or elliptical machine, perhaps you are in the mood for doing yoga or T'ai Chi. Or, perhaps you feel like lifting free weights in front of the television or while you play a favorite CD.

You can change the social context if you find you develop a preference for solitary versus a social exercise setting. This may also change with your growing fitness level. A sedentary woman may begin by walking five minutes a day. Later in her fitness journey, as she gains stamina and increases her level of fitness, she may enjoy walking or exercising with others, or she may welcome the challenge of a planned walk or run for charity.

If your schedule becomes more demanding, you may need to change the timing or location of your activities.

Ultimately, the savvy way to have good nutrition is to consume nutritionally healthy foods. As anyone who has reached the second half of her life knows, healthy eating has its rewards. One patient summed it up for me when she said, after losing 30 pounds: "I used to live to eat; now I eat to live."

RESOURCES

Local public libraries and senior centers often have exercise videos or DVDs that you can borrow to preview or try.

For descriptions of a wide variety of workouts by level, goal, and type, including online fitness video and DVD previews, check Collage Video (www.collagevideo.com). They also have a print catalogue you may request, music to dance or exercise by, and programs for those with long-term physical challenges or restrictions, such as being wheelchair-bound.

Agatston, Arthur, with Joseph Signorile. *The South Beach Diet Supercharged: Faster Weight Loss and Better Health for Life.* New York: Rodale, 2008.

Barnard, Neal. *Breaking the Food Seduction: The Hidden Reasons Behind Food Cravings—and 7 Steps to End Them Naturally.* New York: St. Martin's Press, 2003.

Guttersen, Connie. *The Sonoma Diet Cookbook.* Des Moines, IA: Meredith Books, 2006. This book embodies the Mediterranean diet, a heart-healthy cluster of cuisines. There are excellent recipes and a program to follow regarding portion sizes and balancing different types of foods, but not much guidance about planning meals that don't fit the profile.

Katz, David, with Catherine S. Katz. *The Flavor Point Diet: The Delicious, Breakthrough Plan to Turn Off Your Hunger and Lose the Weight for Good.* Emmaus, PA: Rodale, 2005. This is a fresh approach by a well-qualified physician who has you saturate your taste buds for days with the same flavors. The theory is that if you have cherry muffins for breakfast, followed by a fruit salad with cherries and cherry yogurt for lunch and chicken with cherry sauce for dinner, you will be less likely to overeat because your taste buds are sated by the cherry flavor.

Katzen, Mollie, and Walter Willett. *Eat, Drink, and Weigh Less: A Flexible and Delicious Way to Shrink Your Waist without Going Hungry.* New York: Hyperion, 2006.

Nelson, Miriam, with Sarah Wernick. *Strong Women Stay Slim.* New York: Bantam Books, 1998.

Ornish, Dean. *The Spectrum: A Scientifically Proven Program to Feel Better, Live Longer, Lose Weight, and Gain Health.* New York: Ballantine Books, 2008.

Peeke, Pamela. *Fit to Live: The 5-Point Plan to Be Lean, Strong, and Fearless for Life.* Emmaus, PA: Rodale, 2007.

Prevention Magazine (www.prevention.com). As its title suggests, *Prevention Magazine* does an excellent job of covering preventive health topics, including traditional and alternative medicine approaches. The magazine also offers exercise and nutrition options.

Rolls, Barbara. *The Volumetrics Eating Plan: Techniques and Recipes for Feeling Full on Fewer Calories.* New York: Harper, 2007.

Wansink, Brian. *Mindless Eating: Why We Eat More Than We Think.* New York: Bantam Books, 2006.

Weight Watchers (www.weightwatchers.com). The new version of the program released in December 2008 incorporates additional tools to help you become more aware of the types and quantities of foods you consume, how satisfied you feel after eating them, and how they compare to the amount of energy (calories) you burn during your daily routine. The program may be followed by attending meetings, visiting their website on the Internet, or both. It is updated regularly with information from nutritionists and medical experts. There is leeway to eat more carbohydrates or more protein as you choose, or to follow the program as a vegetarian. *Weight Watchers Magazine* is their monthly print magazine with new recipes, exercises, and approaches to losing weight that is well done.

What Is Metabolic Syndrome? National Heart Lung and Blood Institute Diseases and Conditions Index (www.nhlbi.nih.gov/health/dci/Diseases/ms/ms), April 2007. Last accessed December 13, 2008.

Curbing Your Risk of Cancer

Today, bad news travels fast and negative spin captures our attention. We are drowning in cancer news. Often, the underlying message is: "You could get cancer, it may not be found soon enough, and it may not be curable." It is difficult not to feel helpless in the face of this overwhelming threat. For some of my patients, the fear of getting breast or ovarian cancer is so strong it is palpable. Yet these same women are often unaware of what they can do to decrease their risk of getting cancer. This chapter covers specific ways that you can do just that. While no one can guarantee that these strategies will prevent cancer, research has shown that they do lower your risk. Pursuing these prevention strategies is well worth the effort.

Your Individual Risk Profile

Each of us has our own risk profile based on our personal medical history, family history, physical examination findings, and test results. While our personal medical history and family history cannot be altered, our lifestyle choices can raise or lower the risk of cancer. As an added bonus, many of these lifestyle choices also lower the risk of heart disease and diabetes.

The types of choices that affect your risk of getting cancer include:

- your nutrition (what you do and do not eat)
- your physical activity (how often and how much you move)
- your weight (is it in a healthy range for your age and build, or substantially above that range?)
- whether you smoke
- the number of sexual partners you've had

For example, consuming red meat more than twice a week increases the risk of breast cancer as well as colon (bowel) cancer. Researchers have shown that vegetarians and those who rarely eat meat have a lower risk of breast and colon cancer.

HEREDITY AND FAMILY HISTORY

While no lifestyle change can *eliminate* the risk of cancer, each of us can make choices that will *lower* the risk of certain cancers. The first step in assessing your individual cancer risk is to determine if your family history suggests that you are at higher risk. A woman who has two relatives with breast or ovarian cancer may have a high-risk family history, especially if those relatives include a mother or sister. The closer the relationship of the relatives (such as a mother or sister versus aunt or grandmother), the greater the number of relatives affected, and the younger the age the cancer developed, the higher the risk. Individuals from high-risk families will want to take more aggressive steps (discussed later in this chapter) to lower their risk of cancer. Having a family history of breast or ovarian cancer may mean your risk of getting cancer is greater. It does not, however, mean you will definitely get cancer.

The majority of women who get cancer of the breast, ovary, uterus, or cervix have no family history of these cancers, so none of us should be complacent! In addition to the aggressive measures available to those with high-risk family histories, there are more general measures to help prevent cancer that we can all follow. Examples of these general measures are included later in this chapter.

Some cancers are inherited and others are a result of lifestyle and environmental factors. Still others are due to random mutations or genetic accidents without a recognized pattern. None of these causes of cancer are completely understood, although researchers are making steady progress. Cancer researchers have found that mutations in specific genes increase the chances that an individual will get a certain type of cancer. They also think environmental toxins play a role in causing cancer, as do lifestyle choices such as smoking cigarettes. Still, most cases of cancer are unexplained.

Genes have been identified that are associated with a higher risk of breast and ovarian cancer. The two most well-studied genes are breast cancer antigen 1 and 2 (BRCA1 and 2). Mutations of BRCA are responsible for most hereditary ovarian cancers known today. These mutations, or mistakes in the genes, interfere with the DNA repair process. If a woman has family members who have breast or ovarian cancer and test positive for BRCA1 or 2, she has a higher risk of getting breast or ovarian cancer. Even though her risk of getting these cancers is higher, she may never get these cancers at all. Her risk goes up with a greater number of family members with cancer and if some of the relatives developed the cancer at an earlier age (under 50). Genetic testing is a useful strategy in these families, especially if the testing for BRCA1 and 2 is done on a family member who has already been diagnosed.

❧ THELMA'S STORY ☙

A High-risk Family History

"*I am 42 years old and have two children. My sister was diagnosed with ovarian cancer at age 48. My mother was diagnosed at age 47. My sister never wanted to go to the doctor because she was afraid that she would get bad news. I wanted to be tested for BRCA based upon my family history. When I discussed this with my doctor, she advised formal genetic counseling. My doctor and the genetic counselor agreed that it would be best for my sister to be tested for BRCA since she had the cancer. If she didn't have the BRCA mutation, I would be less likely to have it. My sister tested positive for BRCA. After that I was tested and was also positive for BRCA. My doctor told me that the tubal ligation I had after the birth of my third child lowers my risk of ovarian cancer by 30 to 50 percent. The genetic counselor told me that BRCA muta-*

tions are more common in Ashkenazi Jewish women: they have a one in 40 chance of carrying the mutation. My sister and I have an Ashkenazi Jewish grandmother on my mother's side. Otherwise, outside high-risk groups, the inherited BRCA mutations are pretty rare, and affect only one in 500 individuals.

"Since my family history is high risk, I am considering laparoscopic surgery to remove my tubes and ovaries before they can develop cancer. I am getting another opinion before I make my final decision. I think the second opinion will be helpful because I also found out that just having the BRCA mutation does not mean that I will definitely get ovarian cancer. I have started to tell my 20-year-old daughter about our high-risk family history. My daughter's doctor recommends she start having a CA-125 [Cancer Antigen-125] blood test and a vaginal ultrasound every six months after she turns 35 to keep a close eye on her ovaries and find cancer as early as possible if it does develop. The doctor also advised my daughter to continue taking an oral contraceptive pill because it will lower her risk of ovarian cancer by roughly 50 percent."

N Janice's Story N

No History of Cancer in the Family

"I am 60 years old and was recently diagnosed with ovarian cancer. No one in my family has breast or ovarian cancer. When I grew up, my mother showed us how to put talc on our sanitary pads to keep them fresh. Three months ago I had pelvic discomfort for a month or so and thought it was bloating from something I ate. The bloating didn't go away, so I went to my doctor. When she examined me, she felt an enlarged ovary on one side. A vaginal ultrasound showed that I had a large cyst in that ovary. The features of the cyst concerned the doctor because it was not a simple clear cyst, and was more than three inches wide. She ordered a CA-125 blood test and it was over 400. My doctor sent me to a gynecologic oncologist who specializes in pelvic cancers. The gynecologic oncologist did surgery to remove both tubes and ovaries, and recommended chemotherapy. Now I am back to my part-time job and my usual activities. I asked the oncologist if he would have done a CA-125 test earlier, and he said he would not have, since my family history was negative. I probably had a random mutation. He said the talc I used when I was young may have played a role in increasing my risk of ovarian cancer."

⚘ ROSE'S STORY ⚘

68-year-old Breast Cancer Survivor Diagnosed at Age 39

"I am 68 years old now. Even though no one on my mother's or father's side of the family has breast cancer, I was diagnosed with breast cancer at age 39. I was tested for a mutation in the BRCA1 or 2 gene since my cancer was found at such an early age. Now my daughter Eve is 35 years old and wonders what she should do to protect herself against breast cancer. Eve's doctor told her she is not likely to have a mutation of the BRCA1 or 2 gene since I don't have it. She is trying to find out more about the family history of cancer on her father's side. Even if there are no family members on her father's side with breast cancer, Eve was told she is still at higher risk of getting breast cancer because I had it. Both my doctor and Eve's doctor think she should get genetic counseling to help her fully assess her risk of breast cancer and explore the options to decrease her chances of getting it. I hope they don't tell her to have her ovaries removed or to have both breasts removed, although she may choose one of these options if her risk of breast cancer is high enough."

Discussing your family history of cancer with your doctor is the first step in determining if you have a higher risk of getting those types of cancer. Based upon your family history, your personal risk factors, and your current lifestyle, the doctor can discuss the lifestyle choices that will lower your risk of that cancer (if any). He or she can also suggest screening tests that are helpful and recommend how often they should be done. Before we look at specific screening strategies for the individual cancers, let's take a closer look at what they can and cannot tell you.

Screening versus Diagnosis

Screening is the medical term for procedures designed to find a particular cancer in its earliest stages, before it can be seen or felt, when a cure is most likely. Screening tests, well-suited to finding one type of cancer, are usually not helpful in finding others. For example, a Pap test will detect cancer of the cervix but will not find ovarian or uterine cancer.

There are many forms of screening tests. Mammograms (to detect breast cancer) and Pap smears (to detect cervical cancer) are two well-established screening tests familiar to most women. While neither test enjoys a perfect track record, and both have limitations, the Pap test has helped to reduce substantially the number of women dying from cervical cancer in North America, and mammograms help detect breast cancer early, before a lump can be felt. Unfortunately, accurate, reliable screening tests are not yet available for ovarian or uterine cancers.

Besides your family history and your lifestyle, there are other factors to consider when you and your doctor discuss whether you need more than a mammogram and a Pap smear. These are concerns about changes in your health and the findings on your physical examination. To get the best medical care, list the things about your health that have changed, or that concern you, before seeing your doctor. Bring the list with you. Certain concerns deserve special attention and are best mentioned at the beginning of your appointment. If you have pain or bloating, put it at the top of your list. If you have postmenopausal bleeding, that is a priority for discussion.

Sometimes a woman asks her doctor for specific tests. For example, she may ask for the blood test for CA-125 because she has heard it is a good way to check for ovarian cancer. It isn't helpful for most women. The ideal time to discuss appropriate testing is after you update your medical and family history and have your physical examination. If the history or physical examination findings suggest the CA-125 test will be helpful, the doctor will order it.

Why not do a CA-125 on everyone so no ovarian cancers are missed? There are two reasons. Finding early ovarian cancers in

Present the facts first. Tell your doctor what's going on with your health before you share your own conclusions about the causes or ask for specific tests to be done.

the general population is not feasible yet; the screening process for ovarian cancer is not refined or well established. It produces too many false alarms and even side effects without identifying those at risk. Ovarian cancer is rare enough in the general population that these methods will not find it. In high-risk families identified by history or BRCA1 or 2 testing, the yield is higher, and the tests have a better chance of finding early cancers. If I am looking for a needle in a haystack, I am not likely to find it. Arbitrarily examining individual straws of hay is not a well-designed process and has a low yield. However, if I lose a needle in my sewing kit, I have a good chance of finding it, especially if I use a magnet. My search is confined, the probability of finding the needle is greater, and my tools are better suited to the task.

The second reason for not requesting a CA-125 as a screening test is because it is unlikely to be the best way to address your concerns. It may play a role, depending upon the information garnered from your current medical history and physical examination. In the absence of a high-risk family history, the doctor's best recommendations for helpful testing are made after the history and examination findings are analyzed. If the CA-125 was a good screening test and identified ovarian cancer reliably in the general population, gynecologists would be ordering CA-125 tests as routinely as they do Pap smears and mammograms.

You have read about the role of CA-125 in evaluating a large ovarian cyst found on examination. Your doctor may order this test if he or she has a concern that emerges from your medical history that a CA-125 test can shed light on.

Jumping to Conclusions

"I am 63 years old. I use the Internet sparingly compared to my friends, but I read a lot of magazines. Recently I read that bloating is a sign of ovarian cancer. I have noticed that my tummy is more bloated over the past few months and began to worry that it may mean I have ovarian cancer. I jumped to conclusions, called my gynecologist's office, and asked to have a blood test for CA-125 before my visit. The staff said that the doctor would want to see me first. That miffed me because I didn't want to wait. If I had ovarian cancer I wanted to know as soon as possible. The office staff called me when a cancelled appointment became available.

"I was surprised how many questions the doctor asked about the bloating before doing my examination. She wanted to know:

'Do you have the bloating daily or just certain days each month?

Have you noted the bloating over weeks or over months?

Have you noticed any changes in your bowel habits?

Is the bloating worse after meals?'

"She wanted to evaluate other possible causes for the bloating in addition to the possibility of ovarian cancer. It turned out that I had diverticulitis, a condition of the large intestines where pockets of colon protrude and food and debris get stuck in them and infected. After a course of antibiotics to treat this condition, the bloating resolved. If I had gone ahead with the blood test that I requested, the diverticulitis would have gotten much worse and I might have needed surgery to treat it instead of antibiotics. I was also relieved when the pelvic ultrasound I had done did not show any ovarian cysts."

If I show you a jigsaw puzzle without the cover picture and tell you there is water in the design, you might assume that all of the blue pieces represent water. But some of the blue pieces may belong in the sky. I only gave you limited information, not the "big picture." If you ask for a CA-125 test, and that is all the doctor orders (per your request), other studies that show a different reason for your concerns may not be done. The big picture may not emerge.

Doctors spend years learning what tests in their specialties will
be most helpful as well as the best sequence in which to conduct
them to give you the most accurate and complete results.

Helpful Tests

Medical testing has become increasingly complex over
the past two decades. Often the distinction between screening tests
and diagnostic tests is obscured. Yet, this distinction is critical to
getting quality medical care. Tests designed for screening are not
usually valuable diagnostic tests. And diagnostic tests are not usually helpful screening tools.

Screening tests are designed to check large numbers of patients
who seem healthy: they have not noticed changes in their health,
and do not have new findings on their physical examinations. A
good screening test finds something wrong before the individual is
aware of it. Good screening tests must be sensitive and specific. In
medicine sensitivity and specificity have unique meanings.

The sensitive screening test sniffs out trouble reliably, much like
a seasoned detective. A test with 100 percent sensitivity is like a hy-
pothetical detective with a perfect track record: he finds the culprit
every time. He does not leave any criminals on the street, and he
does not falsely accuse anyone of being a criminal. A perfect detective does not exist, nor does a perfect cancer screening test. However, it's nice to get as close as possible to the ideal and a test with
high sensitivity will identify as many individuals as possible who
have a certain cancer. We don't want the test to miss identifying
anyone with cancer. Nor do we want the test to have a false result,
indicating that someone who is actually healthy has cancer. Just as

the detective looks for criminals, the sensitive screening test looks for individuals with cancer.

Let's say 10 women out of 100 in a clinic are known to have cervical cancer. If we are trying to find out the sensitivity of a test for this cancer, we want to know how many of the 10 women with cervical cancer the test can identify. If it identifies 8 of 10, it has 80 percent sensitivity.

A good screening test also needs to be specific. Specificity is concerned with correctly identifying the healthy individuals. In the group of 100 women in the clinic, 90 are actually healthy and cancer-free. The screening test with the best specificity will accurately identify the greatest number of healthy women. The more of the 90 healthy women the test can correctly identify, the more specific (and helpful) it is.

There are different types of false alarms screening tests can create when they are not "perfect." They can falsely reassure someone with cancer that she is healthy, or they can falsely label a healthy person as having cancer. Neither is desirable. The best tests minimize the chances of both types of false alarms.

So the screening tests that work best find enough cancers to be helpful without producing too many false alarms. But there is more to it, especially in the case of CA-125. The ability of a test to predict who has cancer also depends upon how common that cancer is in the group of women being tested. Women from high-risk families can benefit from tests that are not helpful in the general population. The women from these families are at higher risk and there are many more cancers to find. The test has a greater likelihood of identifying early ovarian cancer in this group. However, in the general population, with no physical findings and no high-risk family history, CA-125 is not a good screening test for ovarian cancer. There will be too many false alarms without identifying those women truly at risk.

The predictive value of a screening test cannot be assessed in a vacuum; the qualities of the group being tested make a difference. A meteorologist who develops a new technique for predicting the timing and severity of a snowstorm is not going to test his technique in Hawaii. The likelihood he can refine his technique is too remote.

Reducing the Risk of Ovarian Cancer

Some ovarian cancers are from mutations that can be inherited. The most-well-understood hereditary pattern is found with BRCA1 and 2. Women who inherit this genetic mutation are at higher risk of getting breast and ovarian cancers. It is possible, however, to have the gene and never get either of these cancers. In addition to inherited mutations, there are other factors that influence the risk of getting ovarian cancer.

Ovarian cancer is more common in women who:

- are sedentary, obese, or both
- have not given birth to a biologic child and were exposed to continuous ovulation
- use or have used talc on sanitary pads
- drink more than two glasses of cow's milk a day. Preliminary research by Dr. Dan Cramer of Brigham and Women's Hospital in Boston shows an increase in ovarian cancer in women who drink more than two glasses of cow's milk a day. Other dairy products, such as yogurt, are not risk factors for ovarian cancer. Other studies have not confirmed Dr. Cramer's results but they may prove valid in the future. For now, my advice is to keep milk consumption to two glasses a day or less to be on the safe side.

Lifestyle choices that decrease the risk of ovarian cancer include:

- taking oral contraceptives or using Nuva Ring (suppresses ovulation)
- tubal ligation (decreases the risk by 30 to 50 percent)
- hysterectomy with the ovaries preserved (decreases the risk by 30 to 50 percent)

The underlying theory for the decrease in ovarian cancer risk with tubal ligation is that environmental toxins (exactly which ones are still unknown) can no longer reach the ovaries and influence them to develop cancer. Similarly, having a vaginal, abdominal, or laparoscopic hysterectomy with preservation of the ovaries decreases the risk of ovarian cancer, even though the ovaries remain in the body. The theory behind this is the same as for the tubal ligation.

Those with a clear and worrisome family history of ovarian cancer, particularly in a mother or sister, should discuss the pros and cons of more aggressive strategies, such as surgical removal of the tubes and ovaries, to lower their risk of ovarian cancer.

Detecting Ovarian Cancer

It is not uncommon for a woman to experience bloating and abdominal discomfort. Many women notice bloating that comes and goes with their cycle each month, especially during perimenopause. It is difficult for women and their doctors to know when the bloating may signify ovarian cancer. One ovarian cancer researcher is looking at the duration of symptoms such as bloating and nausea to help determine when they may signal ovarian cancer. Her preliminary findings are that symptoms occurring every other day for 6 to 12 months are more likely to be found in women with ovarian cancer as opposed to women who have these symptoms only occasionally or for a shorter time.

Share your concerns, how you feel, and any physical changes you notice with your doctor. Then be open to his or her suggestions about how to approach the detective work and medical testing needed to interpret your medical concerns, while still being sure that you are satisfied. If you are concerned about ovarian cancer, you may ask your doctor directly: "How can you be certain that I do not have ovarian cancer?" This approach allows the doctor to use his or her expertise and understanding of your personal history, family history, and lifestyle to select tests that will give you the most accurate answer to your question.

More about Cancer Antigen-125

Cancer Antigen-125, or CA-125 for short, is an example of a diagnostic test women often request as a screening test. If CA-

125 were a good screening test to check for ovarian cancer, my colleagues and I would order it for each of our patients, just as we order a screening mammogram or Pap smear. But numerous studies have shown that CA-125 is *not* a good screening test for ovarian cancer. At this time, a good screening test for ovarian cancer is not available. Researchers are working diligently to develop one.

CA-125 is not a good screening test for two reasons. First, there are many types of ovarian cancer that CA-125 does not find. The CA-125 test can be normal, but falsely reassuring. The test says "no problem," but the ovarian cancer is present and not identified by the test. Second, there is an overwhelming number of false positives, or false alarms, with CA-125.

There are more than a dozen other medical causes for an elevated CA-125 test. The large number of false positive results is one reason CA-125 is not a good screening test for ovarian cancer. A wide variety of medical conditions can trigger a falsely elevated CA-125, ranging from benign, noncancerous gynecologic entities such as a fibroid to non-gynecologic conditions. These trigger false alarms and worry women and their doctors that the high CA-125 signals ovarian cancer when in fact it doesn't.

Endometriosis, a common noncancerous gynecological condition, can cause an elevated CA-125. Inflammation in the lung can produce an elevated CA-125 as well.

At times, a CA-125 test can play a role in determining the status of a woman's ovaries, but it is not a good routine screening test for ovarian cancer. A gynecologist can best advise each woman on an individual basis whether a CA-125 is appropriate for her. For women who have ovarian cancer, CA-125 levels can be used to judge how effective treatment has been. The levels decrease with effective medical or surgical treatment.

A woman at high risk for getting ovarian cancer, such as someone with a first-degree relative (mother, sister, or daughter) who has ovarian cancer, can benefit from having a blood test for CA-125 every six months. If the woman is still perimenopausal, the test is best scheduled after her menstrual period. This test provides monitoring for a woman with a high-risk family history until a better screening test becomes available. In addition, for a woman at high risk, a vaginal ultrasound may be done to check the status of the ovaries and look for abnormal ovarian cysts every 6 to 12 months. This use of the CA-125 is a stop-gap measure because, at present, there isn't a good test available to check high-risk women for ovarian cancer.

In the future, CA-125 will most likely be partnered with other blood tests to screen for ovarian cancer. Since there are many tissue types of ovarian cancer, a combination of at least six tests, only one of which will be the CA-125, should be more helpful.

⚜ ERICA'S STORY ⚜

A False Alarm

Erica, a 42-year-old single woman who has never been pregnant, suffers from PMS (premenstrual syndrome). "I have bloating the week before my period each month. I read about the CA-125 test for ovarian cancer on the Internet, and some of my friends had the test done. I wanted the test to be certain that the bloating did not signify ovarian cancer. I read that women who never had children are at higher risk for ovarian cancer, and that the routine annual pelvic examination usually does not find the cancer. When I saw my gynecologist, he did not recommend that I get a CA-125. I wasn't certain if he was being cost-conscious or if he was not up-to-date about this test, so I got another opinion. I went to my friend's doctor and had the test. My CA-125 level came back elevated at 80. I panicked. The doctor was also concerned. I thought she would recommend a hysterectomy. Instead, she advised I get a pelvic ultrasound to see if any ovarian cysts or abnormalities could be detected. The ultrasound identified a cyst roughly one inch wide. I returned to my regular gynecologist to discuss this. He thought the cyst was probably just related to my menstrual cycle and would dissolve on its own. He did not think it was responsible for the elevated CA-125 result. He suggested repeating the CA-125 test after my next menstrual period. I did have the repeat blood test, and it was low and normal. In retrospect, the timing of the test before my period created a false alarm. My regular menstrual period made the CA-125 go up."

Reducing the Risk of Breast Cancer

Breast cancer is the leading cancer that affects women in the United States today. However, it is not the leading cause of death. That "distinction" goes to heart disease, as you read earlier in this book.

The two most common risk factors for getting breast cancer are female gender and increasing age. Only one percent of breast cancers occur in men. The average age of a woman diagnosed with breast cancer is 61. The risk of getting breast cancer increases up to age 79. After that the data is harder to interpret, and less data is available for women in their eighties and beyond, so it is difficult to predict whether the risk continues to increase further or not. (Many experts think it does continue to increase.) So there is not a clear consensus on the age to discontinue having mammograms. The age to start having mammograms to screen for breast cancer, in a woman with no risk factors or family members with early breast cancer, is 40 years old, and most medical specialty groups recommend that women have annual mammograms from this age forward.

Age and gender are examples of fixed risks and cannot be altered. Other risk factors can be modified to lower the risk of getting breast cancer during one's lifetime. All risk factors are not created equal.

These fixed risk factors significantly increase the risk of breast cancer:

- more than one family member with breast cancer on Mom's side or Dad's side
- relatives who developed breast cancer under age 50
- a male relative with breast cancer
- genetic mutations, including BRCA1 and 2
- personal history of breast cancer, atypical hyperplasia, or lobular carcinoma in situ on breast biopsy (atypical hyperplasia is a precancerous change in the tissue where the nucleus of the cell looks less normal and the cell is more likely to turn into cancer; lobular carcinoma of the breast originates in breast tissue that contains milk-producing glands)

- high-dose radiation to the chest (such as for Hodgkins' disease)

The following fixed risk factors do not increase the risk of breast cancer as much:

- dense breast tissue on mammogram
- extra number of years getting menstrual cycles
  - getting a first menstrual period at a younger age
  - getting a final menstrual period at an older age

Modifiable risk factors that produce a mild increase in breast cancer risk include:

- reproductive factors
  - whether you gave birth
  - late age at first birth, over 30
- being overweight
- being physically inactive
- drinking alcohol
- taking hormones, especially higher doses for many years

Now that the risk factors for breast cancer have been introduced, it is time to discuss screening for breast cancer and diagnosing early cancers.

Mammograms and Breast Cancer Detection

Today, mammograms are still the gold standard to screen for breast cancer. The false negative rate (or falsely reassuring rate) is roughly 15 percent. If 100 women with breast cancer undergo mammograms, the mammograms will find the cancer in 85 of the women and miss cancer in 15 of the women. Or, to put it another way, mammograms detect 85 percent of breast cancers.

Many cancers are found by mammograms before a woman or her doctor can feel a lump. The false negative rate of 15 percent is the reason that women who have a breast lump should not ignore it, even if they have had a negative, reassuring mammogram. Breast

lumps deserve investigation, even if the mammogram does not identify them as cancerous.

Upgrades for Mammograms: Computer-aided Detection and Digital Mammography

Computer-aided detection, or CAD, is a technology where the computer is used to double read the images, or mimic a second reader. It is a virtual second opinion. An expert physician "reader" (a radiologist) interprets the films and then can compare the computer reading with the expert reading.

Another recent upgrade is digital mammography, a technique that stores digital images on the computer, rather than on x-ray film, and uses increased contrast resolution to help evaluate dense breasts. This is particularly helpful in younger women, those taking oral contraceptives or other hormones, or those with "dense" breast tissue. In fact, digital mammography has been found to be 28 percent more effective in detecting early cancers in dense breast tissue than traditional mammography. The other benefit of digital mammography is that it enables the images to be manipulated, or flipped, on the screen, much like flipping drawings on a sketchpad. While digital mammography is a technology that enhances interpretation of mammograms in premenopausal and perimenopausal women, it has not been shown to offer an advantage over traditional mammogram for postmenopausal women who don't have dense breasts.

Both CAD and digital mammography can enhance the radiologist's ability to detect breast cancer early. At times, specialized mammography views are used as diagnostic tools to magnify an area of concern after it has been identified on a screening mammogram study. This can allow a radiologist or surgeon to mark an area for biopsy using the magnification of the X-ray on the mammogram to identify the area of concern.

Ultrasound

An ultrasound of the breast can be done to check an ab-normal area on the mammogram to see if it is a cyst. Breast ultra-sound may also be used to check a mass that is palpated on breast examination to see if it is cystic. The mammogram and the ultrasound are not interchangeable tests. Each plays a different role. While the mammogram will detect most early microscopic solid cancers, the ultrasound can confirm the presence of a cyst. At this time, ultrasounds are not used as screening tests for breast cancer for a number of reasons. One reason is that ultrasounds are not helpful in visualizing small calcium deposits that can signify cancerous or precancerous changes.

MAGNETIC RESONANCE IMAGING

Magnetic resonance imaging (MRI) is now being used as an additional diagnostic tool to identify hard-to-pinpoint breast cancers. Another newer use is to check women with a very high risk of getting breast cancer at an early age, such as someone with a mother or a sister who was diagnosed with premenopausal breast cancer under age 50. Younger premenopausal women have denser breasts that are harder to image and interpret with a mammogram. An MRI may help those with a high-risk family history get an earlier detection of a breast cancer. MRI has not yet been shown to be a useful screening tool for the general population. A breast MRI study may find a cancerous or precancerous area by the contrast solution that is used. The solution shows areas with increased blood flow that can be associated with abnormally rapid cell growth indicative of a cancer or precancer.

✈ PAULETTE'S STORY ✈

Alternative Screenings

"I'm 31. My mother died of breast cancer at age 38. I know from my research that mammograms in women under age 35 are not easy to interpret and are not as accurate in detecting breast cancer. My doctor advised me to have breast exams every six months. He also ordered a mammogram to be done once a year, each January, and advised me to have a breast MRI once a year, each July, six months after the mammogram. In my case, the MRI may detect a breast cancer before the mammogram. This plan makes sense for me, because my risk of getting

breast cancer at a young age is higher. For another woman without a high-risk family history, the MRI would produce too many false alarms to be helpful in screening for cancer."

RISK FACTORS FOR BREAST CANCER AND WAYS TO REDUCE IT

A woman who exercises regularly has a lower risk of breast cancer than her sedentary counterpart.

Excess alcohol consumption increases the risk of breast cancer. The precise threshold or number of drinks a week that will increase the risk has not been determined. One estimate is that more than one alcoholic drink a day will increase the risk. Others speculate that fewer than seven drinks of beer, wine, or liquor a week will increase a woman's risk of breast cancer. One theory is that alcohol is metabolized or processed in the liver, where estrogen is also metabolized. Extra alcohol affects estrogen metabolism, causing excess estrogen to linger in the blood, which exposes breast tissue to excess estrogen and increases the risk of breast cancer.

Testosterone supplementation may increase the risk of breast cancer, as it is converted to estrogen.

Having one's first child over the age of 30, or not bearing any children, increases the risk of breast cancer as well as ovarian cancer.

Nursing an infant decreases the risk of breast cancer. This is probably related to reduced estrogen and fewer ovulations that are one result of breast-feeding.

⚜ MARGARET'S STORY ⚜

Breast Lump after a Normal Mammogram

"I have an annual gynecologic exam, including a breast exam, faithfully. Since I turned 40, six years ago, I have also had an annual mammogram. My mother developed breast cancer at age 70. My sister, who is 10 years older than I am, has not had any abnormal mammograms or breast lumps. I recently found a lump in my breast while showering. I haven't had a menstrual period for the past three months.

I used to get breast lumps a week or so before my period, and then they would go away as soon as I started to bleed. This time the lump didn't go away. My last mammogram, which was six months ago, was negative. My doctor repeated the breast exam and agreed that I had a soft lump about two inches in diameter. She ordered an ultrasound that showed a breast cyst. She numbed a small area of skin over the cyst and used a syringe to remove all of the fluid from the cyst. Then, she ordered another mammogram, which showed the cyst was gone, but there were abnormal changes in the number of calcium spots—there were more of them and they were more irregular in shape. My doctor recommended that I have them biopsied in the radiology department (called a needle localization biopsy), and it showed an early local breast cancer developing. A breast surgeon was able to remove the abnormal tissue and then I had radiation. I have done well since. I am glad I did not assume the normal mammogram I had six months before I found the lump meant that the lump could be ignored."

DETECTING BREAST CANCER

Some scenarios may seem very similar when recounted to you by friends, family, or co-workers, yet their medical outcomes are vastly different. There are subtleties to taking a medical history that doctors refine over many years of study and training prior to acquiring their clinical experience in practice. These subtleties are invariably lost in translation when women share experiences that, on the surface, seem comparable.

Sometimes when women talk about their medical experiences, they draw conclusions about what should be done for a woman who seems to be in the same "situation." In medicine, however, many medical findings can sound similar but actually signify different diagnoses or entities based on context. In one woman, a bloody nipple discharge could be a sign of a breast cancer, in another it could signal a benign milk duct tumor, and in still another it could represent a skin condition such as psoriasis.

Doctors have to work with their patients to determine the significance of a particular concern or physical finding based upon how long it has been present as well as placing the concern in the context of that person's personal and family history, physical examination, and study results.

Sometimes doctors can't be positive if a mass is cancerous or not until it has been removed and biopsied.

Different Breast Problems Dictate Different Medical Approaches

Evaluating breast problems and identifying breast cancer early is a complex process that varies with each individual. What she finds on her self breast exam, her doctor's physical examination findings, and her test results may be different than what someone else with a similar problem may discover. While a comprehensive overview of breast disease is beyond the scope of this chapter, I thought it would be helpful to give you examples of various ways breast cancer may be found, and how different doctors might approach the diagnosis. In real life, mammograms often pinpoint areas of concern that do *not* turn out to be cancerous, so these examples are not representative of what will happen to a woman who has an abnormal mammogram. The differential diagnosis of breast cancer is made when a biopsy sample of the abnormal area of breast tissue is analyzed. There are many common breast problems that do not turn out to be breast cancer. The examples that are provided do not represent benign breast disease, which is more common. The majority of the stories focus on demonstrating various scenarios that lead to the diagnosis of breast cancer.

⚡ KATHY'S STORY ⚡

Spot Compression, Needle-guided Biopsy

"I am 64 years old and had normal mammograms for the past 15 years. I have also had normal breast examinations at my doctor's office for many years. This year, however, I got a call from the radiology department stating that there was a change on the mammogram. They wanted to do another more specialized mammogram called a spot compression, or a magnified view of a smaller area. I was extremely worried;

my co-worker who needed this extra mammogram view turned out to have cancer. When I went for the magnification view, the radiologist who read the film told me that there was an abnormal area on the film. The calcium spots they had seen in previous years now had more 'worrisome' features. There were more of them, they were clustered together, and the shape had changed.

"The radiologist used the magnification view to place a wire in the area with the abnormal calcium spots. A breast surgeon did a biopsy of the tissue around the wire. It showed an early cancer. The surgeon scheduled a surgical procedure to remove the cancerous tissue around the calcium spots so that the margins were clear of cancer. She also checked a representative lymph node with a dye study, and sampled it [a sentinel lymph node biopsy]. Fortunately, the lymph node did not show that any cancer had spread. I went on to have radiation, to decrease the risk that the cancer would spread or recur. I've done well since."

⚜ Lydia's Story ⚜

Mammogram, Cyst Drainage, Repeat Mammogram

Lydia, 49 and perimenopausal, felt a breast mass. "I found a lump two weeks ago. I thought it would go away after my menstrual period. When it persisted, I scheduled an appointment with my doctor. After speaking with me and doing a breast examination, she agreed that I probably had a breast cyst but advised further tests, even though I have no family history of breast cancer. I thought I would need a mammogram as soon as possible. Instead, the doctor recommended I see a breast specialist to remove the fluid and see if the lump would go away completely, and then do the mammogram to see if any abnormalities remained. The mammogram showed an abnormal area behind the collapsed cyst. The radiologist did a core needle biopsy of the area after locating it on a special mammogram view and numbing the area. The biopsy showed breast cancer. I could have chosen to have only the lump removed, and then have radiation. For personal reasons, I did not want to get radiation, so I have chosen to have a simple mastectomy with reconstruction."

❧ CHRISTINA'S STORY ❧

Bloody Nipple Discharge in a 61-year-old

Christina, 61 and postmenopausal, noticed bloody discharge coming from her nipple. "I did not feel a lump, but noticed a bloody discharge from my nipple and dark brown staining on the inside of my bra. I was frightened and was certain I had breast cancer, even though I could not feel a lump. I had just had a mammogram and breast exam at the doctor's office 10 months earlier. I thought my doctor would want another mammogram. Instead, after doing another exam, she checked the bloody discharge for cancer cells. Then she ordered a dye study of the milk ducts in the breast called a ductogram. It turned out there was a noncancerous growth in the milk duct. Once that was surgically removed, the bloody discharge stopped. The scar was at the edge of the nipple and barely visible. My doctor told me that a bloody discharge can be a sign of cancer. I was lucky. In my case it was just a benign tumor in the nipple duct."

❧ CORAL'S STORY ❧

Lump Removed and Biopsied

"I am 55 years old and still menstruating. I found a lump while I was showering. It felt like the thickening I get before my menstrual period, but it did not go away after my period. Even though I had a normal mammogram three months ago, I made an appointment with my doctor. I thought he would order a mammogram or an ultrasound. Instead, he recommended a different test. When I asked him why, he said that we could both see and feel the lump so it would save time to take fluid from the lump to see if it was a cyst or a solid breast mass. He sent me to a breast specialist who numbed the area over the lump and tried to extract fluid. When no fluid came out, he advised the lump be removed *and biopsied. It was an early cancer. In my case another mammogram would not have added additional information and would have delayed my treatment."*

Reducing the Risk of Cervical Cancer

The hereditary pattern for cervical cancer is not well defined, and lifestyle choices such as number of sexual partners and exposure to human papilloma virus (HPV) contribute to the risk. In the past two decades, researchers have learned more about the causes of cervical cancer. Ninety-five percent of cervical cancers are caused by high-risk DNA strains of HPV, or "wart virus."

Reducing the risk of cervical cancer involves several strategies.

1. *Do not smoke.* Smokers have a much higher risk of cervical cancer. Smoking produces nicotine breakdown products that lodge in the cervical cells and alter them. Smoking not only increases a woman's risk of getting cervical cancer, but also its precursor, cervical dysplasia (precancer). The impact of smoking on cervical cancer risk is not just additive; smoking and exposure to the wart virus (high-risk HPV) dramatically increases the risk of cervical cancer. In other words, 2 + 2 does not equal 4 when it comes to smoking and cervical cancer. A woman who smokes and has high-risk HPV DNA does not just have double the risk of getting cervical cancer—together, the smoking and the wart virus increase her risk of cervical cancer even more dramatically.

2. *Limit your exposure to HPV DNA, or the wart virus.* Genital warts or a history of having warts may increase the risk of cervical cancer. If you have had warts, you have been exposed to wart virus, or HPV. However, that does not mean that you were exposed to the high-risk DNA types of wart virus that are more likely to cause cervical cancer. Warts are a physical manifestation of HPV. But you can be exposed to the wart virus without ever developing a visible wart. You can have HPV without knowing it. The virus may remain dormant in the body without showing up in any way, except on a test for HPV exposure. Similarly, your sexual partner could have the

wart virus (HPV), but no genital warts. The virus can become active months, years, or even decades after the person's initial exposure to it. Wart virus can be spread by skin-to-skin contact. It is not necessary to have penile-vaginal intercourse to get wart virus. Therefore, women who have sex or intimate contact with *either* sex are at risk for HPV.

3. *Limit the number of sexual partners you have—and pay attention to the number of sexual partners your partner has had.* A large number of sexual partners increases the risk of cervical cancer. Alternatively, one sexual partner who is high risk by virtue of his or her exposure to high-risk HPV DNA can increase your chance of getting cervical cancer. A woman can acquire a high-risk strain of HPV after a single unprotected sexual encounter with a male or female partner. Condoms reduce the risk of getting HPV but do not eliminate it because it is transmitted by skin-to-skin contact.

4. *Use condoms.* If you have a new partner, or more than one partner, use condoms even if you have another form of contraception or are not fertile. Condoms decrease your chances of getting warts and HPV DNA. Although condoms reduce the risk of getting HPV, they do not eliminate it because it is transmitted by skin-to-skin contact. If your partner has warts, abstain from intercourse until the warts are completely treated and no longer visible. Any warts a woman has on her body should also be promptly treated so that they do not spread; they are very contagious.

5. *Get Pap smears.* Follow your gynecologist's recommendations for the frequency of Pap smears and HPV DNA testing. They will be based upon your personal medical history and current partner situation. If you have a new or different partner or multiple partners, inform your gynecologist so that the testing recommendations are tailored to your lifestyle and exposure to the virus. If you bleed after sexual intercourse, or bleed between menstrual periods, a gynecologist should examine your cervix for changes even if the Pap smear is normal.

A weakened immune system increases the risk of cervical cancer because you cannot fight the wart virus as vigorously and are more susceptible to getting cervical cancer. The immune system can be weakened (compromised) in someone who is taking anti-rejection drugs following an organ transplant, in someone who has HIV or AIDS, those taking steroids, and in other circumstances.

More than 100 different DNA types of HPV have been identified so far. Each has a different cancer-producing potential. Some types, such as HPV5 and 6, are more innocent and are usually associated with benign genital warts. Other types, such as HPV15 and 16, are more aggressive and are associated with precancer and cancerous lesions of the cervix (and throat and anus) more often. High-risk HPV DNA can also increase the risk of getting cancer of the vulva or vagina.

If you are positive for high-risk HPV DNA, you should have a gynecologist do a careful speculum examination each year to be certain there are no warts or other lesions on the vulva or in the vagina. If they are, they should be diagnosed and treated. Even if you have had a hysterectomy and no longer have a uterus, an examination of the vulva and vagina is in order, particularly if you remain sexually active.

Debates are under way regarding the precise role of HPV DNA testing to help women avoid cervical cancer. These debate points will shift as researchers develop targeted treatment for different DNA types of the HPV. At present, each woman's gynecologist can offer her the best screening approach for her based on her personal history, pelvic examination, and Pap smear results.

THE CERVICAL CANCER VACCINE

Warts were first described during the Greek and Roman eras. In the 1980s, researchers identified various DNA types of wart virus and clarified that some were more dangerous promoters of cervical cancer than others. Today, researchers have identified more than 100 distinct DNA types of wart virus. Only a few are particularly worrisome. Most are more innocent and are associated with annoying warts that may be unsightly or uncomfortable, but are not precancerous.

Currently, there is a vaccine available to prevent infection from four types of HPV DNA, Types 6 and 11 (benign types that cause only the common variety of genital warts) and Types 16 and 18 (more worrisome types that are associated with severe dysplasia or precancer of the cervix and frank cervical cancer). The commercial name for the quadrivalent vaccine available now is Gardasil. If a woman (or girl—the vaccine often is given young) has not yet been exposed to that particular DNA type of wart virus, the vaccine will prevent her from getting that type for four or five years or even longer. The vaccine is a prevention strategy, not a treatment for warts or wart virus (HPV).

At this time the vaccine is being promoted for young girls and women between the ages of 9 and 26. The thinking is that the vaccine will decrease their susceptibility to the wart virus before their first sexual exposure. Even after the first sexual exposure, young women will probably not have been exposed to all four HPV DNA types in the vaccine, so they will still derive protection from some of the types, lowering their risk of cervical cancer. Mature women are more likely to have been exposed to the four HPV DNA types in the vaccine. A different type of vaccine will be needed to help women who have already been exposed to HPV.

There is still no treatment that addresses individual types of wart virus. Visible warts on the hands or feet or genital area may be treated with freezing or chemical solutions or laser. At present, doctors can treat visible warts that may appear in the genital area or rectal area of either sex, but they cannot treat the virus itself. Vaccines to treat wart virus when there are no visible warts are in the research and development stage. Identifying the presence of high-risk wart virus helps to identify those women who need closer observation and those who are at increased risk for getting cervical cancer associated with the virus.

A woman's biologic response to being infected with HPV will vary over her lifetime. In her teens or early twenties, a woman who acquires high-risk HPV DNA through intercourse may be able to fight it off on her own, without medical treatment. The precancerous cervix changes caused by the HPV DNA appear only transiently, then resolve spontaneously and the cervix returns to normal. This is HPV leaving its footprint in the snow. When a doctor sees these footprints, he or she assesses whether the Big Bear is still in the woods nearby or if it has already left. If only footprints remain, and the Big Bear is gone, you continue your walk in the snow without concerns. If the Big Bear is still nearby, representing an active threat, it is another matter. In mature women the Big Bear is more likely to be lurking nearby, poised for attack. The precancerous changes are less likely to resolve spontaneously as they so often do in teenagers.

HPV DNA testing may be done at the same time as a Pap smear is performed. It can also be performed by swabbing the cervix to get a sample to analyze for HPV DNA types alone, without doing a Pap smear. Women who test positive for high-risk HPV DNA types are at higher risk of getting cervical cancer going forward, but it may take years for the cervical cancer to show up. On the other hand, a woman with high-risk HPV DNA may never get cervical cancer. Regardless of whether an individual woman gets cervical cancer, today doctors can only treat precancers and cancers of the cervix. Currently, there is no treatment or antidote for addressing high-risk HPV DNA.

Women who develop visible warts on the cervix, in the vagina, or on the vulva (outer skin) should seek treatment from their doctor. The doctor can use a solution, freezing, laser, or Aldara, a prescription cream to treat warts. The same applies to the woman's sexual partner. If the partner is not treated in a time-sensitive manner, the warts may spread quickly on the woman and her partner(s). Warts may also appear in the throat for those who have oral sex and come in contact with untreated, visible warts.

Using condoms decreases the risk of acquiring HPV or warts, but does not eliminate it entirely. A woman who has low-risk HPV DNA, such as Type 6 or 11, is more likely to develop visible warts, but does not have a high risk of getting cervical cancer.

Abnormal Pap Smears

The Pap test has been available since its introduction in 1941 to screen women for cervical cancer. Pap smears have enabled North American physicians, and others, to drastically reduce the number of cervical cancers. In the past 10 years, the technology for performing and interpreting the Pap test has been upgraded to make it an even better screening tool to check for cancer of the cervix. The Pap test checks cells that shed off of the cervix and can find abnormal cells that have not yet turned into cancer, enabling a gynecologist to treat precancerous conditions before the cell changes progress to cancer. But remember, the Pap smear only checks for cancer of the cervix; it will not detect cancer of the uterus or ovary.

The Pap smear is an excellent screening tool, but it is not foolproof. If a gynecologist sees an abnormal area on a woman's cervix, a biopsy is in order, even if the results of the Pap smear are normal. That is why visual inspection of the cervix is important during the annual pelvic examination, even if a Pap smear is not planned for that visit. Screening recommendations for the frequency of Pap smears vary with a woman's medical history and her partner(s)' exposure, as well as her own Pap smear history. A woman who has had precancer of the cervix or visible warts is likely to need an annual Pap smear, as is a woman with more than one partner or a woman who smokes cigarettes.

In contrast, a woman who is a nonsmoker, has been exclusive with the same partner for 10 years or more, and does not have high-risk HPV DNA may need less frequent Paps if her recent Pap smears have been normal. If she has never had warts or wart virus, she may be told by her doctor that a Pap smear every three years is safe (provided she has three negative annual Pap smear results in a row and her history remains low-risk). The downside of this recommendation is that this has been misinterpreted to mean that the woman does not need a pelvic examination and inspection of her cervix every year, which is *not* accurate. You *do* need an annual exam by your gynecologist.

Sometimes precancerous cell changes go away spontaneously, without medical intervention. Or they may linger. They may also progress to cancer that can advance and spread to other parts of the body.

A woman who has an abnormal Pap smear that shows precancerous cells may or may not benefit from merely repeating the Pap smear. The severity of the abnormality points the way. If the

Pap smear abnormality is very mild, and likely to resolve without medical intervention, such as an ASCUS (atypical squamous cells of uncertain significance), HPV DNA may be tested to learn if there is a higher chance of a more serious change lurking beneath the identified abnormal cells. If the HPV DNA test shows a woman has high-risk types of HPV DNA, she is at higher risk of having severe dysplasia (precancer).

Colposcopy

Severe dysplasia or precancer represents abnormal cell changes that are less likely to revert to normal without treatment; they are more likely to progress to cancer over months or years. To determine whether treatment is warranted, a test that is more specific than a Pap smear is needed. Colposcopy is a more specific, *diagnostic* test that provides information used to plan treatment.

A colposcopy is a microscope examination that pinpoints where the changes in the cervical tissue are taking place as well as what those changes are. By performing a tissue sample of those specific areas, or a biopsy, the deeper tissue can be analyzed for severe precancer and cancer. If severe dysplasia or precancer is identified, that specific area may be "spot treated" or removed. A colposcopy is not a suitable screening test because it would subject too many women to biopsies that they do not need. It is, however, a superb test to clarify the degree of abnormal cervical changes in a woman who has an abnormal Pap smear.

Women with only a mild change on their Pap smear, such as ASCUS, may not need a colposcopy, particularly if their HPV DNA is "low risk." In the past, there was a great deal of confusion surrounding ASCUS results and their management. At that time, at medical conferences someone might quip: "Ask Us (for ASCUS), and we will not tell you (what to do)." Now, with the advent of HPV DNA testing, and the increased understanding of how most cervical cancer develops from persistent high-risk HPV DNA virus, we do have the answer. So, go ahead—ask us—we *can* tell you what to do.

While the criteria for the age at which to start doing Pap smears in young women have been established, criteria to determine at what age to stop doing Pap smears are less clear. One recommendation is to stop doing Pap smears at age 70 if a woman is a nonsmoker with no other risk factors for cervical cancer, has had previous normal Pap smears over the past 10 years, and is negative for high-risk HPV DNA, but more data is needed to solidify this recommendation.

Reducing the Risk of Uterine Cancer

Risk factors for uterine cancer include:

- high blood pressure
- obesity
- a sedentary lifestyle
- diabetes

Sedentary women and those who are overweight have more adipose (fatty) tissue where the weak estrogen, estrone, is converted in the fat cells. Excess amounts of estrone, common in these women, exposes the uterine lining to an imbalance of hormone and stimulates the glands in the lining to grow too aggressively. In contrast, women who exercise regularly and maintain a healthy body weight are less likely to get uterine cancer.

Detecting Uterine Cancer

At present there is no good screening test to identify uterine cancer. The best tool gynecologists have is an accurate medical history, which is why keeping a menstrual calendar is so important. Abnormal bleeding can be a clue. Any bleeding during postmenopause is abnormal and should be investigated. In perimenopause, the distinctions are more subtle.

While there is no equivalent Pap test to check for abnormal cells in the uterine lining, when suspected, endometrial (uterine lining) cancer can be identified by performing a biopsy of the uterine lining tissue. Alternatively, a dilatation and curettage (D&C) procedure will produce a tissue sample that can be analyzed for cancer or precancerous changes. While pelvic ultrasound can provide more detailed information about the uterus and ovaries, it is not a screening test for uterine cancer. It is simply not practical or productive to use ultrasounds to check for uterine cancer because there are too many common benign findings that would appear to look like an endometrial cancer (as discussed in Chapter 5).

For example, a strategically placed benign fibroid protruding into the uterine lining may cause it to look thick and worrisome on an ultrasound, mimicking a uterine lining cancer. Alternatively, a polyp (soft tissue growth similar to a skin tag) may protrude into the uterine lining and thicken it, causing a worrisome ultrasound finding. Since polyps or fibroids may mimic uterine cancer on an ultrasound, ultrasound is not a definitive diagnostic test to either prove or disprove that a woman has uterine cancer.

Ultrasound often does play a helpful role in clarifying the anatomy of the uterus and ovaries, including their dimensions and other features. The ultrasound can flag a problem with the lining by measuring the thickness and issuing a warning label that essentially reads, "danger, there may be uterine lining cancer here," but further investigation is warranted to confirm the diagnosis.

That investigation must involve a tissue sample from the uterine lining, such as an endometrial biopsy or a D&C. Today, many gynecology experts may also recommend a hysteroscopy, or direct examination of the lining with a microscope, to check for subtle abnormalities of the blood vessels that may not appear on an ultrasound image. In a postmenopausal woman not taking estrogen, a lining thickness of more than 5 millimeters (0.20 inch) is a red flag to look for cancer or other causes of the thick lining. A biopsy can clarify if it is a benign—an innocent polyp or fibroid—or endometrial cancer.

RESOURCES

American Cancer Society (www.cancer.org). This organization has resources that include information about prevention and treatment of various cancers.

Dana-Farber Cancer Institute (www.Dana-Farber.org). This world-class cancer hospital is associated with Harvard Medical School. It offers free information for all types of cancer treatment as well as trials for new protocols.

Genetic Testing for BRCA1 and BRCA2: It's Your Choice. National Cancer Institute Fact Sheet (www.cancer.gov/cancertopics/factsheet/risk/ brca). This has common questions and answers about BRCA gene mutations, testing, and its ramifications. Last accessed December 15, 2008.

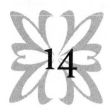

14

Your Doctor Visit

For women who are too busy to see a doctor, self-diagnosis is tempting. However, even well-educated women can mislead themselves about their health. It is not uncommon for me to see, or to hear about, a patient who waited too long to get to the doctor. I don't want to scare you unnecessarily with horror stories, but this is something you do not want to experience. Both self-diagnosis and denial can interfere with your ability to take care of your health. The good news is that regular doctor visits, preventive care, screening and diagnostic tests, and healthy lifestyle choices can help us "live long and prosper."

⚜ ABIGAIL'S STORY ⚜

"This Lump Can't Be Cancer"

Abigail was a slender, energetic, 40-year-old single lawyer. When it came to issues like smoking, eating, and exercising, Abigail made healthy lifestyle choices, but she did not get regular gynecologic exams or mammograms. When she developed a breast lump, she convinced herself it was just a cyst. After all, she reasoned, "No one in my immediate family has had breast cancer." She rationalized that her healthy lifestyle would prevent her from developing breast cancer. After living with the lump for years, Abigail consented to having the cyst aspirated to reduce its size, but she postponed getting a breast biopsy. The lump continued to grow. Not only was Abigail too busy, she was in denial. By the time Abigail finally got a breast biopsy, the breast cancer had spread to her bones. She died at age 46.

One Patient, Many Doctors

As recently as 20 years ago, one doctor could meet most of your medical needs. Preventive health was not well established, so you only saw your doctor when something bothered you. Communities used to be smaller and more stable, so you may have had the same doctor for many years.

Today the patterns and structure of medical care, and our society, have changed dramatically. Women are not just seeing their doctors to fix a broken bone; they are trying to prevent their bones from breaking. Because of ongoing discoveries about chronic illnesses and age-related problems, preventive medical care is now an important part of a medical visit. It's important to visit the doctor even when you're healthy in order to stay healthy.

Preventive health is a positive trend, but it is taking place in a more complex setting. Patients move, doctors relocate, and a change of insurance carriers may force a change of physicians. Multiple health care providers are involved in the care of one patient, and there are more medical decisions to make regarding diagnosis, treatment, and prevention strategies.

These days, achieving continuity of care is increasingly complex. Ten to 15 percent of patients change doctors every year. In any given year, about 20 to 25 percent of patients change their health plans. Continuity of care becomes a challenge when both patients and their doctors are trying to coordinate care from previous doctors with one or more current health care providers.

At midlife and beyond, a woman may be interacting with several doctors to get routine medical tests each year. For example, a healthy woman age 50 or older with no worrisome family history or physical problems needs, at the minimum, a blood pressure check, a breast exam, a pelvic exam, and a mammogram every year. She also needs a

Pap smear to check for cervical cancer every one to 3 years, a blood test for cholesterol every 5 years, and a colonoscopy to check for colon cancer every 10 years. To accomplish all of these preventive screening tests, as well as care for any problems that arise, she will need an internal medicine physician (or a family doctor) as well as a gynecologist. A gastroenterologist will perform her colonoscopy when she reaches age 50, and periodically thereafter. If she develops arthritis, she may acquire a rheumatologist. If she develops any thyroid issues, she may consult an endocrinologist. If she has blocked arteries, she'll need a cardiologist. Different providers deliver these separate services at different locations.

ᚤ Sally's Story ᚥ

77-year-old, Dealing with Multiple Medical Problems

"I'm 77 years old, and at this age one can expect to have some medical problems. But I have a lot of problems: diabetes, thyroid disease, and rheumatoid arthritis as well as acid reflux, heart disease, and osteoporosis. My doctors tell me that my medical care has become increasingly complex. This is an understatement. They don't live with these conditions every day, and it is a real juggling act. It is difficult for me to follow through on one specialist's recommendations, because the advice I get for one problem doesn't always mesh with the advice I get from other specialists for my other medical problems.

"I take thyroid medication daily on an empty stomach, medication for arthritis three times a day with food, heart medication twice a day, medication to control blood sugar three times a day, calcium with food twice a day, and osteoporosis medication once a week on an empty stomach. Just reciting this list makes me feel sick. And of course every time I go to a doctor they make me go through the entire list again. It is hard to think past the next pill I have to take. If I get a new medication, I worry that it may interact with one of my other ones. Recently, I was surprised to learn that I wasn't absorbing the calcium I was taking because the medicine for acid reflux was blocking my calcium absorption. I realized that I shouldn't just see my rheumatologist for my arthritis, *my endocrinologist for my thyroid problem, and my cardiologist for my heart. My primary care doctor has a role to play. He offered to help me keep track of all the specialists' recommendations and make certain that the medications didn't 'fight' one another. He also suggested switching to a once-a-month medication for osteoporosis instead of once a week so I didn't have to disrupt the timing of taking my thyroid medication, since it also is taken on an empty stomach."*

This common scenario highlights the need for a primary care doctor, such as an internist or family physician, to oversee the care of the whole person. This primary care doctor sorts out what won't work and what is doable. The primary care doctor may streamline the regimen, simplifying it so that it is livable. Further, the primary care doctor may ensure that the patient's input and personal preferences are part of her medical care plan. Cobbling together a group of medical specialists without a primary care doctor in charge is no more desirable than making a movie with superb actors and no director.

These changes in the fabric of medical care, including the increased complexity of medical tests and the requisite team of health care providers, make it imperative for you to provide accurate, up-to-date information to every doctor at every visit. Your health and well-being depend on it.

There is important, specific information you should have at your fingertips when you see a doctor. Without this essential information, you will not receive optimal care. Remember the health alliance I spoke about in Chapter 1? Without access to all the facts, your doctor is handicapped. On the other hand, when you share thorough, current, accurate information about your personal and family health histories, medications, allergies, and so on, you'll find that the time you spend with your doctor is more pleasant as well as more productive. In addition to building trust, you will be contributing to an effective doctor-patient relationship.

This chapter covers three types of visits:

1. a comprehensive "new patient" visit to a gynecologist
2. an annual or yearly visit to a gynecologist

3. a "problem" visit to the gynecologist — one that is spurred by a troublesome symptom

Each type of visit offers unique opportunities to interact with your doctor. By understanding the way your doctor typically approaches each kind of visit, you can improve your own medical experiences as well as the care you receive. As you will see, your role in the doctor-patient relationship is critical. While there are wide differences among physicians as well as patients, this chapter will give you some ideas about how to get more out of your trips to the doctor.

A Comprehensive "New Patient" Visit to the Gynecologist

Let's assume you have moved to a new state and located a new doctor. Appointments for new patients are generally given more time, which allows you and the doctor to establish a baseline for future care.

By taking time to pull together useful information in advance of your "new patient" visit, you'll have more time to talk about what's important and to tell your doctor if you have any current concerns. This will influence the time he or she spends on different areas of your medical history and examination, so your visit will meet your needs.

WHAT PREPARATIONS DO YOU TAKE ON A REGULAR BASIS?

Some people hate to take even an aspirin, while others are quick to use pills and other remedies. Some refuse to take prescription medications, but will take natural medicinal preparations from the health food store. Other people are exactly the opposite, and prefer traditional Western medicine. Before your doctor visit, make a list of *everything* you take regularly, whether it's once a day or once a month.

Over-the-counter Remedies

Your doctor needs to know about anything you use or take on a regular basis, whether you think it counts as a medication or not.

- over-the-counter medications for pain relief, including aspirin, ibuprofen (Advil), acetaminophen (Tylenol)
- over-the-counter remedies for heartburn
- hormonal preparations from the health food store, such as DHEA (dehydroepiandrosterone) supplements or progesterone cream
- homeopathic medicines
- digestive aids
- coffee, tea, or soda
- herbal remedies or medicinal teas from the health food store
- vitamin pills, particularly if you take high-dose supplements
- Chinese herbs
- weight-loss pills
- sleep aids
- nutritional supplements

Look around your kitchen; check the medicine cabinet. If an over-the-counter preparation contains many ingredients (or mysterious ones), bring the bottle to your visit. You never know if one of those items could make the difference when the doctor is trying to put together the complex puzzle that represents your total health picture.

In the first chapter of this book, the importance of the patient-doctor team was introduced. Cassandra, a healthy 58-year-old who recently became postmenopausal, has developed a healthy collaboration with her gynecologist and her internist, as shown here.

⚜ CASSANDRA'S STORY ⚜

Reducing Blood Pressure Naturally

"I recently became postmenopausal and was pleased that my transition was smooth. I am controlling my hot flashes with paced respiration, regular exercise, and reducing the amount of coffee I drink. Since I have been using vaginal lubricants, the vaginal dryness I experienced has improved enough that I have not needed to try the vaginal estrogen my gynecologist offered to prescribe.

"Although I have gained 15 pounds, I am still fit. My waist measurement is 36 inches, only a little over the healthy guidelines, so I am not planning to diet at this point. I thought I was doing well for my age, especially compared to so many of my friends. At a recent checkup, my internist wanted to prescribe medication to lower my blood pressure. My diastolic blood pressure has gone up more than 15 points, despite all of my healthy routines. In addition, my cholesterol is now over 250. I read that garlic is good for heart disease and wanted to use a natural approach. I cook with garlic regularly, and thought that adding a garlic supplement should do the trick. I couldn't think of a reason my internist wouldn't go along with this, since I have a healthy lifestyle and exercise regularly.

"At first I was put off that my doctor was not receptive to my taking garlic alone to treat my blood pressure and high cholesterol. I thought she was just not as up to date on natural remedies as she is on prescription medications. The thought even crossed my mind that she might favor the pharmaceutical companies because they influence her to prescribe their latest medications. I was concerned about the potential side effects of both prescription blood pressure medications and cholesterol-lowering medications.

"I was pleasantly surprised by our discussion, even though the outcome was not what I preferred. The doctor explained that the studies about the benefits of garlic to lower the risk of heart disease were in the earliest phases. Garlic is good for the heart and blood vessels, but its exact contribution has not yet been identified. It may not be enough to lower my blood pressure and cholesterol into a healthy range before I get a heart attack or stroke. Until the studies show exactly which supple-

ments, in which amounts, affect exactly which aspects of heart disease, she advised me to continue to eat garlic in my diet, but also to take prescription medication proven to bring cholesterol and blood pressure down into the normal range. While she agreed that I had done well to only put on 15 pounds, and that I was more active than most women my age, I still could benefit from additional exercise and a weight-loss program to shed the extra pounds, especially around my waist. If I successfully remove the extra pounds, there is a good chance I will be able to stop taking the medications in the future. I hadn't realized that natural remedies like garlic were being formally studied and that it wasn't enough to know generally that it helps heart disease; it needs to address my particular problems effectively so I can lower my risk of heart attack and stroke in the near future. My doctor said she will let me know when the newer studies clarify whether garlic helps to prevent high blood pressure or high cholesterol or both."

Prescription Medications

What prescription medications do you take? Think of all the medications you pick up at the pharmacy, whether you take them every day or only occasionally. Obviously, the doctor needs to know what medicines have already been prescribed for you, not only because this helps explain your health status, but also because some medications cause side effects that could be relevant. Remember to include:

- birth control pills
- antidepressants or anti-anxiety medications
- hormones
- heart or blood pressure medications
- heartburn or ulcer medications

Make a list that includes the name of the drug as printed on the prescription bottle, the dosage, and the frequency. If you don't have time to or don't want to write down your prescription information, bring the pill bottle(s) with you to your visit. Many preparations

UNDERSTANDING YOUR PRESCRIPTION MEDICATIONS
Brand Name or Generic?

Modern medicine has brought us an abundance of new medications, in addition to upgrades of the tried-and-true staples. Within one category, there are often dozens of choices. For example, there are a dizzying number of brands of birth control pills on the market, as well as numerous hormone preparations for postmenopause.

When a company goes to the trouble and expense of creating and marketing a new drug, it generally is given patent protection for a set number of years, meaning that company has the sole right to manufacture and sell the brand-name version of the drug. The rationale for this is that the drug company needs a window of opportunity during which it can recoup the initial expenses associated with bringing a drug to market. After the patent expires, other companies can introduce generic versions of the medication that are less expensive because they are not associated with the same startup costs (which these days are likely to include enormously expensive direct-to-consumer advertising campaigns).

New generic formulations are continuously being introduced into the marketplace and are released without advanced notification to doctors. When your doctor writes a prescription, he or she can designate that you must receive the brand-name drug if you so choose. Otherwise, a generic preparation may be substituted. If no generic version of the medication is available at the time the original prescription is written, the doctor might not specify either way. What happens next is that, even though your doctor prescribed a brand-name medication, 6 to 12 months later your pharmacist may substitute a newly available generic formula because the pharmacy is permitted to do so as soon as it becomes available to them. When you return to your doctor, you may have a different name on your prescription bottle or package, even though the doctor never rewrote or changed the prescription.

Insurance companies encourage these substitutions to save money. Sometimes there is no medical reason to keep using a brand-name medication, but other times it is not advisable to switch to a generic drug. It depends upon you, your diagnosis, and your experience with a particular formulation.

A generic drug is required by the Food and Drug Administration to be chemically equivalent to the brand-name drug it is replacing but there is leeway in matching the "bioequivalence" of the generic drug to the original brand product. The additives may differ, and the precise amount of the active ingredients may differ. If you are taking a medication on a regular basis, it's possible for you to receive a different generic version of the drug when you refill different prescriptions, depending on what your pharmacist has available. The effectiveness of the different generic formulations may vary slightly each month. Technically you could get a version that is slightly less effective one month and slightly more effective the next. Most of the time this is not considered a problem, but there may be situations in which the consistent use of a brand-name drug is preferable.

If your medication stops working the way it used to, and the color or packaging of the medication has changed, you may be receiving a generic preparation, and you may not be getting the same benefits as you did from the brand-name prescription. Discuss your concerns with your doctor to determine if they are related to the generic version of your medication or some other cause.

have names that sound alike, and pills for different, unrelated conditions often look alike, so don't rely on recollection alone.

❧ Yvonne's Story ☙

Switching from Brand Name to Generic . . . and Back Again

"Last year I visited my doctor months before my scheduled annual exam because of debilitating hot flashes and irregular menstrual periods. I am 47 years old, suffer from PMS [premenstrual syndrome], and experienced headaches before my period. I don't want to have any more children, and I don't smoke. My doctor prescribed a low-dose birth control pill to decrease the hot flashes, even out my irregular menstrual periods, and provide contraception. With the control of these symptoms, my concerns about PMS decreased. I took the pill he prescribed, and was pleased with the results. Each month I returned to the pharmacy and picked up my prescription. By the time I started taking my pills for the next month, I had already thrown away the container for the last month, so it never occurred to me that the pills could be different.

"At my next annual exam, I complained that some of my old problems had returned, including the premenstrual headaches. Fortunately I had brought the pill packet with me, and my doctor confirmed that the pharmacist had substituted a newly available generic version of the pill, and

I did not tolerate it as well as the original prescription medication. We discussed alternatives. I could continue to take a generic pill preparation, or, if I was willing to pay a higher co-pay with my health maintenance organization, I could go back to the brand-name preparation with the doctor specifying 'No Substitution' on the prescription. I decided to return to the brand preparation of birth control pills, and when I did my headaches subsided again. I saved myself months of headaches—literally—by bringing the pill pack to my doctor visit so we could solve the problem together."

ALLERGIES OR SENSITIVITIES TO MEDICATIONS

Allergies are extremely individual. Some people seem to be OK with any kind of medication, while others are acutely allergic. It is not uncommon for people to be allergic to antibiotics in the penicillin and sulfa categories. If you have ever had an allergic reaction to a medication, be sure to mention this to your doctor. What type of reaction did you have? Did you get hives, or a rash, or itching? Were you short of breath? You also may have sensitivities to certain medications—for example, cold preparations make you feel dizzy, or certain pain medications make you feel nauseated.

In addition, the doctor may check for allergies to iodine (used in dyes for certain types of diagnostic X-rays), Betadine (a topical disinfectant commonly used during surgery), or latex (rubber). If you are allergic to latex, your doctor will use latex-free gloves for your examination. Latex allergies are becoming so common that some health care facilities and operating rooms are moving toward being 100 percent latex-free.

YOUR MEDICAL HISTORY

Next, your doctor will inquire about different aspects of your medical history. He or she is intent on understanding your total health picture, and the past influences the present.

Have You Had Any Previous Surgeries or Surgical Procedures?

Your doctor will want to know what surgeries you have had and when. The approximate year of the surgery is helpful, or at least your age when you had the surgery. Have you had your appendix, tonsils, gall bladder, uterus, or ovaries removed? Have you had a cesarean section, a tubal ligation (sterilization procedure), or a dilatation and curettage (D&C)? Have you had bladder surgery, or any breast biopsies or breast surgery? It's important for you to mention any office or out-patient procedures, such as a biopsy, a laparoscopy, a colonoscopy (a colon exam using a scope), or a colposcopy (a vaginal exam using a microscope to check the cervix).

Surgical procedures you have had in the past may play a role in how you are currently feeling. For example, your surgical history can help the evaluation process if you are experiencing pain. If you have pain in the right lower area of your abdomen, it could be your intestines, your appendix, or your ovaries, among other possibilities. It is helpful to know if your appendix has already been removed! Your doctor also wants to determine whether you could have any problems with anesthesia or with excess bleeding. In some cases the doctor may request a copy of the operation notes from a previous surgery or the pathology report that analyzed any tissue that was removed.

What Are Your Health Issues?

After inquiring about surgeries, your doctor will probably note any health problems you have had or continue to have, such as:

- any past or chronic illnesses (cancer, heart disease, high blood pressure, chronic fatigue syndrome, diabetes, arthritis, and so on)
- exposure to the human immunodeficiency virus (HIV) or symptoms of AIDS; history of blood transfusions
- emotional health issues (including any depression, anxiety, or panic attacks)
- any hospitalizations (for example, if you were hospitalized with pneumonia or a heart problem)

- any heart problems (including a history of heart murmur, mitral valve prolapse, heart palpitations, or chest pain)
- any blood clots, such as pulmonary embolus or deep-vein thrombosis (deep vein clots in the lungs or legs)
- any thyroid problems
- a history of asthma, bronchitis, pneumonia, or a recurrent cough
- any stomach problems (including heartburn, acid reflux, nausea, or ulcers)
- any intestinal problems (episodes of diarrhea, constipation, or irritable bowel syndrome lasting more than two weeks at a time)
- any kidney or bladder problems (including pyelonephritis, kidney infections, kidney stones, urinary infections)
- gallbladder disease

What Is Your Obstetric and Gynecological History?

Your surgical history provided some clues, but here is your chance to provide more information about your gynecologic health:

- any births, miscarriages, ectopic pregnancies, or pregnancy terminations
- any breast cysts or ovarian cysts
- any issues involving the cervix (including abnormal Pap smears, evidence of cervical dysplasia, precancer or cancer of the cervix, colposcopy, freezing or cryosurgery, cone biopsy, or loop excision)
- any problems involving the uterus (such as fibroids or endometrial hyperplasia)
- exposure to diethylstilbestrol, or DES (whether your mother took it when she was pregnant with you, or you took it yourself)
- problems with the vulva (vulvar dystrophy or dysplasia), ovaries, or fallopian tubes
- any sexually transmitted diseases, including herpes, genital warts, gonorrhea, Chlamydia, or pelvic inflammatory disease (PID)

What Is the Status of Your Menstrual Cycle?

In addition to assessing your phase of menopause, your gynecologist uses your past menstrual history to form a picture of your gynecologic risk profile. For example, if you started your menstrual period at a very young age, had no biologic children, and had your final menstrual period at age 58, you had prolonged estrogen exposure and are at higher risk for getting breast cancer. By virtue of that history, you would also be at higher risk for ovarian cancer. The doctor will want to know:

- How old were you when you got your first period?
- Do you still have periods?
  - How many days do you bleed (three, five, more)?
  - Are your menstrual periods heavy—that is, do you bleed and soak through more than a regular pad or a tampon in an hour?
  - Do you bleed or spot between periods (break-through bleeding)?
  - Do you spot or bleed before your period, after your period, or between periods?
  - What is the cycle length—that is, how many days usually pass between Day One of your period to Day One of the next period?
- Have your periods stopped?
  - When was the last time you noticed any bleeding? Include even a scant amount of bleeding, pink or brown staining, or clots.
  - How often did you menstruate before your periods stopped?

YOUR SOCIAL HISTORY

Next the doctor will inquire about your social history, which includes:

- your level of education
- whether or not you work and the type of work you do; how many hours a week you work

- who lives with you—parents, siblings, children, grandchildren, spouse or partner
- what your hobbies, interests, or homemaking priorities are
- if you have a spouse, significant other, or partner; if so, how long you have been in that relationship

Your social history is a broad category, and how many questions you will be asked in this area varies a great deal from doctor to doctor. The doctor will ask about your lifestyle choices, such as:

- *What about your sexual activity?* Do you have intercourse with men, women, both, or neither? If you are sexually active, are you in a mutually exclusive relationship? Do you experience any pain or related problems? If you are in a relationship with a man and are perimenopausal, what method of birth control do you use?
- *Do you smoke?* If so, how long have you smoked? How many cigarettes do you smoke per day? If you used to smoke, how many years did you do so, and how long ago did you quit?
- *Do you drink alcohol?* Note if you often have more than three drinks of beer, wine, or liquor a week. Also tell the doctor if you have a history of alcoholism and/or rehabilitation.
- *Do you use recreational drugs?* If so, what kind and how often? Mention if you have used intravenous drugs, or if you had a sexual partner who has used them.
- *Do you exercise regularly?* If so, what types, how much, and how often?

In order to understand every aspect of your health, your doctor needs to know things you might find embarrassing. Chances are your doctor has heard it all before. His or her role is not to judge your lifestyle choices, but to try to keep you as healthy as possible.

YOUR FAMILY HISTORY

Your family history is important because you may have a genetic predisposition to certain problems. People who were adopted often know very little about their family history. If you have a sense of the genetic strengths and vulnerabilities of your family, consider yourself lucky!

Relevant family members include your biologic mother and father, siblings, grandparents on both your mother's side and your father's side, and aunts and uncles. Include only blood relatives. Is there a history of breast, ovarian, prostate, colon, or intestinal cancer in these family members? Do any of these individuals have a history of heart disease, high blood pressure, stroke, diabetes, or osteoporosis? Are there family members who have suffered heart problems before age 60? Heart attacks or strokes in female relatives under age 69, or male relatives under age 50, raise a red flag. What about arthritis and Alzheimer's disease?

When it comes to breast cancer, some people have the impression that only the mother's side of the family is important, but that is not the case. If any female relatives on either side developed breast cancer before age 50, this suggests premenopausal breast cancer, which poses a higher risk and calls for more aggressive screening.

Your Physical Examination

At some point you will probably be asked to take off your clothes and put on a gown so the doctor can do a physical exam. You may choose to have a nurse or medical assistant present in addition to the doctor.

A complete gynecological examination for an adult woman should include examination of the breasts, abdomen, and pelvis. The doctor will check for lumps or cysts or thickened areas in both breasts by palpation. He or she will also check in the armpits, where the lymph nodes drain. Your abdomen will be palpated next, starting below your ribs. Many doctors also percuss, or tap over the upper organs, including the liver and the spleen, to see if they are enlarged. The doctor also is feeling for masses in your lower abdomen, such as a protuberant, enlarged uterus. He or she will note any scars from prior surgeries you may have had, and check in your groin area for tenderness or lumps along the panty line.

The Pelvic Exam

By this time in your life, you have most likely had a pelvic examination. If you haven't, it is never too late. Twenty-six years ago I did a first pelvic examination on an 80-year-old woman who came to the emergency room hemorrhaging from a large mass in her pelvis. She had never been to the doctor, and had never given birth. Fortunately, her pelvic mass was not cancerous and after it was surgically removed she went home in a dress that was four sizes too big. (I hope that by this point in your life, your first pelvic exam is many years behind you. You should not wait until you are 80 to have your first gynecological checkup!)

The first part of the pelvic exam involves examining the vulva, which is the skin outside the vagina, to look for anything unusual, such as changes in the skin color or texture. The second part of the exam is an inspection of the vagina and cervix using a speculum, an instrument that keeps the vaginal walls apart so the doctor can examine the walls for changes and see the cervix at the top of the vagina. Once the speculum is opened, the doctor looks at the cervix and, if a Pap smear is being done, uses a small, soft brush to sweep the surface of the cervix and gather cells for analysis. Analyzing the cells on the Pap smear allows early detection of precancerous conditions as well as cancer of the cervix.

The doctor may also test for sexually transmitted diseases by using a cotton swab in the cervical opening. While examining the vaginal canal, the gynecologist checks for the health of the tissue inside. Is it red—possibly from infection or lack of estrogen? Is there a normal or abnormal amount and type of discharge present?

After the speculum is removed, the gynecologist manually palpates the uterus and ovaries to check whether they feel enlarged or are tender. The doctor also can check if there is a cystocele, or dropped bladder (this occurs when the floor of the bladder, and supporting roof of the vagina, get saggy). The doctor also may determine if you leak urine when you cough. If there is leakage, the doctor may recommend additional testing.

The Rectal Exam

If you are 50 years old or older, the doctor will perform a rectal exam to check for any masses and to evaluate the support of the rectum. The roof of the rectum borders on the floor of the vagina, and sometimes the rectum can herniate into the vagina (a condition that is called a rectocele). The doctor may also check for hidden blood in the rectum by taking a stool sample. The rectal examination and stool guaiac test may help to find early rectal or bowel cancer. Colonoscopy, a microscopic examination of the inner walls of the intestines, is a thorough way to check for intestinal polyps, cancers, and precancers as well as other conditions of the gastrointestinal tract. It is recommended at age 50 and then every 5 to 10 years if there are no other worrisome findings. For those with a high-risk family history of colon cancer, an earlier or a more frequent colonoscopy screening may be recommended. Check with your internal medicine doctor or family doctor as well as your gynecologist for their recommendations.

THE DOCTOR'S ASSESSMENT

At the conclusion of your physical examination the doctor may want to order laboratory tests. For example, he or she may order a blood test, urine sample, mammogram, or bone density test, or, as you just read, you may be told to schedule a colonoscopy.

After making plans for testing, the doctor begins his or her assessment. The assessment is a key component of every medical visit. During the assessment, the doctor pulls together all of the information gleaned from your history, physical exam, and any available laboratory tests to paint a medical picture of your health status. The assessment is like assembling the pieces of a jigsaw puzzle to get the big picture. It drives the plan that the doctor will formulate with you.

The doctor will make a comprehensive list that includes:

- any concerns you mentioned during the visit
- any concerns he or she has, based upon your physical examination and entire history

- tests that should be done and that will warrant follow-up
- any prescriptions you will be receiving
- when you should schedule your next visit
- preventive care goals, to keep you as healthy as possible for as long as possible

As you decide on your next steps going forward, collaboration between you and the doctor is essential. Ask questions so you understand the reasoning behind your doctor's recommendations. The doctor needs your feedback and reaction to his or her recommendations before the end of the visit. If the doctor suggests an approach you don't like, speak up. This is the time to indicate whether you would like to discuss other approaches because if you are not committed to a particular treatment plan, it is unlikely to be effective. Your input is essential. For example, if the doctor prescribes a medication, but you are reluctant to take it, you are not getting the best medical advice for you. The recommendation needs to be tailored further to your preferences whenever possible so you will feel comfortable following through with it.

Most likely, the doctor will plan to see you again. A final assessment may be made at a later visit, after your test results are available. If you are starting a new medication or treatment, the doctor may want to see you in a few weeks or months to evaluate how well it is working for you. If you are healthy, up to date with your medical tests, and have no particular worries, the doctor may suggest an appointment for another checkup in a year.

An Annual Visit to the Gynecologist

Your annual exam is a modified version of the comprehensive "new patient" visit. It is scheduled on a regular basis, independent of any health concerns or problems that come up during the year. In perimenopause and postmenopause, it is important to have breast and pelvic exams every year. Even if you are not due for a Pap smear, it is important for you to have a pelvic exam and a rectal exam annually after you are over age 50.

During your annual exam, update any information from your initial visit. Inform the doctor of any changes in your health or lifestyle, and let him or her know what is working for you and what isn't. The purpose of the annual exam is to ensure that your medications and lifestyle choices match your current state of health. This is also the time to get new information from the doctor. Updated information may influence you to stop taking a particular medication or supplement, or to exchange it for a newer version that is more effective. New symptoms may make it advisable to start taking hormones, or to adjust the levels you are taking.

Preventive care should be an aspect of your annual checkup every year. You and your doctor can discuss the latest prevention strategies to help you avoid medical problems such as diabetes, heart disease, or osteoporosis.

⚡ Betty's Story ⚡

Betty's Annual Gynecology Visit—Fortuitously Not Cancelled

"I am 57 years old and done with menopause-related changes. I almost skipped my annual gynecologic examination as many of my friends did this year. Usually my doctor asks me if I booked my mammogram yet, examines my breasts to check for lumps, does a pelvic examination with a Pap smear, and sends me on my way. I forgot to cancel the appointment, so I went.

"The doctor asked me about the supplements I am taking. I had already researched them on the Internet and wasn't planning to mention them. I am glad that I did. I found out that the women's multivitamin that I was taking is not the best one for me, despite the advertising. The iron it includes is preventing me from absorbing the calcium it contains. Since I am no longer bleeding, and I am not anemic, I don't need the iron; but I do need the calcium for my bones, and I wasn't getting it. Now I am changing to a multivitamin for seniors, which has no iron, even though I do not think of myself as a 'senior.'

"After asking if I had developed any new allergic reactions to medications, the doctor asked about changes in my physical health. She also *wanted to know if there were any changes in my work situation, my family, or my current relationship, and whether I was having any problems with sex. I would not have brought it up, but I told her that my partner and I have both noticed a decrease in my sex drive. The doctor said we could discuss this further at a subsequent appointment if this concern remains, or causes a problem for me or my partner.*

"Finally, the doctor mentioned that I had gained weight, and asked how I felt about it. When I told her about the over-the-counter weight-loss supplement I had purchased, she explained that it was not a healthy choice. There is a risk of getting an irregular heartbeat due to the stimulants in the preparation, and that is even riskier for a postmenopausal woman over 50. Sure enough, the next month I read on the Internet that the weight-loss supplement was taken off the market. I am glad I kept my appointment.

A "Problem" Visit with the Gynecologist

In between your annual exams, you may visit the gynecologist for a focused or "problem" visit to:

- check your progress after a new medication, treatment, or lifestyle change
- evaluate healing after a surgical procedure, and discuss treatment options
- discuss something unexpected

For example, I instruct my postmenopausal patients to schedule an appointment if they notice any bleeding (see Chapter 5). Even if a woman's last gynecologic checkup was normal, unexpected vaginal bleeding calls for a prompt visit to the doctor.

WHAT IS YOUR MAIN CONCERN?

When doctors say your "complaint is stomach pains," they don't actually mean you are complaining. In medical jargon, the reason you are seeing the doctor is called your "chief complaint."

Before you call for an appointment, clarify your main concern.

If you are in pain, the receptionist or nurse may ask how severe it is and how long you have had it. Having this information helps with scheduling a timely appointment. Some doctors and nurses use a pain scale to assess the severity of your pain. On a scale of 1 to 10, excruciating pain is a 10. You may be asked where your pain falls on the intensity scale. If you are calling a physician you have not seen before, the office may recommend that you schedule a comprehensive evaluation.

Prior to your medical appointment, write down any information you have about your most pressing medical concern. Bring up your "chief complaint" at the beginning of the visit. Helpful information for the doctor includes:

- How often does this problem occur?
- When did it first develop?
- Does it vary with your menstrual cycle (if you still have one)?
- What was the date of your last menstrual cycle (if you still have one)?
- Does this problem occur after eating, or between meals on an empty stomach?
- What is the severity of the symptoms?
- Is this problem painful?
- Is the pain sharp, achy, or cramping?
- Is it associated with nausea, vomiting, or diarrhea?
- Does it occur with activity or at rest?
- How long does it last, and how often do you get it?
- Does it ever wake you up at night?

When I am a patient myself, or accompanying a family member to his or her doctor visit, I find it helpful to have a short written list of questions or concerns I want to discuss. Without a list, I've found it's too easy to get sidetracked during the office visit and forget the things I wanted to mention.

THE SOAP FORMAT

Doctors use the acronym SOAP to structure a problem visit.

- *"S" stands for Subjective.* These are the concerns that you, the patient, report. Symptoms are subjective because they are experienced by you. This category also includes information the doctor elicits regarding what you are feeling.
- *"O" stands for Objective.* This includes signs the doctor can observe and information the doctor can acquire. This category includes the findings from your physical exam, as well as laboratory reports, ultrasounds, x-ray studies, bone density reports, mammogram results, colonoscopy conclusions, and so on.
- *"A" stands for Assessment.* Here, the doctor pieces together the subjective and objective information to determine what's going on. Ideally, the doctor's preliminary assessment is cross-checked with the patient herself in case she has additional information or concerns. Sometimes the assessment is completed after additional pieces of the jigsaw puzzle are on the table. For example, an ultrasound may be ordered and the results used to clarify the final assessment at the next visit.
- *"P" stands for Plan.* This is the "where do we go from here?" piece. The best medical plans are those that accommodate your individual preferences. Ideally, you have input into the plan and feel comfortable with it. A medical plan that does not fit your lifestyle or personal philosophy is useless. If the doctor assembles the pieces of your health puzzle into a picture you don't appreciate, the pieces go back in the box.

The doctor will use *differential diagnosis* to generate various possible explanations for the particular features of your health history, physical exam, and lab results that are in play at this visit. He or she will make a mental list that ranges from the best-case scenario to the worst-case scenario, or from the most common reasons for your complaint to the most serious or life-threatening reasons—the "do not miss" causes. Balancing these two extremes is the art of practicing medicine. If a doctor leaps to the dire causes too readily, you may be needlessly alarmed. On the other hand, if the doctor fails to consider the most serious possibilities, you could end up with a problem that could have been avoided or diagnosed sooner.

⚐ OFELIA ⚐

Ovarian Cancer or Ovarian Cyst?

Ofelia is 45 years old. After experiencing pelvic pain on her left side for three months, she scheduled a doctor's appointment. "My doctor took a comprehensive history and performed a gynecologic exam. I told her that my maternal aunt had ovarian cancer in her mid-forties. The pelvic exam showed that my left ovary was enlarged and tender. I was very worried, and my doctor later told me she felt like she needed to walk a tightrope between diagnosing what was probably a benign harmless cyst and being certain that she was not ignoring an early sign of ovarian cancer. She needed to communicate her awareness that the cyst could be ominous while simultaneously reassuring me it was most likely an innocent cyst.

"She ordered an ultrasound, which revealed a cyst in my left ovary that was just under two inches in diameter. Because of my family history, she ordered a blood test called CA-125. This test checks for some, but not all, of the many types of ovarian cancer. To help avoid a false alarm, the doctor told me to have the blood drawn for the CA-125 test after the end of my next menstrual period. The results of the test were reassuring, and an ultrasound two months later showed that the ovarian cyst had completely resolved—that is, it was reabsorbed by my body.

"The doctor and I discussed ways to decrease my risk of ovarian cancer, including low-dose oral contraceptives or a tubal ligation. Although birth control pills could have been a safe choice for me, I had experienced headaches in the past with two different birth control pill preparations and was not eager to try this approach again. Once I learned that it would decrease my risk of ovarian cancer by 30 to 50 percent, I elected to have a tubal ligation. Because I had only one relative with ovarian cancer, and it was my aunt, not my mother or sister, the doctor felt I did not have to consider removal of my ovaries to prevent ovarian cancer."

How Your Doctor Thinks

Doctors are trained to consider problems from various points of view. This can be compared to using different lenses to look at the same situation. By categorizing your problem, your doctor helps to narrow down the immense number of treatment options that are available.

- *Is this problem acute or chronic?* Acute problems are recent, discrete episodes. In contrast, a chronic problem persists over months or years.
- *Is this problem persistent or recurrent?* Persistent problems never completely resolve after the initial intervention. In contrast, a recurrent problem may resolve completely with treatment, but then return. A persistent problem is continuous (imagine a constant stream of water from a hose), while a recurrent problem is episodic (the stream of water is turned on and off at intervals).
- *Does this situation call for treatment or prevention, or both?* Treatment is important for acute or persistent problems. Preventive measures are used to keep a problem from occurring or recurring, but they cannot always be used when the problem is severe or ongoing. Treatment strategies do not always match prevention strategies.

Some doctors are better than others at staying up to date about treatment and prevention strategies. One reason I wrote this book is to make sure you have the most recent information available. Although medical care of perimenopausal and postmenopausal women has drastically improved in the past two decades, there is still a lot to learn. There are questions that will be answered by studies that have not yet been completed. There are medications we would like to be able to prescribe that have not yet been approved by the Food and Drug Administration and are not yet available in this country. Try to be open to any new options your doctor suggests because every year the medications improve in ways designed to provide more benefit with fewer risks or side effects. With ongoing visits, your doctor can constantly fine-tune your treatments to meet your changing needs.

The Role of the Internet

The Internet inserted itself into our lives before we could figure out how we wanted to embrace it. I have seen Internet use sabotage doctor-patient relationships. This can occur when a well-meaning patient prints out dozens of pages of research on topics that do not actually pertain to her. Sometimes a patient will present her medical conclusions—based on her Internet research—before the doctor has had a chance to review her current history, perform a physical exam, get any laboratory results, make an assessment, and draw his or her own conclusions. Internet information that has been gathered before a doctor's diagnosis has been obtained is often misleading. It can do more harm than good. If you want to do Internet research, I suggest that, whenever possible, you wait until you know the specific problem or procedure on which to focus your investigation.

The Internet can unduly frighten people who use it to self-diagnose. It is not a good idea to reach conclusions about what is causing your problem before allowing your doctor to filter your concerns through the medical sieve of your history, exam, and lab findings. This sieve is a tried-and-true tool that successfully filters out false alarms. For example, a 52-year-old woman who has abdominal bloating may conclude from her Internet research that she has ovarian cancer. Her history, exam, and laboratory tests may show that she has simply become lactose-intolerant.

Another hazard of Internet use is that it requires some expertise to locate the best information. Basically, anybody can post anything they want on the Internet. Some people have a hidden agenda, such as promoting a certain procedure or selling a certain supplement. Sometimes information is out of date or provided by an unreliable source. The Pew Internet and American Life Project tracked the behavior of Americans using the Internet to learn about their health. They found that 85 million of the 113 million adults who search for health information online do not consistently check the source and date of the health information that they find. This means their Internet research may be no more helpful than going to a library and reading an out-of-date medical textbook.

The Internet *can* play a very supportive role if you use it in the right context. Medical information from the Internet can be extremely valuable once you have a specific diagnosis made by your physician. Your physician may also be able to provide up-to-date, reliable websites for some aspects of your care. If you are not certain about the accuracy of the site, or whether it has current information, remember this: don't believe everything you read!

I *do* encourage you to visit the U.S. Department of Health and Human Services website at www.hhs.gov/familyhistory/. You will find a helpful free tool for creating your own "Family Health History" record. This information will be of great help to you and your doctor as you work together to achieve and maintain your optimal health.

RESOURCES

Groopman, Jerome. *How Doctors Think*. Boston: Houghton Mifflin, 2007. This Harvard medical professor is a respected cancer researcher and master clinician. The book contains insights about doctors' reactions to their patients, and patients' reactions to their doctors.

Harvard Women's Health Watch. © Harvard University (www.health .harvard.edu/newsletters/Harvard_Womens_Health_Watch). You may subscribe to this newsletter in print, electronic form, or both. The editor-in-chief, Celeste Robb-Nicholson, M.D., is an assistant professor of medicine at Harvard Medical School and the founding editor-in-chief of the newsletter. There is helpful information on current medical topics. It is apparent that the editor wants her readers to be informed and share in the decision-making process with their doctors.

Roizen, Michael, and Mehmet Oz. *You, the Smart Patient: An Insider's Handbook for Getting the Best Treatment*. New York: Free Press, 2006. The book provides in-depth coverage of how best to work with your doctor and how to assemble the information he or she needs. There is also information about evaluating your care and getting second opinions.

References

Chapter 1. You and Your Doctor: The Health Alliance

Lewis J, et al. Caution on the use of saliva measurements to monitor absorption of progesterone from transdermal creams in postmenopausal women. *Maturitas* 41 (2002): 1–6.

Life Expectancy Tables. National Vital Statistics System, www.efmoody .com/estate/lifeexpectancy.html. Last accessed December 10, 2008.

Risk of Breast Cancer by Age. Department of Health and Human Services Centers for Disease Control and Prevention. www.cdc.gov/cancer/ breast/statistics/age.htm. Last accessed May 6, 2009.

Santoro N, et al. Helping midlife women predict the onset of the final menses: SWAN, the Study of Women's Health Across the Nation. *Menopause* 14, no. 3 (2007): 415–424.

Chapter 2. Handling Hot Flashes without Hormones

Avis N, et al. A randomized, controlled pilot study of acupuncture treatment for menopausal hot flashes. *Menopause* 15, no. 6 (2008): 1070–1078.

Bair Y, Gold E, et al. Use of complementary and alternative medicine during the menopause transition: longitudinal results from the Study of Women's Health Across the Nation (SWAN). *Menopause* 15, no. 1 (2008): 45–62.

Brett K, Keenan N. Complementary and alternative medicine use among midlife women for reasons including menopause in the United States. *Menopause* 14, no. 2 (2002): 300–307.

Butt DA, Lock M, Lewis JE, et al. Gabapentin for the treatment of menopausal hot flashes: a randomized controlled trial. *Menopause* 15, no. 2 (2008): 310–318.

Cant M, Johnstone R. Reproductive conflict and the separation of reproductive generations in humans. *Proceedings of the National Academy of Sciences* 105, no. 14 (2008): 5332–5336.

Cheng G, Wilczek B, et al. Isoflavone treatment for acute menopausal symptoms. *Menopause* 14, no. 3 (2007): 468–473.

D'Anna R, et al. Effects of the phytoestrogen genistein on hot flushes, endometrium, and vaginal epithelium in postmenopausal women: a 1-year randomized, double-blind, placebo-controlled study. *Menopause* 14, no. 4 (2007): 648–655.

Komesaroff PA, Black CV, Cable V, Sudhir K. Effects of wild yam extract on menopausal symptoms, lipids and sex hormones in healthy menopausal women. *Climacteric* 4, no. 2 (2001): 144–150.

Liske E, et al. Physiological investigation of a unique extract of black cohosh (Cimicifugae racemosae rhizome): a 6-month clinical study demonstrates no systemic estrogenic effect. *Journal of Women's Health and Gender-Based Medicine* 11, no. 2 (2002): 163–174.

Lock M. Ambiguities of aging: Japanese experience and perceptions of menopause. *Culture, Medicine and Psychiatry* 10, no. 1 (1986): 23–46.

Nelson HD, Vesco KK, Haney E, et al. Nonhormonal therapies for menopausal hot flashes: systematic review and meta-analysis. *Journal of the American Medical Association* 295, no. 17 (2006): 2057–2071.

Newton KM, Reed SD, et al. Treatment of vasomotor symptoms of menopause with black cohosh, multibotanicals, soy, hormone therapy, or placebo: a randomized trial. *Annals of Internal Medicine* 145, no. 12 (2006): 869–879.

Pandya KJ, Morrow GR, Roscoe JA, et al. Gabapentin for hot flashes in 420 women with breast cancer: a randomized double-blind placebo-controlled trial. *Lancet* 366, no. 9488 (2005): 818–824.

Pruthi S, et al. Pilot evaluation of flaxseed for the management of hot flashes. *Journal of the Society for Integrative Oncology* 5, no. 3 (2007): 106–112.

Randomized trial of black cohosh for the treatment of hot flashes among women with a history of breast cancer. *Journal of Clinical Oncology* 19, no. 10 (2001): 2739–2745.

Shanafelt T, et al. Pathophysiology and treatment of hot flashes. *Mayo Clinic Proceedings* 77 (2002): 1207–1218.

Treatment of menopausal vasomotor symptoms. *The Medical Letter* 46, nos. 1197/1198 (2004): 98–99.

Wild yam. American Cancer Society, www.cancer.org. Last accessed December 3, 2008.

Chapter 3. Taking Hormones in Menopause

Boothby L, et al. Bioidentical hormone therapy: a review. *Menopause* 11, no. 3 (2004): 356–367.

Compounded bioidentical hormones. *ACOG Committee Opinion* no. 322, November 2005.

Department of Health and Human Services, U.S. Food and Drug Administration, Center for Drug Evaluation and Research. *2006 Limited FDA Survey of Compounded Drug Products,* www.fda.gov/cder/pharmcomp/survey_2006.htm. Created January 28, 2003, updated March 5, 2008. Last accessed December 7, 2008.

Grodstein F, et al. Postmenopausal hormone therapy and stroke. Role of time since menopause and age at initiation of hormone therapy. *Archives of Internal Medicine* 168 (2008): 861–866.

Manson JE, et al. Estrogen therapy and coronary-artery calcification. *New England Journal of Medicine* 356, no. 25 (2007): 2591–2602.

Morch L et al. Hormone therapy and ovarian cancer. *Journal of the American Medical Association* 302, no. 3 (2009): 298–305.

Rossouw JE, Anderson GL, Prentice RL, et al. Writing Group for the Women's Health Initiative investigators. Risks and benefits of estrogen plus progestin for healthy postmenopausal women. *Journal of the American Medical Association* 288 (2002): 321–333.

Rossouw JE, Ross PL, Manson JE, et al. Postmenopausal hormone therapy and risk of cardiovascular disease by age and years since menopause. *Journal of the American Medical Association* 297, no. 13 (2007): 1465–1477.

Salpeter S, Walsh J, et al. Brief report: coronary heart disease events associated with hormone therapy in younger and older women. A meta-analysis. *Journal of General Internal Medicine* 21 (2006): 363–366.

Shaffer L, Krantz C. Hormone therapy and cardiovascular risk. *Journal of the American Medical Association* 298, no. 6 (2007): 623–624.

Stefanick ML, Anderson GL, Margolis KL, et al., for the Women's Health Initiative Investigators. Effects of conjugated equine estrogens on breast cancer and mammography screening in postmenopausal women with hysterectomy: The Women's Health Initiative. *Journal of the American Medical Association* 295 (2006): 1647–1657.

Wren BG, et al. Effect of sequential transdermal progesterone cream on endometrium, bleeding pattern, and plasma progesterone and salivary progesterone levels in postmenopausal women. *Climacteric* 3 (2000): 155–160.

Wren BG, et al. Transdermal progesterone and its effect on vasomotor symptoms, blood lipid levels, bone metabolic markers, moods, and quality of life for postmenopausal women. *Menopause* 10 (2003): 13–18.

Chapter 4. Heart Disease: The Risk of Doing Nothing

Arsenault B, et al. Visceral adipose tissue accumulation, cardiorespiratory fitness, and features of the metabolic syndrome. *Archives of Internal Medicine* 167, no. 14 (2007): 1518–1525.

Barnard ND, et al. A low-fat vegan diet improves glycemic control and cardiovascular risk factors in a randomized clinical trial in individuals with Type 2 diabetes. *Diabetes Care* 29 (2006): 1777–1783.

Barnard ND, Scialli AR, et al. Effectiveness of a low-fat vegetarian diet in altering serum lipids in healthy premenopausal women. *American Journal of Cardiology* 85 (2000): 969–972.

Canto J, Goldberg R, Hand M, et al. Symptom presentation of women with acute coronary syndromes: myth versus reality. *Archives of Internal Medicine* 167, no. 22 (2007): 2405–2413.

Church T, et al. Effects of different doses of physical activity on cardiorespiratory fitness among sedentary, overweight or obese postmenopausal women with elevated blood pressure. A randomized controlled trial. *Journal of the American Medical Association* 297 (2007): 2081–2091.

Clarkson, T. Estrogen effects on arteries vary with stage of reproductive life and extent of subclinical atherosclerosis progression. *Menopause* 14, no. 3 (2007): 373–384.

Heidemann C, Schulze M, Franco O, et al. Dietary patterns and risk of mortality from cardiovascular disease, cancer, and all causes in a prospective cohort of women. *Circulation* 118 (2008): 230–237.

Johannes C, et al. Relation of dehydroepiandrosterone and dehydroepiandrosterone sulfate with cardiovascular disease risk factors in women: longitudinal results from the Massachusetts Women's Health Study. *Journal of Clinical Epidemiology* 52, no. 2 (1999): 95–103.

Katcher H, Legro R, et al. The effects of a whole grain–enriched hypocaloric diet on cardiovascular disease risk factors in men and women with metabolic syndrome. *American Journal of Clinical Nutrition* 87 (2008): 79–90.

Mosca L, et al. Evidence-based guidelines for cardiovascular disease prevention in women. *Circulation* 109 (2004): 672.

Wang L, et al. Whole- and refined-grain intakes and the risk of hypertension in women. *American Journal of Clinical Nutrition* 86 (2007): 472–479.

Welty F, et al. Effect of soy nuts on blood pressure and lipid levels in hypertensive, prehypertensive, and normotensive postmenopausal women. *Archives of Internal Medicine* 167 (2007): 1060–1067.

Young D, et al. The effects of aerobic exercise and T'ai Chi on blood pressure in older people: results of a randomized trial. *Journal of the American Geriatrics Society* 47 (1999): 277–284.

Chapter 5. Understanding Unexpected Bleeding

American College of Obstetricians and Gynecologists Committee Opinion Number 440, The role of transvaginal ultrasonography in the evaluation of postmenopausal bleeding. *Obstetrics and Gynecology* 114, no. 2 (2009): 409–411.

Antunes A, et al. Endometrial polyps in pre- and postmenopausal women: factors associated with malignancy. *Maturitas* 57 (2007): 415–421.

Kelly P, et al. Endometrial hyperplasia involving endometrial polyps: report of a series and discussion of the significance in an endometrial biopsy specimen. *British Journal of Obstetrics and Gynaecology* 114 (2007): 944–950.

Moschos E, et al. Saline-infusion sonography endometrial sampling compared with endometrial biopsy in diagnosing endometrial pathology. *Obstetrics and Gynecology* 113, no. 4 (2009): 881–887.

Pinto I, Chimeno P, Romo A, et al. Uterine fibroids: uterine artery embolization versus abdominal hysterectomy for treatment—a prospective, randomized, and controlled clinical trial. *Radiology* 226, no. 2 (2003): 425–431.

Tabor A, et al. Endometrial thickness as a test for endometrial cancer in women with postmenopausal vaginal bleeding. *Obstetrics and Gynecology* 99 (2002): 663–670.

Trost L, et al. The diagnosis and treatment of iron deficiency and its potential relationship to hair loss. *Journal of the American Academy of Dermatology* 54 (2006): 824–844.

Chapter 6. Common Concerns

Hussain A, Harrison S. Neuromodulation for lower urinary tract dysfunction—an update. *Scientific World Journal* 7 (2007): 1036–1045.

Rittenmeyer H. Sacral nerve neuromodulation (InterStim®) part I: review of the InterStim® system. *Urologic Nursing* 28, no. 1 (2008): 15–20.

Rittenmeyer H. Sacral nerve neuromodulation (InterStim®) part II: review of programming. *Urologic Nursing* 28, no. 1 (2008): 21–25.

Chapter 7. Smoother Sex

Barnhart K, et al. The effect of dehydroepiandrosterone supplementation to symptomatic perimenopausal women on serum endocrine profiles, lipid parameters, and health-related quality of life. *Journal of Clinical Endocrinology and Metabolism* 84 (1999): 3896–3902.

Basson, R. Sexuality and sexual disorders in women. In *Women's Mental Health: A Life-Cycle Approach,* edited by Sarah E Romans and Mary V Seeman, 205–220. Philadelphia: Lippincott Williams and Wilkins, 2005.

Basson R. Female sexual response: the role of drugs in the management of sexual dysfunction. *Obstetrics and Gynecology* 98, no. 2 (2001): 350–353.

Basson R. The female sexual response. A different model. *Journal of Sex and Marital Therapy* 26 (2000): 51–65.

Basson RB, Berman J, Burnett A, et al. Report of the international consensus development conference on female sexual dysfunction: definitions and classifications. *Journal of Urology* 163 (2000): 888–893.

Basson R, McInnes R, Smith MD, et al. Efficacy and safety of Sildenafil in estrogenized women with sexual dysfunction associated with female sexual arousal disorder. *Obstetrics and Gynecology* 95 (2000): 51–54.

Dennerstein L, et al. Hormones, mood, sexuality and the menopausal transition. *Fertility and Sterility* 77 (Supplement 4) (2002): 42–48.

Dennerstein L, et al. Sexuality and the menopause. *Journal of Psychosomatic Obstetrics and Gynaecology* 15, no. 1 (1994): 59–66.

Gracia CR, et al. Predictors of decreased libido in women during the late reproductive years. *Menopause* 11, no. 2 (2004): 144–150.

Graziottin A. Hormones and libido. In *Progress in the Management of the Menopause: Proceedings of the 8th International Congress on the Menopause, Sydney, Australia, November 1996,* edited by Barry G. Wren, 393–401. New York: Parthenon, 1997.

Laumann E, Das A, Waite L. Sexual dysfunction among older adults: prevalence and risk factors from a nationally representative U.S. probability sample of men and women 57–85 years of age. *Journal of Sexual Medicine* 5 (2008): 2300–2311.

Leder BZ, et al. Effects of oral androstenedione administration on serum testosterone and estradiol levels in postmenopausal women. *Journal of Clinical Endocrinology and Metabolism* 87 (2002): 5449–5454.

Modelska K, Cummings S. Female sexual dysfunction in postmenopausal women: systematic review of placebo-controlled trials. *American Journal of Obstetrics and Gynecology* 188 (2003): 286–293.

Nair KS, et al. DHEA in elderly women and DHEA or testosterone in elderly men. *New England Journal of Medicine* 355 (2006): 1647–1659.

Reed SD, et al. Night sweats, sleep disturbance, and depression associated with diminished libido in late menopausal transition and early post menopause: baseline data from the Herbal Alternatives for Menopause Trial (HALT). *American Journal of Obstetrics and Gynecology* 196, no. 6 (2007): 593.e1–7.

Riley AR, Riley E. Controlled studies on women presenting with sexual drive disorder, I: endocrine status. *Journal of Sex and Marital Therapy* 26 (2000): 269–283.

Rosen R, Brown C, Heiman J, Leiblum S, et al. The Female Sexual Function Index (FSFI): a multidimensional self-report instrument for the assessment of female sexual function. *Journal of Sex and Marital Therapy* 26 (2000): 191–208.

Rosenbaum T. The role of physical therapy in female sexual dysfunction. *Current Sexual Health Reports* 5 (2008): 97–101.

Sarrel P. Effects of hormone replacement therapy on sexual psychophysiology and behavior in postmenopause. *Journal of Women's Health and Gender-Based Medicine* 9 (Supplement 1) (2000): S25–S32.

Shifren JL, Braunstein GD, Simon JA, et al. Transdermal testosterone treatment in women with impaired sexual function after oophorectomy. *New England Journal of Medicine* 343 (2000): 682–688.

Speroff, L. Special feature: measuring testosterone. *Ob/Gyn Clinical Alert* (2003).

Chapter 8. Compatible Contraception

Franco E, Duarte-Franco E. Ovarian cancer and oral contraceptives. Comment. *Lancet* 371 (2008): 277.

Henshaw SK. Unintended pregnancy in the United States. *Family Planning Perspectives* 30 (1998): 24–29.

Chapter 9. Moods, Memory, and Mental Health

Allen J, et al. The efficacy of acupuncture in the treatment of major depression in women. *Psychological Science* 9 (2001): 397–401.

Brody D, et al. Identifying patients with depression in the primary care setting. A more efficient method. *Archives of Internal Medicine* 158 (1998): 2469–2475.

Cyranowski J, Frank E, et al. Adolescent onset of the gender difference in lifetime rates of major depression. A theoretical model. *Archives of General Psychiatry* 57 (2000): 21–27.

DeKosky ST, Williamson JD, Fitzpatrick AL, et al. Ginkgo biloba for prevention of dementia. *Journal of the American Medical Association* 300, no. 19 (2008): 2253–2262.

Dunn A, et al. Exercise treatment for depression. Efficacy and dose response. *American Journal of Preventive Medicine* 28, no. 1 (2005): 1–8.

Farmer M, Locke B, et al. Physical activity and depressive symptoms: The NHANES I epidemiologic follow-up study. *American Journal of Epidemiology* 128 (1988): 1340–1351.

Grimley EJ, Malouf R, Huppert F, van Niekerk JK. Dehydroepiandrosterone (DHEA) supplementation for cognitive function in healthy elderly people. *Cochrane Database of Systematic Reviews* 2006, issue 4. art. no.: CD006221.

Josselson R, Apter T. *Best Friends: The Pleasures and Perils of Girls' and Women's Friendships.* New York: Crown Publishers, 1998.

Kessler R, et al. The use of complementary and alternative therapies to treat anxiety and depression in the United States. *American Journal of Psychiatry* 158 (2001): 289–294.

Miller JM. *Toward a New Psychology of Women.* Boston: Beacon Press, 1976.

Mortola J. Estrogens and mood. In *Estrogen and the Brain. Journal of the Society of Obstetricians and Gynaecologists of Canada (SOGC) Supplement* (1997): 1–5.

Mulrow C, et al. Case-finding instruments for depression in primary care settings. *Annals of Internal Medicine* 122 (1995): 913–921.

Noble R. Depression in women. *Metabolism Clinical and Experimental* 54 (Supplement 1) (2005): 49–52.

Phenninx B, Rejeski WJ, et al. Exercise and depressive symptoms: a comparison of aerobic and resistance exercise effects on emotional and physical function in older persons with high and low depressive symptomatology. *Journal of Gerontology: Psychological Sciences* 57B, no. 2 (2002): P124–P132.

Quah-Smith JI, et al. Laser acupuncture for mild to moderate depression in a primary care setting—a randomized controlled trial. *Acupuncture in Medicine* 23, no. 3 (2005): 103–111.

Rubinow D, Schmidt P, Roca C. Estrogen-serotonin interactions: implications for affective regulation. *Biological Psychiatry* 44 (1998): 839–850.

Singh N, et al. The efficacy of exercise as a long-term antidepressant in elderly subjects: a randomized controlled trial. *Journal of Gerontology* 56A, no. 8 (2001): M497–M504.

Tsang P, Shaner T. Age, attention, expertise, and time-sharing performance. *Psychology and Aging* 13, no. 2 (1998): 323–347.

Walker E, et al. Women and stress. In *Women's Mental Health: A Life-Cycle Approach,* edited by Sarah Romans and Mary Seeman, 35-47. Philadelphia: Lippincott Williams and Wilkins, 2006.

Chapter 10. Successful Sleep

Bixler EO, Vgontzas AN. Sleep disorders in perimenopausal and menopausal women. Diagnosis and clinical management. In *Management of the Perimenopause,* edited by Margery Gass and James Liu, 77–89. New York: McGraw-Hill, 2006.

Dennis K. Postmenopausal women and the health consequences of obesity. *Journal of Obstetric, Gynecologic and Neonatal Nursing* 36 (2007): 511–519.

Gangwisch JE, et al. Inadequate sleep as a risk factor for obesity: analyses of the NHANES I. *Sleep* 28, no. 10 (2005): 1217–1220.

Harsch IA, et al. Insulin resistance and other metabolic aspects of the obstructive sleep apnea syndrome. *Medical Science Monitor* 3 (2005): RA70–75.

Knutson KL, et al. The metabolic consequences of sleep deprivation. *Sleep Medicine Reviews* 11, no. 3 (2007): 163–178.

Phillips BG, et al. Increases in leptin levels, sympathetic drive, and weight gain in obstructive sleep apnea. *American Journal of Physiology Heart and Circulatory Physiology* 279 (2000): H234–H237.

Prinz P. Sleep, appetite, and obesity—what is the link? *Public Library of Science Medicine* 1, no. 3 (2004): e61.

Spiegel K, et al. Leptin levels are dependent on sleep duration: relationships with sympathovagal balance, carbohydrate regulation, cortisol, and thyrotropin. *Journal of Clinical Endocrinology and Metabolism* 89 (2004): 5762–5771.

Taheri S, et al. Short sleep duration is associated with reduced leptin, elevated ghrelin, and increased body mass index. *Public Library of Science Medicine* 1, no. 3 (2004): e62.

Vorona R, et al. Overweight and obese patients in a primary care population report less sleep than patients with a normal body mass index. *Archives of Internal Medicine* 165 (2005): 25–30.

Chapter 11. Better Bones

Bilezikian J. Osteonecrosis of the jaw—do bisphosphonates pose a risk? *New England Journal of Medicine* 355, no. 22 (2006): 2278–2281.

Bischoff-Ferrari H, Giovannucci E, Willett W, Dietrich T, Dawson-Hughes B. Estimation of optimal serum concentrations of 25-hydroxyvitamin D for multiple health outcomes. *American Journal of Clinical Nutrition* 84 (2006): 18–28.

Brannon P, Yetley E, Regan B, Bailey R, Picciano M. Overview of the conference "Vitamin D and Health in the 21st Century: an Update." *American Journal of Clinical Nutrition* 88, no. 2 (2008): S483–S490.

Cranney A, Weiler HA, O'Donnell S, Puil L. Summary of evidence-based review on vitamin D efficacy and safety in relation to bone health. *American Journal of Clinical Nutrition* 88 (Supplement) (2008): S513–S519.

Dawson-Hughes B. Serum 25-hydroxyvitamin D and functional outcomes in the elderly. *American Journal of Clinical Nutrition* 88 (Supplement) (2008): S537–S540.

Dawson-Hughes B, Tosteson A, Melton L, et al. Implications of absolute fracture risk assessment for osteoporosis practice guidelines in the USA. *Osteoporosis International* 19 (2008): 449–458.

Finigan J, Greenfield D, et al. Risk factors for vertebral and nonvertebral fracture over 10 years: a population-based study in women. *Journal of Bone and Mineral Research* 23, no. 1 (2008): 75–85.

Holick MF. Vitamin D deficiency. *New England Journal of Medicine* 357 (2007): 266–281.

Kanis J, Burlet N, et al. on behalf of the European Society for Clinical and Economic Aspects of Osteoporosis and Osteoarthritis (ESCEO). European guidance for the diagnosis and management of osteoporosis in postmenopausal women. *Osteoporosis International* 19 (2008): 399–428.

Kuehn B. New tool measures 10-year fracture risk. *Journal of the American Medical Association* 299, no. 14 (2008): 1651–1652.

Marini H, et al. Effects of the phytoestrogen genistein on bone metabolism in osteopenic postmenopausal women. A randomized trial. *Annals of Internal Medicine* 146 (2007): 839–847.

Pinkerton J, Dalkin A. Combination therapy for treatment of osteoporosis: a review. *American Journal of Obstetrics and Gynecology* 4 (2007): 559–565.

Roux C, et al. Assessment of non-vertebral fracture risk in postmenopausal women. *Annals of Rheumatic Diseases* 66 (2007): 931–935.

Siris E, Delmas PD. Assessment of 10-year absolute fracture risk: a new paradigm with worldwide application. *Osteoporosis International* 19 (2008): 383–384.

Tucker K, Morita K, et al. Colas, but not other carbonated beverages, are associated with low bone mineral density in older women: The Framingham Osteoporosis Study. *American Journal of Clinical Nutrition* 84 (2006): 936–942.

Voukelatos A, et al. A randomized, controlled trial of Tai Chi for the prevention of falls: the central Sydney Tai Chi trial. *Journal of the American Geriatric Society* 55 (2007): 1185–1191.

WHO Scientific Group on the Assessment of Osteoporosis at Primary Health Care Level. Summary Meeting Report. Brussels, Belgium, May 5–7, 2004. www.shef.ac.uk/FRAX. Last accessed June 4, 2008.

Woo SB, et al. Systematic review: bisphosphonates and osteonecrosis of the jaws. *Annals of Internal Medicine* 144 (2006): 753–761.

Chapter 12. Lifestyle Choices for Living Longer

Anderson JW, Konz EC, et al. Long-term weight-loss maintenance: a meta-analysis of US studies. *American Journal of Clinical Nutrition* 74 (2001): 579–584.

Berkow S, Barnard N. Vegetarian diets and weight status. *Nutrition Reviews* 64, no. 4 (2006): 175–188.

Bloom S. Hormonal regulation of appetite. *Obesity Reviews* 8 (Supplement 1) (2007): 63–65.

Boyce T. The media and obesity. *Obesity Reviews* 8 (Supplement 1) (2007): 201–205.

Bravata D, et al. Using pedometers to increase physical activity and improve health. A systematic review. *Journal of the American Medical Association* 298, no. 10 (2007): 2296–2304.

Dhingra R, et al. Soft drink consumption and risk of developing cardiometabolic risk factors and the metabolic syndrome in middle-aged adults in the community. *Circulation* 116 (2007): 480–488.

Feskanich D, et al. Walking and leisure-time activity and risk of hip fracture in postmenopausal women. *Journal of the American Medical Association* 288 (2002): 2300–2306.

Gardner C, et al. Comparison of the Atkins, Zone, Ornish, and LEARN diets for change in weight and related risk factors among overweight premenopausal women. The A TO Z weight loss study: a randomized trial. *Journal of the American Medical Association* 297 (2007): 969–977.

Hare-Bruun H, et al. Glycemic index and glycemic load in relation to changes in body weight, body fat distribution, and body composition in adult Danes. *American Journal of Clinical Nutrition* 84 (2006): 871–879.

Holm S. Obesity interventions and ethics. *Obesity Reviews* 8 (Supplement 1) (2007): 207–210.

Holt SHA, et al. Satiety index of common foods. *European Journal of Clinical Nutrition* 49 (1995): 675–690.

James GA, et al. Interaction of satiety and reward response to food stimulation. *Journal of Addictive Diseases* 23, no. 3 (2004): 23–37.

Johnson J, et al. Exercise training amount and intensity effects on metabolic syndrome (from studies of a targeted risk reduction intervention through defined exercise). *American Journal of Cardiology* 100 (2007): 1759–1766.

Johnson-Taylor WL, et al. The change in weight perception of weight status among the overweight: comparison of NHANES III (1998–1994) and 1999–2004 NHANES. *International Journal of Behavioral Nutrition and Physical Activity* 5 (2008): 9.

Kip K, et al. Clinical importance of obesity versus the metabolic syndrome in cardiovascular risk in women. A report from the Women's Ischemia Syndrome Evaluation (WISE) study. *Circulation* 109 (2004): 706–713.

Lampinen P, et al. Changes in intensity of physical exercise as predictors of depressive symptoms among older adults: an eight-year follow-up. *Preventive Medicine* 30 (2000): 371–380.

Lanou AJ, Barnard ND. Dairy and weight loss hypothesis: an evaluation of the clinical trials. *Nutrition Reviews* 66, no. 5 (2008): 272–279.

Linde JA, et al. Self-weighing in weight gain prevention and weight loss trials. *Annals of Behavioral Medicine* 30 (2005): 210–216.

Lorenzo A, Gobbo V, et al. Normal-weight obese syndrome: early inflammation? *American Journal of Clinical Nutrition* 85 (2007): 40–45.

Manson JE, et al. Walking compared with vigorous exercise for the prevention of cardiovascular events in women. *New England Journal of Medicine* 347 (2002): 716–725.

McMillan-Price J, Brand-Miller J. Low-glycaemic index diets and body weight regulation. *International Journal of Obesity* (London) 30 (Supplement 3) (2006): S40–S46.

Mitrou P, et al. Mediterranean dietary pattern and prediction of all-cause mortality in a US population. Results from the NIH-AARP diet and health study. *Archives of Internal Medicine* 167, no. 22 (2007): 2461–2468.

Nordmann A, et al. Effects of low-carbohydrate vs low-fat diets on weight loss and cardiovascular risk factors. *Archives of Internal Medicine* 166 (2006): 285–293.

Ogden CL, et al. Prevalence of overweight and obesity in the United States, 1999–2004. *Journal of the American Medical Association* 295, no. 13 (2006): 1549–1555.

Pischon T, Nothlings U, Boeing H. Obesity and cancer in the Symposium on Diet and Cancer. *Proceedings of the Nutrition Society* 67 (2008): 128–145.

Prentice R, Thomson C, et al. Low-fat dietary pattern and cancer incidence in the Women's Health Initiative dietary modification randomized controlled trial. *Journal of the National Cancer Institute* 99 (2007): 1534–1543.

Rolls ET. Understanding the mechanisms of food intake and obesity. *Obesity Reviews* 8 (Supplement 1) (2007): 67–72.

Turner-McGrievy G, Barnard N, Scialli A. A two-year randomized weight loss trial comparing a vegan diet to a more moderate low-fat diet. *Obesity* 15 (2007): 2276–2281.

Turner-McGrievy GM, Barnard ND, Scialli AR, Lanou AJ. Effects of a low-fat vegan diet and a Step II diet on macro- and micronutrient intakes in overweight postmenopausal women. *Nutrition* 20 (2004): 738–746.

Ulijaszek SJ. Obesity: a disorder of convenience. *Obesity Reviews* 8 (Supplement 1) (2007): 183–187.

Verheijden MW, Bakx JC, et al. Role of social support in lifestyle-focused weight management interventions. *European Journal of Clinical Nutrition* 59 (Supplement 1) (2005): 179–186.

Wadden T, et al. Lifestyle modification for the management of obesity. *Gastroenterology* 132 (2007): 2226–2238.

Wilding JPH. Treatment strategies for obesity. *Obesity Reviews* 8 (Supplement 1) (2007): 137–144.

Young D, et al. The effects of aerobic exercise and T'ai Chi on blood pressure in older people: results of a randomized trial. *Journal of the American Geriatric Society* 47 (1999): 277–284.

Chapter 13. Curbing Your Risk of Cancer

Alaszewski A, Horlick-Jones T. How can doctors communicate information about risk more effectively? Education and debate. *British Medical Journal* 327 (2003): 728–731.

Calle E, et al. Overweight, obesity, and mortality from cancer in a prospectively studied cohort of U.S. adults. *New England Journal of Medicine* 348 (2003): 1625–1638.

Collaborative Group on Epidemiological Studies of Ovarian Cancer. Ovarian cancer and oral contraceptives: collaborative reanalysis of data from 45 epidemiological studies including 23257 women with ovarian cancer and 87303 controls. *Lancet* 371 (2008): 303–314.

Cramer DW, Kuper H, Harlow BL, Titus-Ernstoff L. Carotenoids, antioxidants and ovarian cancer risk in pre- and postmenopausal women. *International Journal of Cancer* 94, no. 1 (2001): 128–134.

Cramer DW, Liberman RF, Titus-Ernstoff L, Welch WR, Greenberg ER, et al. Genital talc exposure and risk of ovarian cancer. *International Journal of Cancer* 81, no. 3 (1999): 351–356.

Cui X, et al. Dietary patterns and breast cancer risk in the Shanghai Breast Cancer Study. *Cancer Epidemiology Biomarkers and Prevention* 16, no. 7 (2007): 1443–1448.

Editorial. The case for preventing ovarian cancer. *Lancet* 371 (2008): 275.

Elmore J, Gigerenzer G. Benign breast disease—the risks of communicating risk. *New England Journal of Medicine* 353 (2005): 297–299.

Fairfield KM, Hunter DJ, Colditz GA, Fuchs CS, Cramer DW, et al. A prospective study of dietary lactose and ovarian cancer. *International Journal of Cancer* 110, no. 2 (2004): 271–277.

Ferdowsian H, Barnard ND. The role of diet in breast and prostate cancer survival. *Ethnicity and Disease* 17 (Supplement 2) (2007): S2-18–S2-22.

Fletcher S, Elmore J. Mammographic screening for breast cancer. *New England Journal of Medicine* 348, no. 17 (2003): 1672–1680.

Invasive Female Breast Cancer (Invasive), Age-Adjusted Surveillance Epidemiology and End results (SEER) Incidence Rates by Year, Race, and Age. www.seer.cancer.gov/csr/1975_2005/results_merged/sect_04_breast.pdf. Last accessed May 6, 2009.

Joura E, et al. Efficacy of a quadrivalent prophylactic human papillomavirus (types 6, 11, 16, and 18) L1 virus-like-particle vaccine against high-grade vulval and vaginal lesions: a combined analysis of three randomized clinical trials. *Lancet* 369 (2007): 1693–1702.

Kuper H, Cramer DW, Titus-Ernstoff L. Risk of ovarian cancer in the United States in relation to anthropometric measures: does the association depend on menopausal status? *Cancer Causes Control* 13, no. 5 (2002): 455–463.

Lin J, et al. Intakes of calcium and vitamin D and breast cancer risk in women. *Archives of Internal Medicine* 167 (2007): 1050–1059.

Loong TW. Understanding sensitivity and specificity with the right side of the brain. *British Medical Journal* 327 (2003): 716–719.

Mayrand JH, Duarte-Franco E, Rodrigues I, et al. for the Canadian Cervical Cancer Screening Trial Study Group. Human papillomavirus DNA versus Papanicolaou screening tests for cervical cancer. *New England Journal of Medicine* 357. no. 16 (2007): 1579–1588.

Moss E, Hollingworth J, Reynolds T. The role of CA125 in clinical practice. *Journal of Clinical Pathology* 58 (2005): 308–312.

Paley P. Screening for the major malignancies affecting women: current guidelines. *American Journal of Obstetrics and Gynecology* 184 (2001): 1021–1030.

Pisano E, et al. for the Digital Mammographic Imaging Screening Trial (DMIST) Investigators Group. Diagnostic performance of digital versus film mammography for breast-cancer screening. *New England Journal of Medicine* 353, no. 17 (2005): 1773–1783.

Rebbeck TR, et al. Prophylactic oophorectomy in carriers of BRCA1 or BRCA2 mutations. *New England Journal of Medicine* 346, no. 21 (2002): 1616–1622.

Reeves G, Pirie K, Beral V, et al. for the Million Women Study Collaborators. Cancer incidence and mortality in relation to body mass index in the Million Women Study: cohort study. *British Medical Journal* 335, no. 7630 (2007): 1134.

Renehan A, et al. Body-mass index and incidence of cancer: a systematic review and meta-analysis of prospective observational studies. *Lancet* 371 (2008): 569–578.

Schrag D, Kuntz K, Garber J, Weeks J. Decision analysis—effects of prophylactic mastectomy and oophorectomy on life expectancy among women with BRCA1 or BRCA2 mutations. *New England Journal of Medicine* 336, no. 20 (1997): 1465–1471.

Singletary SE. Rating the risk factors for breast cancer. *Annals of Surgery* 237, no. 4 (2003): 474–482.

Smith R, Editor. Communicating risk: the main work of doctors. Editor's choice. *British Medical Journal* 327, no. 7417 (2003).

Trock B, Hilakivi-Clarke L, Clarke R. Meta-analysis of soy intake and breast cancer risk. *Journal of the National Cancer Institute* 98 (2006): 459–471.

Van Calster B, et al. Discrimination between benign and malignant adnexal masses by specialist ultrasound examination versus serum CA-125. *Journal of the National Cancer Institute* 99 (2007): 1706–1714.

Chapter 14. Your Doctor Visit

Ackermann R, Mulrow C, et al. Garlic shows promise for improving some cardiovascular risk factors. *Archives of Internal Medicine* 167 (2007): 813–824.

Boyd CM, Durer J, Boult C, et al. Clinical practice guidelines and quality of care for older patients with multiple comorbid diseases. *Journal of the American Medical Association* 294, no. 6 (2005): 716–724.

Charlson M, McFerren M. Garlic, what we know and what we don't know. Editorial. *Archives of Internal Medicine* 167 (2007): 325–326.

Gardner C, Lawson L, et al. Effect of raw garlic vs commercial garlic supplements on plasma lipid concentrations in adults with moderate hypercholesterolemia. *Archives of Internal Medicine* 167 (2007): 346–353.

Holmboe E, Lipner R, Greiner A. Assessing quality of care, knowledge matters. *Journal of the American Medical Association* 299, no. 3 (2008): 338–340.

Kim D, Pickhardt P, Taylor A, et al. CT colonography versus colonoscopy for the detection of advanced neoplasia. *New England Journal of Medicine* 357, no. 14 (2007): 1403–1412.

Weiss CO, Boyd CM, Yu Q, Wolff JL, Leff B. Patterns of prevalent major chronic disease among older adults in the United States. *Journal of the American Medical Association* 298, no. 10 (2007): 1160–1162.

Women: Stay Healthy at Any Age, Your Checklist for Health, February 2007, www.ahrq.gov/ppip/healthwom.htm. This is the U.S. Preventive Services Task Force's (USPSTF) site that reviews screening tests for cancer and gynecologic conditions and lists healthy guidelines. Last accessed December 14, 2008.

Index

medications for, 243, 248–56; and natural bone formation, 224–25; and osteopenia, 222–24, 233; and osteoporosis, 222–23; promotion of, 240; research technologies and, 258–60; and risk factors for osteoporosis, 227–30; ultrasound measures of, 238–39; vitamin D for, 228, 234, 240, 242, 246–47. *See also* Osteoporosis

Bone mineral density (BMD), 231–38, 247

Bone remodeling, 224–26

Boniva, 250–51, 257

BRCA1 and 2 gene mutations, 300–301, 302, 304, 308, 312

Breast biopsy, 317, 319, 321, 331–32

Breast cancer, 2, 5, 38, 312–17, 331–32; age-related risk of, 312; alcohol and, 313, 316; BRCA gene mutations and, 300, 308, 312; computer-aided detection of, 314; detection of, 317–18; differential diagnosis of, 318–21; estrogen vaginal ring after, 147; exercise and, 313, 316; family history of, 299–300, 302, 312, 346; hormone therapy and, 46, 48, 49, 50–51, 54, 62, 64, 69, 313; mammograms in detection of, 49, 51, 54, 303, 313–14, 332; medications to lower risk of, 254; mortality from, 67–68; MRI detection of, 315–16; oral contraceptives and, 168; radiation for, 317, 319; reducing risk of, 312–17; soy and, 30, 38; surgery for, 317, 319–21; ultrasound detection of, 314–15, 317

Breast cyst, 317, 319, 331

Breast disease, benign, 48, 49

Breast examination, 332, 346

Breast tenderness, 10

Breathing: paced respiration for hot flashes, 25–26, 28; sleep-disordered, 207, 210, 213–16

Bulimia, 228, 229

CA-125, 301–5, 307, 309–11, 354

CAD, 314

Caffeine: bone effects of, 228, 240, 253; hot flashes and, 28–29; incontinence and, 117, 118, 142; PMS and, 188; for sleep deprivation, 208, 209, 211; sleep effects of, 28, 217–18

Calcium, 187, 240–46; art of taking, 244–45; for bone health, 226, 228, 230, 234, 240–46, 253, 255–56; food sources of, 243, 245–46; in food vs. supplements, 245; kinds of, 245; recommended intake of, 243; vitamin D and, 246

Calorie requirements, 278, 288

Cancer, 2, 5, 66, 298–329; depression and, 194; family history of, 299–302, 346; individual risk for, 298–302; lifestyle and, 299, 300; mortality from, 67–68; response to diagnosis of, 178–79; screening tests for, 303–7. *See also specific cancers*

Cancer antigen-125 (CA-125) blood test, 301–5, 307, 309–11, 354

Candida vulvovaginitis, 123

Carbohydrates, 277–81, 284, 288, 289–90

Cardiac exercise, 275–76

Cardiovascular disease (CVD), 2, 5, 17, 18, 66–81; age and, 76–77; aspirin and, 80–81; cholesterol and, 71; diabetes and, 70, 263–64; diet and, 69; family history of, 69, 346; forms of, 71–72; gender and, 73–76; hormone therapy and, 44–45, 47, 48, 49, 50, 57; metabolic syndrome and, 264–66; mortality from, 68; obesity and, 69–70; prevention of, 67–68; risk factors for, 68–71; sedentary lifestyle and, 69; smoking and, 68–69

Catapress, 39, 62

CBT. *See* Cognitive behavioral therapy

Celiac sprue disease, 229

Central sleep apnea (CSA), 214

seling/psychotherapy for, 196, 197; drug-induced, 193; estrogen therapy for, 198; exercise for, 198; family history of, 193, 195; gender and, 179, 190–91, 192; hot flashes and, 190; insomnia and, 211, 212, 213; medical causes of, 193–94; osteoporosis and, 229, 230; in perimenopause, 191; in postmenopause, 191–92; postpartum, 174, 191, 195; risk factors for, 174, 191–92; role overload and, 190–91; serotonin and, 175; sexual effects of, 138; St. John's wort for, 195–96; susceptibility to, 173, 175; symptoms of, 192–93

DES, 343

DHEA, 158, 336

Diabetes, 2, 5, 17, 66, 262, 263–64; cardiovascular disease and, 70, 75, 76, 263–64; dementia and, 202; medications for, 333; metabolic syndrome and, 264–66; obesity and, 70, 263–64; osteoporosis and, 229; sex and, 136, 140; sleep apnea and, 214

Diaphragm, contraceptive, 164–65

Diethylstilbestrol (DES) exposure, 343

Diet/nutrition, 18, 262–63, 277–93; assessment of, 294, 295; and calcium, 243, 245–46; and calories, 278, 288; cancer risk and, 299; and carbohydrates, 277–81, 284, 288, 289–90; cardiovascular disease and, 69, 77, 79; and cranberry juice, 115; definition of, 283; and fats, 279; and fiber, 29, 142, 188, 244, 281; and foods to avoid, 280–81; high-sodium, 230, 240; hot flashes and, 20, 29–31; to lower cholesterol and blood pressure, 73; low-fat, 79, 188, 284–85, 291; low-sodium, 286, 288; and nutrient-dense foods, 278–79; osteoporosis and, 228, 240, 290; for PMS or PMDD, 187–88; and portion sizes,

277–78, 280–81, 284, 291, 292–93; and protein, 279, 288; sleep and, 217; and soy products, 30–31, 38; and stress eating, 281–83; vegetable-based, 20, 29, 288–89, 291–92; and vitamin D, 228, 234, 240

Diets for weight loss, 77, 262, 278, 283–93; Atkins diet, 287, 288, 289–90; to begin, 283–84; behavioral strategies of, 287–88; DASH diet, 286; evaluation of, 285–88; Flavor Point diet, 291; Jenny Craig, 286–87; maintenance phase of, 287; and pressure to be thin, 283; Sonoma (Mediterranean) diet, 77, 285–86, 290, 293; South Beach diet, 77, 286, 287, 290, 292–93; vegetarian, 291–92; Volumetrics, 290–91; Weight Watchers, 77, 282, 283, 287, 290, 292

Differential diagnosis, 353–54

Digital mammography, 314

Dilantin, 229

Dilatation and curettage (D&C), 87, 88, 91–92, 95, 96, 98, 99, 100, 109, 328, 329

Diuretics, 137

Diverticulitis, 305

Doctor-patient team, 1–7, 17–18, 349

Doctor visits, 331–57; annual checkups, 349–51; comprehensive new patient visit, 335–49; doctor's assessment of, 348–49, 355–56; Internet research and, 356–57; with multiple specialists, 332–33; for specific problem, 351–54

Dong quai, 35, 36, 112

Douching, 132

Dual Energy X-ray Absorptiometry (DXA), 223, 231–38, 257, 260; of arm, 237–38; as assessment of treatment for osteoporosis, 256–57; limitations of, 234–36; after prior fracture, 235, 237; thinnest area of bone on, 233–34; T score for, 232–35, 256; Z score for, 235, 236

DVT, 254

DXA. *See* Dual Energy X-ray Absorptiometry

Dyslipidemia, 264–66. *See also* Cholesterol, high

Early menopause, 15–16; hormone therapy and, 55; surgical, 16–17

Eczema, 128

E-diets, 282

Effexor, 37, 38, 62, 196

EKG, 75

Electrical stimulation, for urge incontinence, 118

Electrocardiogram (EKG), 75

"Empty nest," 153, 172, 177, 195

Endometrial ablation, 88, 91, 102–6; for adenomyosis, 96, 103, 104; cryoablation, 104; fertility after, 103, 105; hydrothermal, 104; NovaSure method, 103, 105–6; Thermachoice balloon method, 104; uterine cancer after, 102–3

Endometrial biopsy, 84, 87, 88, 90, 95, 96, 328, 329

Endometrial cancer. *See* Uterine cancer

Endometrial hyperplasia, 82–86, 92–93, 96–99; diagnosis of, 96, 97–98; hysterectomy for, 97, 110; lifestyle and, 97, 99; progesterone for, 93, 96–99

Endometriosis, 310

Epinephrine, 180

Erectile dysfunction, 136–37

Essure™, 170

Estraderm, 56

Estradiol, 10, 11, 15, 56, 64, 270

EstraTest, 59, 157

Estring vaginal ring, 146–47

Estrogen levels, 8, 9; endometrial hyperplasia and, 97; fibroids and, 101; heart disease risk and, 76; in menstrual cycle, 9, 10; mood and, 174–75;

oxytocin and, 181; in perimenopause, 9–10, 101; PMS and, 184–85; in postmenopause, 10–11, 15, 147; sex and, 135, 159; sleep and, 209; vaginal dryness and, 122, 143, 144–47

Estrogen receptors, 174–75

Estrogen therapy: alcohol and, 52, 54; breast cancer and, 46, 48, 49, 51, 54, 62, 64; dementia and, 204–5; for depression, 198; after early menopause, 55; heart disease and, 44–45, 48, 49; for hot flashes, 58–61; after hysterectomy, 55–56; for low sex drive, 160; precautions for, 54; to prevent osteoporosis, 253–54; skin patch, cream, lotion, or gel forms of, 56, 60–61, 64, 144–46; stopping, 61–63; stroke and, 48; sun sensitivity and, 54; uterine cancer and, 47–48; vaginal, 57, 144–47; when pills stop working, 60–61; who may safely start, 53; who should avoid, 46, 48–49, 52–53. *See also* Hormone therapy

Estrone, 11, 97, 159, 270, 328

Evamist, 56

Evening primrose oil, 36, 188

Evista, 243, 254, 256, 260

Exercise, 2, 18, 21, 262–63, 269–77, 345; aerobic/cardiac, 275–76; assessing progress in, 294–95; balance, 276–77; to begin program of, 271–72; benefits of, 270, 271; for bone health, 228, 230, 240, 242, 247–48; breast cancer and, 313, 316; cancer risk and, 299; choosing activities for, 270–71, 295; cognitive benefits of, 203; for constipation, 142; for depression, 198; for endometrial hyperplasia, 97, 99; goals for, 271; for heart health, 69, 73, 77, 78, 79; hot flashes and, 20, 31; importance of, 269–70; increasing amount of, 272; Kegel exercises, 117, 119–20; motivation to, 272, 274;

to lower risk of, 266–68; risk factors for, 265; weight-loss diets for, 285–86
Metamucil, 142, 244
MI. *See* Myocardial infarction
Micro magnetic resonance imaging (micro MRI) of bone, 259–60
Million Women Study, 52, 64
Mood, 8, 10, 15, 172–77; age-related changes affecting, 176–77; "blue," 175; and depression, 189–98; genetics and, 175; hormones and, 174–77; insomnia and, 211, 212, 213; in PMDD, 186–89; in PMS, 182–85; serotonin and, 174, 175, 183, 187, 189, 196
"Morning-after" pill, 165
MRI, 259–60, 315–16
Multiple sclerosis, 193
Multitasking, 199
Multivitamins, 244
Muscle mass loss, 269–70, 277, 294
Myocardial infarction (MI), 72; depression and, 194; gender and, 73–75, 180
Myomectomy, 107–8

Naps, 218
National Health and Nutrition Examination Survey (NHANES), 366, 367, 370
National Osteoporosis Foundation (NOF), 222, 231
Natural remedies: abnormal bleeding due to, 112; for high blood pressure, 337–38; for hot flashes, 31–36; informing doctor about use of, 335–38; interaction with oral contraceptives, 33, 34; for PMS, 188; safety and effectiveness of, 31–33
Neurontin, 39–40, 62
NHANES (National Health and Nutrition Examination Survey), 366, 367, 370
Niacin, 22

Night sweats, 5, 6, 22, 190, 207; caffeine and, 28–29; estrogen levels and, 10; after stopping hormone therapy, 61. *See also* Hot flashes
Nipple discharge, bloody, 320
NOF, 222, 231
Non-rapid eye movement (NREM) sleep, 208
NovaSure endometrial ablation, 103, 105–6
NREM sleep, 208
Nurses' Health Study, 50, 181
Nutrition. *See* Diet/nutrition
Nuva Ring, 170

Obesity/overweight, 2, 5, 45, 46, 262; abdominal, 11, 264–66, 267–68, 270, 281; cancer risk and, 299, 313; cardiovascular disease and, 69, 75, 77; cystocele or rectocele and, 121; endometrial hyperplasia and, 97, 99; health risks of, 263; incontinence and, 117; metabolic syndrome and, 263–66; sleep apnea and, 214; sleep deprivation and, 210–11, 293; uterine cancer and, 328
Obstetrical/gynecological history, 343
Obstructive sleep apnea (OSA), 214
Odor, vaginal, 122, 124, 128
Ogen, 56
Omega-3 fatty acids, 36
Oophorectomy, bilateral, 16, 56
Oral contraceptives, 167–69; for abnormal bleeding, 107; breast cancer and, 168; early menopause and, 16; for heavy periods, 95; for hot flashes, 7, 57–58, 169; interaction of, with natural remedies, 33, 34; "morning-after" pill, 165; ovarian cancer and, 168, 308, 354; for PMS or PMDD, 189, 340–41; smoking and, 69, 167; who should not take, 167
Orgasms, 134, 150

Ortho Evra skin patch, 169
Ortho Prefest, 59, 64
OSA, 214
Osteoarthritis, 282–83
Osteonecrosis of jaw, 252
Osteopenia, 222–24, 233
Osteoporosis, 2, 5, 17, 66, 222–23, 262; Atkins diet and, 290; bone thinning in, 225–27; DXA measures in, 223, 231–38; ethnicity and, 230; family history of, 227; Fracture Risk Assessment tool for, 235, 239–40; fractures due to, 18, 222–23, 226; importance of, 223; Lupron and, 106; prevalence of, 221; prevention of, 221; research technologies and, 258–60; risk factors for, 227–30; as silent problem, 224; Type 2 (senile), 226; ultrasound measures in, 238–39. *See also* Bone health
Osteoporosis medications, 243, 248–56, 333; bisphosphonates, 250–53; estrogen and hormone therapy, 253–54; parathyroid hormone, 255; selective estrogen receptor modulators, 254
Ovarian cancer, 2, 67, 308–9; BRCA gene mutations and, 300–301, 302, 304, 308; CA-125 blood test for, 301–5, 307, 309–11, 354; detection of, 309; family history of, 299–301, 309; hormone therapy and, 52; hysterectomy and, 308, 309; oral contraceptives and, 168, 308, 354; reducing risk of, 308–9; talc and, 301, 308; tubal ligation and, 171, 300–301, 308–9, 354
Ovarian cyst, 139, 301, 311, 354
Ovaries, 8–9; hormones produced by, 8; after hysterectomy, 16–17, 56; in perimenopause, 9–10; in postmenopause, 14, 15; surgical removal of, 16, 56; after uterine artery embolization, 108

Ovulation, 9, 14
Oxytocin and stress, 180–82

Paced respiration, 25–26, 28
Pain: during sex, 15, 57, 149–50, 151; while urinating, 114–15
Pap smear, 88, 93, 126–27, 303, 322–23, 333, 347; abnormal, 325–27; age to stop having, 327–38; frequency of, 326; with HPV DNA testing, 325
Parathyroid hormone (PTH), 255
Parkinson's disease, 193
Patient-doctor team, 1–7, 17–18, 349
Paxil, 37, 196
Pelvic examination, 332, 347
Pelvic fracture, 222
Pelvic inflammatory disease (PID), 343
Pelvic ultrasound, 88, 91
Per Diem, 142
Perimenopause, 7, 176–77; abnormal bleeding in, 82, 83, 85–87; depression in, 191; duration of, 10, 12–14; fertility in, 7, 11–12; follicle-stimulating hormone and, 13; hormones in, 9–10; memory problems in, 200–205; menstrual bleeding in, 8, 12; mood, memory, and mental health in, 172–73; sleep problems in, 207–20
Peripheral vascular disease (PVD), 78
Pessary, 117, 119, 121
Pets, 220
Physical examination, 346–48; annual, 349–51; for specific problem, 351–54
Phytoestrogens, 30
PID, 343
Pilates, 274, 276, 277
Plan B, 165
Plant-derived hormones, 63–64
PMDD. *See* Premenstrual dysphoric disorder
PMS. *See* Premenstrual syndrome
PMS Escape, 188
Polycystic ovarian disease, 214

Stages of menopause, 7–8

Starvation response, 278

Statins, 4

STDs. *See* Sexually transmitted diseases

Sterilization: female, 170–71; male, 171

Strengthening exercises, 247–48, 271, 275

Stress: cognitive effects of, 203; cortisol and, 180; estrogen and, 175; "fight or flight" response to, 178, 181; gender and response to, 178–82; health consequences of, 180; hot flashes and, 27; oxytocin and, 180–82; PMS and, 185; sex and, 147–48; sources of, 172; stages of response to, 178; tend and befriend response to, 178–79, 181; vulnerability to, 173, 175, 197

Stress eating, 281–82

Stress incontinence, 116–17

Stress reduction strategies, 282

Stretching, 274

Stroke, 5, 18, 66, 67, 72; depression and, 194; diabetes and, 70, 263–64; hemorrhagic, 72; hormone therapy and, 45–46, 48; inactive lifestyle and, 69; ischemic, 72; metabolic syndrome and, 265–66; obesity and, 70; risk factors for, 68–71; smoking and, 69, 78. *See also* Cardiovascular disease

Study of Women's Health Across the Nation (SWAN), 359

Sun: exposure to, 247; sensitivity to, 54

Surgical history, 342

Surgical menopause, 16–17; depression and, 191; hormone therapy for, 55–57

Swab test of cervix, 88

SWAN, 359

Swimming, 242

Syndrome X, 263, 264. *See also* Metabolic syndrome

T'ai Chi, 31, 274, 276, 295

Talc, ovarian cancer and, 301, 308

Tamoxifen, 22–23, 254

Testosterone, 8, 15, 155; breast cancer and, 316; for hot flashes, 59; for low sex drive, 155–58; measurement of, 156; side effects of, 156; topical and oral forms of, 156; who should not take, 156

Thermachoice balloon endometrial ablation, 104

Thyroid disease, 6–7; abnormal bleeding due to, 83, 111–12; blood tests for, 23, 24, 25, 90, 100; depression and, 193; hot flashes and, 22, 23–25; medication for, 333; osteoporosis and, 229; vs. PMS, 183; sex and, 141; weight loss and, 293

TIA, 71, 204

Tibolone, 254

Trabecular bone, 224–25; loss of, 226, 236

Transient ischemic attack (TIA), 71, 204

Transvaginal ultrasound, 88, 91, 301

Triamcinolone, 129

Trichomonas, 128

Triglycerides, 71, 265–66

Tryptophan, 183, 188, 217

Tubal ligation, 170–71; ovarian cancer and, 171, 300–301, 308–9, 354

Tums, 245

UAE, 88, 108–9

Ultrasound, 88, 91; and bone strength, 238–39; and breast cancer, 304–15, 317; and ovarian cancer, 301, 354; and uterine cancer, 328–39; pelvic and transvaginal, 88, 91

Urethrocele, 116

Urge incontinence, 117–18

Urinary problems, 4, 113–20; cystocele, 119–20; incontinence, 15, 113, 116–18, 141; infections, 114–16; Kegel exercises for, 117, 119–20; medication-related, 119; sex and, 141

of, 210; supplements for, 351; support for, 282
Weight Watchers, 73, 77, 282, 283, 287, 290, 292
Wellbutrin, 196
WHI. *See* Women's Health Initiative
WHIMS, 204
WHO, 239, 264
Whole grains, 277, 279, 281, 290
Wild yam cream, 33–34
WISDOM, 204
Withdrawal contraceptive method, 163
Women's Health Initiative (WHI), 1, 40, 43–54, 69, 247, 253; halting of, 44; hormones studied in, 47–48; interpreting findings of, 44–46, 50–54; participants in, 47; Premarin study results, 48–49, 51; Prempro study results, 49–51. *See also* Hormone therapy

Women's Health Initiative Memory Study (WHIMS), 204
Women's International Study of Long Duration Estrogen after Menopause (WISDOM), 204
World Health Organization (WHO), 239, 264
Wrist fracture, 222

Yaz, 189
Yeast infection, 87, 121, 122, 123–26, 137; diabetes and, 140; vs. lichen sclerosis, 130; sex and, 137, 140
Yoga, 31, 274, 276, 295
Youth-centered culture, 21, 190

Zoledronate, 250, 252